T0293361

Highlights of Interdisciplinary Care in Rheumatology

Editors

ANISHA B. DUA
JEFFREY A. SPARKS

RHEUMATIC DISEASE CLINICS OF NORTH AMERICA

www.rheumatic.theclinics.com

Consulting Editors
MICHAEL H. WEISMAN
JEFFREY A. SPARKS
ANISHA B. DUA

August 2024 • Volume 50 • Number 3

ELSEVIER

1600 John F. Kennedy Boulevard • Suite 1800 • Philadelphia, Pennsylvania, 19103-2899
http://www.theclinics.com

RHEUMATIC DISEASE CLINICS OF NORTH AMERICA Volume 50, Number 3
August 2024 ISSN 0889-857X, ISBN 13: 978-0-443-34365-0

Editor: Joanna Gascoine
Developmental Editor: Nitesh Barthwal

Rheumatic Disease Clinics of North America (ISSN 0889-857X) is published quarterly by Elsevier Inc., 360 Park Avenue South, New York, NY 10010-1710. Months of issue are February, May, August, and November. Business and editorial offices: 1600 John F. Kennedy Boulevard, Suite 1800, Philadelphia, PA 19103-2899. Periodicals postage paid at New York, NY and additional mailing offices. Subscription prices are USD 384.00 per year for US individuals, USD 100.00 per year for US students and residents, USD 449.00 per year for Canadian individuals, USD 100.00 per year for Canadian students/residents, USD 489.00 per year for international individuals, and USD 230.00 per year for foreign students/residents. For institutional access pricing please contact Customer Service via the contact information below. To receive student/resident rate, orders must be accompanied by name of affiliated institution, date of term, and the *signature* of program/residency coordinator on institution letterhead. Orders will be billed at individual rate until proof of status received. Foreign air speed delivery is included in all *Clinics* subscription prices. All prices are subject to change without notice. **POSTMASTER:** Send address changes to *Rheumatic Disease Clinics of North America,* Elsevier Health Sciences Division, Subscription Customer Service, 3251 Riverport Lane, Maryland Heights, MO 63043. **Customer Service: 1-800-654-2452 (US and Canada). From outside of the US and Canada: 314-447-8871. Fax: 314-447-8029. For print support, e-mail: JournalsCustomerService-usa@elsevier.com. For online support, e-mail: JournalsOnlineSupport-usa@elsevier.com.**

Reprints. For copies of 100 or more of articles in this publication, please contact the Commercial Reprints Department, Elsevier Inc., 360 Park Avenue South, New York, New York, 10010-1710; Tel.: +1-212-633-3874, Fax: +1-212-633-3820, and E-mail: reprints@elsevier.com.

Rheumatic Disease Clinics of North America is covered in *MEDLINE/PubMed (Index Medicus), Current Contents/Clinical Medicine, Science Citation Index, ISI/BIOMED,* and *EMBASE/Excerpta Medica.*

Contributors

CONSULTING EDITORS

MICHAEL H. WEISMAN, MD
Division of Rheumatology and Immunology, Department of Medicine, Stanford University School of Medicine, Palo Alto, California, USA

JEFFREY A. SPARKS, MD, MMSc
Associate Professor, Division of Rheumatology, Inflammation, and Immunity Department of Medicine Brigham and Women's Hospital and Harvard Medical School, Boston, Massachusetts, USA

ANISHA B. DUA, MD, MPH
Associate Professor, Division of Rheumatology Department of Medicine Northwestern University Feinberg School of Medicine, Chicago, Illinois, USA

EDITORS

ANISHA B. DUA, MD, MPH
Associate Professor, Division of Rheumatology Department of Medicine Northwestern University Feinberg School of Medicine, Chicago, Illinois, USA

JEFFREY A. SPARKS, MD, MMSc
Associate Professor, Division of Rheumatology, Inflammation, and Immunity Department of Medicine Brigham and Women's Hospital and Harvard Medical School, Boston, Massachusetts, USA

AUTHORS

CHRISTINE B. CHUNG, MD
Professor, Department of Radiology, University of California, San Diego, VA Medical Center, San Diego, La Jolla, California, USA

KENNETH C. CUMMINGS III, MD, MS
Associate Professor, Department of Anesthesiology, Anesthesiology Institute, Cleveland Clinic, Cleveland, Ohio, USA

M. KRISTEN DEMORUELLE, MD, PhD
Associate Professor of Medicine, Division of Rheumatology, University of Colorado School of Medicine, Aurora, Colorado, USA

WILLIAM S. FRYE, PhD, BCB, ABPP
Pediatric Psychologist, Department of Psychology, Johns Hopkins All Children's Hospital, St Petersburg, Florida, USA

KIMBERLY KALLIANOS, MD
Assistant Professor of Clinical Radiology, Department of Radiology and Biomedical
Imaging, University of California, San Francisco, San Francisco, California, USA

ELLA A. KAZEROONI, MD, MS
Professor, Divisions of Pulmonary and Critical Care Medicine and Cardiothoracic
Radiology, Departments of Internal Medicine and Radiology, University of Michigan,
Ann Arbor, Michigan, USA

DINESH KHANNA, MD, MS
Professor, Scleroderma Program, Division of Rheumatology, Department of Internal
Medicine, University of Michigan, Ann Arbor, Michigan, USA

YE RIN KOH, MD
Chief Resident, Anesthesiology Institute, Cleveland Clinic, Cleveland, Ohio, USA

STEPHEN C. MATHAI, MD, MHS
Associate Professor, Division of Pulmonary and Critical Care Medicine, Johns Hopkins
School of Medicine, Baltimore, Maryland, USA

SCOTT M. MATSON, MD
Assistant Professor of Medicine, Division of Pulmonary, Critical Care and Sleep Medicine,
University of Kansas School of Medicine, Kansas City, Kansas, USA

DIANA MILOJEVIC, MD
Pediatric Rheumatologist, Department of Medicine, Johns Hopkins All Children's
Hospital, St Petersburg, Florida, USA

AUREA VALERIA ROSA MOHANA-BORGES, MD
Post-Doctoral Fellow, Department of Radiology, University of California, San Diego,
La Jolla, California, USA

JUSTIN OLDHAM, MD, MS
Associate Professor, Division of Pulmonary and Critical Care Medicine, Departments of
Internal Medicine and Epidemiology, University of Michigan, Ann Arbor, Michigan,
USA

WIN MIN OO, MD, PhD
Department of Physical Medicine and Rehabilitation, Mandalay General Hospital,
University of Medicine, Mandalay, Mandalay, Myanmar; Rheumatology Department,
Royal North Shore Hospital, Institute of Bone and Joint Research, Kolling Institute,
The University of Sydney, Sydney, New South Wales, Australia

SONAL PRUTHI, MD
Cardiologist, Division of Cardiology, Department of Medicine, NYU Langone Health,
New York, New York, USA

JANELLE VU PUGASHETTI, MD, MS
Clinical Instructor, Division of Pulmonary and Critical Care Medicine, Department of
Internal Medicine, University of Michigan, Ann Arbor, Michigan, USA

SYED RAFAY A. SABZWARI, MBBS, MD
Clinical Cardiac Electrophysiology Fellow, University of Colorado Anschutz Medical
Campus, Aurora, Colorado, USA

EMAAD SIDDIQUI, MD
Division of Cardiology, Department of Medicine, NYU Langone Health, New York,
New York, USA

NATHANIEL R. SMILOWITZ, MD, MS
Assistant Professor of Medicine, The Leon H. Charney Division of Cardiology, NYU Langone Health, NYU School of Medicine, Cardiology Section, Department of Medicine, VA New York Harbor Healthcare System, New York, New York, USA

WENDY S. TZOU, MD, FHRS, FACC
Director, Cardiac Electrophysiology, Associate Professor, Department of Medicine, University of Colorado Anschutz Medical Campus, Aurora, Colorado, USA

Contents

Pulmonary hypertension (PH), a syndrome characterized by elevated pulmonary pressures, commonly complicates connective tissue disease (CTD) and is associated with increased morbidity and mortality. The incidence of PH varies widely between CTDs; patients with systemic sclerosis are most likely to develop PH. Several different types of PH can present in CTD, including PH related to left heart disease and respiratory disease. Importantly, CTD patients are at risk for developing pulmonary arterial hypertension, a rare form of PH that is associated with high morbidity and mortality. Future therapies targeting pulmonary vascular remodeling may improve outcomes for patients with this devastating disease.

Systemic diseases can cause heart block owing to the involvement of the myocardium and thereby the conduction system. Younger patients (<60) with heart block should be evaluated for an underlying systemic disease. These disorders are classified into infiltrative, rheumatologic, endocrine, and hereditary neuromuscular degenerative diseases. Cardiac amyloidosis owing to amyloid fibrils and cardiac sarcoidosis owing to noncaseating granulomas can infiltrate the conduction system leading to heart block. Accelerated atherosclerosis, vasculitis, myocarditis, and interstitial inflammation contribute to heart block in rheumatologic disorders. Myotonic, Becker, and Duchenne muscular dystrophies are neuromuscular diseases involving the myocardium skeletal muscles and can cause heart block.

The majority of connective tissue diseases (CTDs) are multisystem disorders that are often heterogeneous in their presentation and do not have a single laboratory, histologic, or radiologic feature that is defined as the gold standard to support a specific diagnosis. Given this challenging situation, the diagnosis of CTD is a process that requires the synthesis of multidisciplinary data which may include patient clinical symptoms, serologic evaluation, laboratory testing, and imaging. Pulmonary manifestations of connective tissue disease include interstitial lung disease as well as multicompartmental manifestations. These CT imaging patterns and features of specific diseases will be discussed in this article.

Ischemic heart disease (IHD) affects more than 20 million adults in the United States. Although classically attributed to atherosclerosis of the epicardial coronary arteries, nearly half of patients with stable angina and IHD who undergo invasive coronary angiography do not have obstructive epicardial coronary artery disease. Ischemia with nonobstructive coronary arteries is frequently caused by microvascular angina with underlying coronary microvascular dysfunction (CMD). Greater understanding the pathophysiology, diagnosis, and treatment of CMD holds promise to improve clinical outcomes of patients with ischemic heart disease.

Pediatric rheumatic diseases (PRDs) are a heterogeneous group of diseases that can have a chronic unpredictable disease course that can negatively affect mood, functioning, and quality of life. Given the range of difficulties faced in managing PRDs, as well as the psychosocial issues youth with these diseases experience, pediatric psychologists can be well suited to address concerns that arise in care for youth with PRDs including adherence, cognitive assessment, pain management, functional disability, and mood. Potential ways that pediatric psychologists can address these concerns and be embedded within an interdisciplinary treatment plan for youth with PRDs are described.

With the advent of small-molecule immune modulators, recombinant fusion proteins, and monoclonal antibodies, treatment options for patients with rheumatic diseases are now broad. These agents carry significant risks and an individualized approach to each patient, balancing known risks and benefits, remains the most prudent course. This review summarizes the available immunosuppressant treatments, discusses their perioperative implications, and provides recommendations for their perioperative management.

RHEUMATIC DISEASE CLINICS OF NORTH AMERICA

SERIES OF RELATED INTEREST

Emergency Medicine Clinics
Available at: https://www.emed.theclinics.com/
Medical Clinics
Available at: https://www.medical.theclinics.com/

THE CLINICS ARE AVAILABLE ONLINE!
Access your subscription at:
www.theclinics.com

Foreword

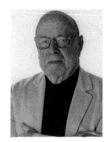
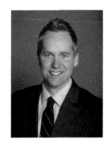
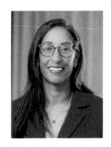

Michael H. Weisman, MD   Jeffrey A. Sparks, MD, MMSc   Anisha B. Dua, MD, MPH
Consulting Editors

Anisha Dua and Jeffrey Sparks have put together a series of critically written and well-annotated review articles that come from our colleague specialists in cardiology, radiology, immunology and allergy, pediatrics, and anesthesiology. Why is this important for us? Typically, we operate in silos and stay within the boundaries of our specialties; what is needed is an ability to synthesize and harmonize among disciplines and form a new approach. We can only do this if we address our complex patients and diseases with the knowledge and perspectives brought to us from our colleagues. This is true in research as well, and the NIH goes out of its way to reward the interdisciplinary nature of projects and programs that supplement each other. The works presented by Anisha

Rheum Dis Clin N Am 50 (2024) xi–xii
https://doi.org/10.1016/j.rdc.2024.05.003
0889-857X/24/© 2024 Published by Elsevier Inc.

rheumatic.theclinics.com

and Jeffrey in this issue will help us solve problems where understanding is beyond the scope of a single discipline. There is a good reason for you to read this collection.

Michael H. Weisman, MD
Division of Rheumatology and Immunology
Department of Medicine
Stanford University School of Medicine
300 Pasteur Dr, Palo Alto
CA 94304, USA

Jeffrey A. Sparks, MD, MMSc
Division of Rheumatology, Inflammation, and Immunity
Department of Medicine
Brigham and Women's Hospital and
Harvard Medical School
60 Fenwood Road #6016U
Boston, MA 02116, USA

Anisha B. Dua, MD, MPH
Division of Rheumatology
Department of Medicine
Northwestern University
Feinberg School of Medicine
Galter Pavilion, 675 N St Clair St Ste 14-100
Chicago, IL 60611, USA

E-mail addresses:
Michael.Weisman@cshs.org (M.H. Weisman)
jsparks@bwh.harvard.edu (J.A. Sparks)
anisha.dua@northwestern.edu (A.B. Dua)

Preface

Highlights of Interdisciplinary Care in Rheumatology

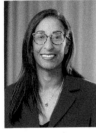   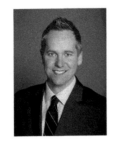

Anisha B. Dua, MD, MPH   Jeffrey A. Sparks, MD, MMSc
Editors

This special issue of *Rheumatic Disease Clinics of North America* was created to highlight some of the most interesting and impactful review articles published in *The Rheumatic Disease Clinics* series over the past two years. As rheumatologists, we are all drawn to and fascinated by the interdisciplinary nature of our field and realize that managing our patients requires critical conversations and insights from other subspecialty areas. While rheumatologists often serve as quarterbacks in the management of complex multiorgan disease patients, some of our best discoveries and work come from collaboration with other fields. From checkpoint inhibitors, to interstitial lung disease complicating many of our rheumatic diseases, to evolving therapeutics and biomarkers, learning from other specialists continues to help us further the field of rheumatology. Scientifically and clinically, we are in a state of evolution that is bolstered by this interdisciplinary exchange. This issue highlights articles from Cardiology, Radiology, Heart Failure, Immunology and Allergy, Geriatrics, Pediatrics, and even Anesthesiology. We include a focus on pulmonary and cardiac manifestations of rheumatologic diseases ranging from biomarkers to imaging modalities. We also have included a section on perioperative considerations in immunocompromised patients as well as evolving prospects in disease-modifying osteoarthritis drugs that may enable our patients to require fewer surgeries in the future.

Rheum Dis Clin N Am 50 (2024) xiii–xiv
https://doi.org/10.1016/j.rdc.2024.05.002
0889-857X/24/© 2024 Published by Elsevier Inc.

rheumatic.theclinics.com

DISCLOSURES

The authors have no conflicts to disclose.

Anisha B. Dua, MD, MPH
Division of Rheumatology
Department of Medicine
Northwestern University
Feinberg School of Medicine
Galter Pavilion, 675 N St Clair St Ste 14-100
Chicago, IL 60611, USA

Jeffrey A. Sparks, MD, MMSc
Division of Rheumatology, Inflammation, and Immunity
Department of Medicine
Brigham and Women's Hospital and
Harvard Medical School
60 Fenwood Road
#6016U, Boston, MA 02116, USA

E-mail addresses:
anisha.dua@northwestern.edu (A.B. Dua)
jsparks@bwh.harvard.edu (J.A. Sparks)

Pulmonary Hypertension Associated with Connective Tissue Disease

Stephen C. Mathai, MD, MHS

KEYWORDS

- Pulmonary hypertension • Connective tissue disease • Epidemiology • Diagnosis
- Outcomes

KEY POINTS

- Pulmonary hypertension commonly complicates connective tissue disease.
- Connective tissue disease predisposes patients to development of all five groups of the World Health Organization clinical classification.
- Pulmonary hypertension of any type portends a poor prognosis in connective tissue disease.
- Advances in therapies for certain forms of pulmonary hypertension have improved outcomes in connective tissue disease patients.

INTRODUCTION

Pulmonary hypertension (PH) is a syndrome characterized by elevated pulmonary pressures leading to increased pulmonary vascular resistance (PVR) that ultimately causes right ventricular (RV) dysfunction, failure, and death.[1] PH can develop in association with many different diseases and can result from processes that primarily affect systems distinct from the pulmonary vasculature, such as the heart, lung parenchyma, liver, and kidneys, in addition to processes that affect the pulmonary vasculature directly, such as thromboembolism.[2] Patients with connective tissue disease (CTD) are at particularly high risk for the development of PH and in certain forms of CTD, such as systemic sclerosis or scleroderma (SSc), pulmonary arterial hypertension (PAH), the most rare form of PH.[3] The presence of PH in any form is associated with increased morbidity and mortality. Unfortunately, patients with CTD-associated PH tend to have poorer survival compared with patients with PH without CTD. The reasons for the increased risk of development of PH, attenuated response to therapy, and poorer outcomes are poorly understood.

This article previously appeared in *Cardiology Clinics* volume 40 issue 1 February 2022.
Division of Pulmonary and Critical Care Medicine, Johns Hopkins University School of Medicine, 1830 E. Monument Street, Room 540, Baltimore, MD 21205, USA
E-mail address: smathai4@jhmi.edu

DEFINITION AND CLASSIFICATION OF PULMONARY HYPERTENSION

According to the most recent consensus guidelines, PH is defined hemodynamically as a mean pulmonary artery pressure (mPAP) greater than 20 mm Hg.[4] This threshold for elevated pulmonary pressures was lowered from 25 mm Hg based on studies demonstrating the normal range of pulmonary pressures in healthy subjects and poor outcomes for patients with mean pulmonary pressures greater than 20 mm Hg.[5–7]

Furthermore, the risk of progression from mild to more severe hemodynamic impairment appears to be high in CTD, with 2 cohort studies suggesting up to one-third of patients with mPAP between 21 and 24 mm Hg progressing to mPAP greater than 25 mm Hg over 3 years.[8,9] Right heart catheterization (RHC) is required to diagnose PH, as mPAP cannot be directly measured by echocardiography. In hemodynamic terms, PH is often divided in to precapillary, postcapillary, and combined precapillary and postcapillary disease based on the pulmonary capillary wedge pressure (PCWP) and PVR.[4] Current guidelines further refine this classification and incorporate hemodynamic criteria with clinical and associated characteristics (**Table 1**).

Because CTD in general can affect multiple organ systems, PH related to CTD can be associated with any of the 5 World Health Organization (WHO) groups (**Fig. 1**).[3,10–17] The most common CTDs associated with PH are listed in **Fig. 1** and include mixed connective tissue disease (MCTD), polymyositis/dermatomyositis (PM/DM), rheumatoid arthritis (RA), Sjogren syndrome (SS), systemic lupus erythematosus (SLE), and SSc. The risk of development of PH of any form varies by underlying CTD; the risk of PAH in particular seems to be higher in certain CTDs, such as SSc. Thus, recommendations for screening for PH in CTD vary by type of CTD. Importantly, it does not appear that the change in mPAP threshold defining PH has had a significant impact on the prevalence of PAH in SSc, as 2 recent cohort studies demonstrated that less than 2% of patients with SSc were reclassified as PAH based on the new definition.[10,18] In general, the presence of PH of any severity complicating any CTD is associated with a poorer prognosis.[11–14]

PATHOPHYSIOLOGY AND PATHOBIOLOGY

The pathophysiology and pathobiology of PH remain poorly understood. PAH develops as a consequence of progressive remodeling of the small- to medium-sized pulmonary vasculature. Plexiform lesions, medial hypertrophy with muscularization of the arterioles, concentric intimal proliferation, and in situ thrombosis are the pathologic hallmarks of the disease.[15] Although the exact mechanisms of this remodeling remain unclear, multiple factors are thought to be involved.[16] Genetic factors demonstrated to predispose to the development of PAH or to the progression of disease and disease severity have not been routinely shown to be present in PAH-CTD.[17]

Table 1 Hemodynamic classification of pulmonary hypertension				
Definition	Mean PAP (mm Hg)	PCWP (mm Hg)	PVR (Wu)	WHO Group
Normal hemodynamics	14.0 ± 3.3	8.0 ± 2.9	0.93 ± 0.38	N/A
Precapillary PH	>20	≤15	≥3	1, 3, 4, 5
Isolated postcapillary PH	>20	>15	<3	2 and 5
Combined precapillary and postcapillary PH	>20	>15	≥3	2 and 5

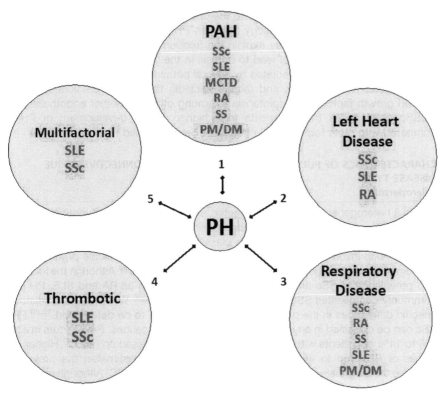

Fig. 1. Types of PH in various CTDs.

Inflammation and autoimmunity are thought to play a central role in the development of PAH, both in the idiopathic pulmonary arterial hypertension (IPAH) and in PAH-CTD.[19,20] Autoimmunity and subsequent immune dysregulation may lead to activation of pathogenic autoreactive B cells and T cells and thus may be involved in the pathobiology of PAH, and in particular, PAH-CTD.

The pathobiology of other forms of PH outside of PAH is less well characterized. Patients with group 2 PH can have either passive PH (due solely to increased pressure downstream of the pulmonary arteries) or reactive/mixed PH (due to a combination of increased downstream pressure and structural and/or functional abnormalities of the pulmonary vasculature).[4] Pathologically, pulmonary veins are enlarged, dilated, and thickened with pulmonary capillary dilatation, interstitial edema, alveolar hemorrhage, and enlarged lymphatics. Distal pulmonary arteries can show evidence of medial hypertrophy, smooth muscle cell proliferation, and eccentric intimal lesions, but do not have classic plexiform lesions. Patients with CTD may be particularly prone to developing group 2 PH because of high prevalence of diastolic dysfunction of the left ventricle; additionally, valvular disorders, particularly those affecting the mitral valve, may also be present in certain CTDs and lead to increased pulmonary venous pressures.[3]

Group 3 PH can result from several entities, including obstructive lung disease, restrictive lung disease, neuromuscular disease, or obstructive sleep apnea. Within this category, PH related to interstitial lung disease (ILD) is most commonly encountered clinically in patients with CTD. Vascular obliteration related to parenchymal destruction and hypoxia contributes to the development of PH related to ILD. There exist commonalities in pathobiology between PH and ILD, and in particular, SSc-related ILD (SSc-ILD), that may explain the frequent copresentation of these 2 entities.[21] The same factors that lead to fibrosis in the vasculature may be influencing fibrosis in the interstitium, mediated by several pathways, including the transforming growth factor-β superfamily, and factors such as the CXC chemokines, platelet-derived growth factor, and angiotensin II, among others. Whether endothelial injury in SSc predisposes these patients to a higher risk of development of PH-ILD compared with other forms of ILD remains to be determined.[22]

CHARACTERISTICS OF PULMONARY HYPERTENSION BY CONNECTIVE TISSUE DISEASE TYPE
Scleroderma

SSc is a heterogeneous disorder characterized by endothelial dysfunction, fibroblast dysregulation, and immune system abnormalities that lead to progressive fibrosis of the skin and internal organs.[23] SSc is classified as limited or diffuse based on the extent of skin involvement. In either form, SSc can involve multiple organ systems, including the heart, lungs, gastrointestinal tract, and kidneys.[24] Although the incidence and prevalence of SSc are lower than other CTDs, such as RA and SLE, PH more commonly complicates SSc compared with other CTDs.[25] Whether this is related to specific differences in the pathobiology of SSc remains to be determined.[19,20] PH in SSc can be classified in any of the 5 WHO group classifications. PAH occurs in about 8% to 14% of patients with SSc when the diagnosis is based on RHC.[11] Higher estimates of PAH (up to 45% in certain series) have overestimated the prevalence because the diagnosis relied on echocardiography and not RHC. Although echocardiography can be useful to suggest the presence of PH and to identify potential causes of PH (eg, valvular disease, left ventricular dysfunction, congenital he art disease), echocardiography cannot establish the diagnosis of PH because of the inaccuracy of the Doppler signal in assessing true RV systolic pressure and the frequent inability to obtain an adequate Doppler signal, particularly in patients with CTD.[26] However, despite the potential for overdiagnosis of PAH based on the limitations of echocardiography, PAH in SSc is still likely to be underrecognized and underdiagnosed as suggested by its lower than expected prevalence in PH registries.

In addition, patients with SSc can develop pulmonary veno-occlusive disease (PVOD, World Symposium on Pulmonary Hypertension [WSPH] group 1.6), a rare form of PAH.[27] PVOD is a severe form of PAH characterized by both pulmonary arterial and pulmonary venule remodeling. In general, PVOD is a rare phenomenon, occurring in an estimated 0.1 to 0.2 persons per million.[28] Although genetic factors contribute to the development of PVOD in some cases, the genetic mutations have yet to be described in CTD patients with PVOD. PVOD can occur in various forms of CTD, including RA, SLE, SS, MCTD, but is most commonly seen in SSc, reported in up to 75% of autopsies in patients with SSc with PAH.[27] Clinically, PVOD is characterized by a low diffusion capacity for carbon monoxide, and classical chest computed tomographic (CT) evidence of mediastinal lymphadenopathy, septal thickening, and centrilobular ground-glass opacities. Patients with PVOD may have a more rapid disease progression and thus require close evaluation and consideration of advanced therapy.

Screening and early detection
Because patients with SSc are at high risk of developing PAH, routine screening for this disease has been recommended.[29] Many support the use of the DETECT algorithm, a 2-step algorithm incorporating pulmonary function testing parameters, serum

biomarkers, clinical characteristics (presence of telangiectasias), and electrocardiogram findings to generate a risk score to determine the need for echocardiography (**Fig. 2**).[29] Subsequent findings on echocardiography (right atrial enlargement, TR jet ≥2.5 m/s) in combination with step 1 score determine the need for RHC. Using this algorithm, the false negative rate for PAH was 4% compared with a nearly 30% false negative rate when using the European Society of Cardiology/European Respiratory Society (ESC/ERS) guidelines for screening in this population. Still, this algorithm

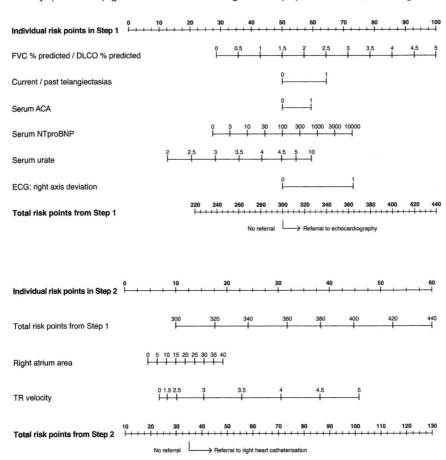

Fig. 2. The DETECT algorithm. Nomograms for the DETECT algorithm. Two-step algorithm for determining referral for RHC or suspected PAH in systemic sclerosis. At step 1 (*top*), risk points for each of the 6 nonechocardiographic variables are calculated and summed. If the total risk points from step 1 are greater than 300, the patient is referred for echocardiography. Similarly, at step 2, risk points for the carried forward and the 2 echocardiographic variables are calculated. If the total risk points from step 2 is greater than 35, the patient is referred to RHC. If a single step 1 variable is missing, it should be assigned 50 risk points, with the exception of current/past telangiectasias, which should be assigned 65 points. If a single step 2 variable is missing, it should be assigned 10 points. The nomograms cannot be reliably used if more than 1 variable out of the 8 total variables is missing. ACA, anticentromere antibody; FVC, forced vital capacity; TR, tricuspid regurgitant jet. (*From* Coghlan JG, Denton CP, Grunig E, Bonderman D, Distler O, Khanna D, et al. Evidence-based detection of pulmonary arterial hypertension in systemic sclerosis: the DETECT study. Ann Rheum Dis 2014 Jul;73(7):1340-9.)

has limitations: (1) it was developed in a high-risk subset of patients with SSc (those with a diffusing capacity for carbon monoxide [DLCO] < 60% predicted and >3 years duration of SSc) and (2) it was designed to detect PH defined as a mean PAP ≥ 25 mm Hg rather than the current definition of PH (mean PAP > 20 mm Hg). Therefore, this approach may not apply to all patients with SSc, nor have the same test characteristics (sensitivity and specificity) for the new definition of PH.

Outcomes
Outcomes in patients with SSc with PAH are poor, particularly in comparison to other forms of PAH. Modern era cohort studies have reported 3-year survival ranging from 50% to 75%.[30–33] The improved survival in the PHAROS registry may reflect inclusion of patients with less severe disease, as more than half of the subjects were in WHO functional class 1 or 2 at enrollment. Prior studies have also demonstrated that survival remains worse in SSc with PAH than in patients with the idiopathic form of PAH, despite seemingly less severe hemodynamic perturbations at diagnosis. This may reflect differences in the RV adaptation to increased afterload. In 1 cohort study, N-terminal pro b-type natriuretic peptide (NT-proBNP) levels were significantly higher in PAH because of SSc compared with IPAH despite less severe hemodynamic impairment; this difference persisted when controlling for potential confounders, such as age and renal function.[34] Because NT-proBNP is released from the ventricles in response to increased wall stress, the observation suggested that responses to increased afterload on the RV may differ between PAH in SSc and IPAH. In line with this, physiologic studies have shown depressed RV function for a similar afterload in compared with IPAH.[35,36] Using pressure-volume measurements in the RV, Tedford and colleagues[36] demonstrated significantly lower contractility in PAH from SSc compared with patients with IPAH, despite similar pulmonary vascular resistive and pulsatile loading characteristics as assessed by resistance-compliance relationships and arterial elastance measures. This may reflect intrinsic differences in RV contractility. Furthermore, Hsu and colleagues[37] demonstrated a "dose-response" relationship in RV contractility assessed using isolated myocyte preparations from RV biopsies between patients with SSc without PAH, patients with SSc with PAH, and patients with IPAH. These findings suggest intrinsic RV dysfunction may contribute to the clinical differences in presentation and outcomes. **Box 1** shows predictors of outcomes in patients with SSc and PAH.

Pulmonary hypertension related to interstitial lung disease and other comorbidities in systemic sclerosis
Patients with SSc can also develop PH related to ILD, but there are limited data describing its prevalence. The presence of PH in SSc-ILD portends a poor prognosis.[11,19] In a cohort of 59 patients with SSc with PH, 20 of whom had significant ILD (defined as a total lung capacity [TLC] < 60% predicted or TLC between 60% and 70% predicted combined with moderate to severe fibrosis on high-resolution CT of the chest), survival was significantly worse in the SSc-ILD cohort with 1-, 2-, and 3-year survival rates of 82%, 49%, and 39% compared with 87%, 79%, and 64% in the PH alone group, respectively (*P*<.01)[11] and presence of ILD portended a 5-fold increased risk of death compared with PAH. Occult left heart disease may also be common in patients with SSc with PH and impacts outcomes. Fox and colleagues[20] demonstrated that nearly 40% of patients with SSc who were diagnosed with PAH based on PCWP ≤ 15 mm Hg actually had postcapillary PH after fluid challenge during RHC. Furthermore, patients with evidence of diastolic dysfunction and

---

Box 1
Predictors of survival in pulmonary arterial hypertension–systemic sclerosis

Male gender[a]

Age[a]

New York Heart Association functional class at diagnosis[a]

Increased NT-proBNP

Right atrial pressure[a]

Mean pulmonary artery pressure[a]

Cardiac index

Stroke volume index

Pulmonary vascular resistance

Renal function

[a] Variable association with survival in PAH-SSc.

---

precapillary PH had a 2-fold increased risk of death compared with patients with PAH-SSc after adjusting for hemodynamic severity of PH.[38]

Other Connective Tissue Diseases

Although PH can complicate other CTDs, these have been less well characterized, largely because of the lower overall prevalence of PH in patients with other CTDs or the lower overall prevalence of these CTDs in the general population.

Mixed Connective Tissue Disease

Patients with MCTD have clinical features of several CTDs, including SSc, SLE, RA, and PM/DM. The characteristic laboratory feature is the presence of antibodies to uridine-rich (U1) RNP polypeptides, which is required to establish the diagnosis.[39] Lung disease in MCTD is common and can manifest as parenchymal disease, pulmonary vascular disease, or both.[14,40] Cohort studies have provided estimates of the prevalence of PAH in MCTD ranging from 1% to as high as 50% and of ILD in up to 50%.[14,41] Thromboembolism may be more common in MCTD; in 1 study, 19.9% of patients with MCTD had venous clots.[41] Whether these patients with venous thrombosis developed chronic thromboembolic disease and PH is unknown.

Patients with MCTD and PAH tend to be diagnosed late in their disease course, with nearly 70% having WHO FC 3 symptoms at diagnosis.[42] Compared with patients with SSc with PAH, patients with MCTD with PAH are younger and more likely to be black or Hispanic. Biomarkers of disease severity in PAH, such as brain natriuretic peptide, are lower, and DLCO is higher in MCTD compared with SSc, suggesting less severe disease. Hemodynamics do not differ significantly between the 2 groups, except that right atrial pressure tends to be lower in MCTD.[42]

Outcomes

PAH appears to be the most common cause of death in patients with MCTD.[41,43] Two cohort studies have reported outcomes in RHC-proven PAH in MCTD. In a national registry from the United Kingdom, survival in PAH from MCTD was similar to PAH from SSc at 1 year (83% vs 77%) but perhaps better at 3 years (66% vs 47%).[44] In the REVEAL registry, 1-year survival did not differ between PAH related to MCTD or SSc (88% vs 82%).[42] However, when compared with other forms of CTD-related

PAH, such as SLE, survival was worse in the MCTD cohorts in both studies. Based on these studies showing the impact of PAH on outcomes, expert consensus recommends screening for PAH in patients with MCTD, particularly those with SSc features.[43]

Systemic Lupus Erythematous

SLE is a multisystem disease that can affect the lungs and lead to several forms of pulmonary vascular disease, including ILD-related PH, PAH, and chronic thromboembolic pulmonary hypertension (CTEPH). In addition, PH can result from SLE-associated cardiomyopathy or from renal failure requiring hemodialysis and placement of arteriovenous fistulas.[45] Thus, PH in SLE can also be classified in any of the 5 PH categories (see **Fig. 1**).

Prevalence estimates of PH in SLE vary widely, from 0.0005% to 14% of patients.[45] Patients who develop the disease tend to be young (average age around 30 at diagnosis) and often have Raynaud phenomenon.[46] Risk factors for the development of PAH related to SLE are not well described, but blacks, those with anti-smooth muscle or anticardiolipin antibodies, and history of pericarditis appear more likely to have PH.

Outcomes

As expected, outcomes in patients with SLE with PH are worse than for those without PH. Cohort studies report survival for PAH in patients with SLE that range from 50% to 75% at 3 years; however, there may be geographic differences in outcomes, as deaths attributable to PAH seem to be lower in European and North American cohorts compared with Asian cohorts.[45,46] Risk factors for poor outcomes have been described in a systematic review and include both PH-specific and SLE-specific parameters.[47] Higher mPAP at diagnosis, vascular manifestations of SLE such as Raynaud phenomenon, pulmonary vasculitis, thrombosis, thrombocytopenia, and presence of anticardiolipin antibodies all portend a poorer prognosis. Interestingly, neither lupus disease activity nor nephritis was associated with poorer outcome.

Sjogren Syndrome

SS is a chronic inflammatory disease characterized by lymphocytic infiltration of exocrine glands and extraglandular tissues. It can present as primary disease or in association with other CTDs, such as RA or SSc, and predominantly affects women.[48] Although the sicca syndrome (xerophthalmia and/or keratoconjunctivitis sicca and xerostomia) is most commonly present in patients with SS, extraglandular involvement of the lungs is common, typically manifesting as ILD. Various types of ILD have been described in SS, including lymphocytic interstitial pneumonia, nonspecific interstitial pneumonitis, usual interstitial pneumonitis, and organizing pneumonia.[48]

In contrast to other CTDs, PAH is rare in SS. Relatively large cohort studies have estimated the prevalence of PH at around 20%; however, the diagnosis of PH was based on echocardiography. In the largest case series of patients with SS-associated PH, Launay and colleagues[49] describe associations between anti-Ro and RNP antibodies and hypergammaglobulinemia in patients with SS with PAH. Survival in this cohort was poor with 1-year and 3-year survival at 73% and 66%, respectively, similar to survival seen in patients with PAH from SSc.

Rheumatoid Arthritis

RA is an autoimmune disease characterized by a symmetric, inflammatory polyarthritis that leads to joint destruction. RA is more prevalent that most other CTDs, occurring in 40 out of 100,000 persons in the United States. Women in the United States have a nearly 4% lifetime risk of developing RA.[50] Extra-articular disease affects multiple organs, and cardiopulmonary involvement is common. There is a high risk of coronary artery disease, myocardial infarction, heart failure, and sudden death compared with age-matched persons without RA. Pulmonary manifestations include ILD, rheumatoid nodules, airways disease with bronchiolitis obliterans and organizing pneumonia, and pleural disease.[50] Lung disease may also result from disease-modifying antirheumatic drugs, with complications such as pneumonitis, fibrosis, obliterative bronchiolitis, infection, and bronchospasm, among others.

PH in RA has been reported in association with left heart disease, ILD, and chronic thromboembolic disease. Isolated PH, that is, PH in the absence of overt left heart disease, ILD, and chronic thromboembolic disease, has been infrequently reported in the literature. In the UK registry, only 12 patients with RA with PAH were identified, whereas in the REVEAL registry, 28 cases of RHC-proven PAH owing to RA were included.[42,44] When compared with patients with SSc-related PAH in the REVEAL cohort, RA patients with PAH tended to be younger (54 ± 15.8 vs 61.8 ± 11.1 years). Raynaud phenomenon was less likely to be present (3.6% vs 32.6% of the cohort); renal insufficiency was less frequent, and b-type natriuretic peptide levels were significantly lower. Functional class at baseline, 6-minute walk distance (6MWD), and hemodynamics were similar. Although spirometry and lung volumes were similar when compared with PAH in SSc, diffusing capacity was higher in the PAH owing to RA cohort. One-year survival in the RA cohort was significantly better than the SSc cohort (96% vs 82%, $P = .01$).

Polymyositis/Dermatomyositis

PM and DM are idiopathic inflammatory myopathies that are characterized by proximal muscle weakness. DM has characteristic skin manifestations, although clinical features of both DM and PM vary among affected individuals. The estimated prevalence of these diseases varies from 5 to 22 per 100,000 persons, with an annual incidence of 2 per 100,000.[51] The most common pulmonary manifestation of PM/DM is ILD, occurring in about 10% of patients, although respiratory symptoms, such as dyspnea and orthopnea, can also arise from muscle weakness affecting the diaphragm.[52]

PH appears to be a rare complication of PM/DM, and if present, may be more related to underlying ILD.[52] In the UK registry, only 7 patients (2% of the entire PAH-CTD cohort) had PAH related to PM/DM, and there were no cases of PAH related to PM/DM seen in the REVEAL registry.[42,44] No clinical demographic or hemodynamic characteristics of these patients were reported in the UK registry; however, the 1- and 3-year survival was 100% for these patients, suggesting better outcomes compared with other PAH-CTD.

DIAGNOSIS

Given the need for precision in the classification of PH phenotype in patients with underlying CTD, a detailed diagnostic algorithm should be followed. Clinical suspicion for PH should be informed by the risk inherent to the underlying CTD. However, in many cases, a thorough evaluation for CTD has not been undertaken before evaluation for PH and thus should be completed. In addition to history and physical examination focusing on identifying features of CTD, serologic evaluation including screening tests for CTD should be completed. Current guidelines recommend anti-nuclear antibody testing using immunofluorescence.[53] If CTD is suggested by results of serologies or if clinical suspicion remains high despite negative screening serologies, additional testing, including anticentromere, antitopoisomerase, anti-RNA polymerase III, double-stranded DNA, anti-Ro, anti-La, and U-1 RNP, antibodies should be sent, and referral to rheumatology should be considered. Furthermore, given the high prevalence of left heart disease, ILD, and thromboembolism in CTD, evaluation for each of these entities should be undertaken before proceeding to RHC given the implications for clinical management. If CTEPH is identified in a CTD patient, further evaluation for thrombophilia should be undertaken.

TREATMENT

Currently, specific pulmonary vasodilator therapy for PH in the setting of CTD is approved by the Food and Drug Administration (FDA) only for patients with PAH, PH due to ILD, and CTEPH. These therapies have been developed by targeting pathways in the putative pathogenesis of PAH and then tested in the PH due to ILD and the CTEPH populations. Randomized clinical trials of novel therapeutics for PAH have included patients with various forms of PAH-CTD, although most patients enrolled likely have SSc. Subgroup analyses in the PAH-CTD cohorts of these studies have not been consistently reported.[54–60] Given the differences in demographic and hemodynamic characteristics between PAH-CTD types, the results from these clinical trials are unlikely to be generalizable to all forms of PAH-CTD and thus should be interpreted with caution in most cases. Still, the PAH therapies discussed later are commonly used in all forms of CTD-PAH, even though the evidence base for diseases other than SSc is minimal.

General Measures

Despite a lack of specific data for PAH of any form, consensus guidelines recommend the use of supplemental oxygen in patients who are hypoxic (peripheral oxygen saturation <90%) at rest or with exercise, largely based on extrapolation of data from chronic obstructive lung disease.[61,62] In addition, diuretics are recommended for the management of right heart failure and volume overload. Digoxin may also be useful for management of refractory right heart failure complicated by atrial arrhythmias. Exercise, and in particular, pulmonary rehabilitation, may also be beneficial as demonstrated in a clinical trial of prescribed exercise in a population of patients with IPAH and PAH-CTD.[63,64]

Anticoagulation

Anticoagulation is recommended in the treatment of IPAH based primarily on retrospective, observational data showing improved survival in patients on warfarin therapy. However, no such data exist for PAH-CTD, and there may be increased risk of harm with anticoagulation.[65] Thus, routine anticoagulation for PAH-CTD in the absence of other comorbidities for which anticoagulation is necessary is not recommended by current expert consensus.[2,66]

Immunosuppression

As discussed previously, inflammatory and immunologic mechanisms are likely involved in the pathogenesis of both CTD and PAH. Given this potential commonality in pathobiology, anti-inflammatory agents have been used in various types of PAH-CTD. However, there are no randomized, clinical trials in patients with PAH-CTD to support its use in this patient population. Still, several case series have suggested efficacy in certain populations within PAH-CTD. In the report by Jais and colleagues,[67] 23 patients with either SLE- or MCTD-associated PAH were treated with combination therapy including cyclophosphamide and glucocorticoids; nearly half of the patients with SLE and patients with MCTD demonstrated clinical improvement in functional capacity and hemodynamics, although patients with SSc did not. Other investigators have reported improvements in functional capacity, hemodynamics, and survival with immunosuppressant therapy.[68–70] A recently completed randomized controlled double-masked trial in patients with SSc with PAH of rituximab, a monoclonal antibody targeting CD20 on B cells, did not meet its primary endpoint of change in 6MWD (NCT01086540).

Pulmonary Vasodilator Therapy

There are now more than a dozen FDA-approved pulmonary vasodilator therapies for PAH, one for CTEPH, and most recently, one for PH-ILD. According to expert consensus, selection of therapy for patients with PAH should be based on risk stratification at diagnosis and follow-up.[66] There are numerous risk-stratification tools that have been developed and applied in various cohorts. A recent comparison of the predictive value of these tools suggests fair to good discrimination, defined as the ability of the model to separate individuals who develop an event from those who do not, across models.[71] However, the relevance of these predictive models in PAH-CTD is less certain, as some of these models were derived from populations that specifically excluded patients with PAH-CTD or had small proportions of PAH-CTD. Specific analyses of the REVEAL 1.0 model and the ESC/ERS model suggest poor to acceptable predictive utility when applied specifically to PAH-CTD.[72,73] Future studies examining risk in PAH-CTD should be undertaken to better inform prediction model development in this population. Regardless, as shown in **Fig. 3**, current treatment recommendations for patients with PAH, including PAH-CTD, depend on risk assessment.

Historically, response to pulmonary vasodilator therapy in PAH-CTD was thought to be less robust than in other PAH populations. An analysis of patient-level data from registration trials for PAH medications reports a higher rate of adverse events in patients with PAH-CTD and attenuated effect on quality of life compared with IPAH.[74] Subsequently, Rhee and colleagues[75] found the treatment effect, as assessed by change in 6MWD, was similar in magnitude between patients with PAH-CTD and patients with IPAH, but patients with PAH-CTD on therapy had minimal improvement. Interestingly, patients with PAH-CTD treated with placebo had a significant decline in 6MWD in contrast to patients with IPAH. Several factors, specific to patients with PAH-CTD, may influence the observed response to therapy, as shown in **Table 2**. Similarly, interpretation of the clinical relevance of response to therapy for a given outcome measure may differ between PAH-CTD and IPAH. Analysis of change in 6MWD from the registration study for tadalafil in PAH suggests that the minimal clinically important difference (MCID), the smallest change in an outcome measure that is noticeable to a patient and would lead to a change in therapy, is smaller for PAH-CTD than IPAH.[76] Thus, although not statistically significant in the context of the clinical trial data, smaller changes in 6MWD may be more clinically relevant for PAH-CTD.

Recent data from combination therapy trials suggest that response to therapy may not differ significantly between PAH-CTD and IPAH.[77] This may be particularly true when considering morbidity outcomes, such as time to clinical worsening. In the GRIPHON study of selexipag in combination with other PAH therapy, outcome event rates were similar between PAH-CTD and IPAH groups.[59] Furthermore, although adverse events were numerically higher in the PAH-CTD group, there were no significant differences in rates between groups. This trial also offered the unique opportunity to examine responses in patients with SLE with PAH. Importantly, no difference in magnitude of response between SLE and other PAH-CTD or IPAH was seen. Robust data from the AMBITION study also support the use of initial combination therapy with phosphodiesterase inhibitors and endothelin receptor antagonists in PAH-CTD to improve time to clinical worsening.[60] In a 36-week open-label study of newly

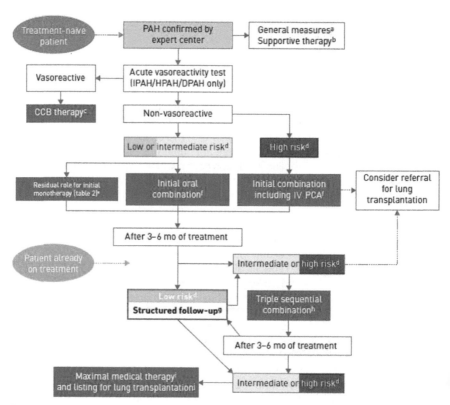

Fig. 3. Treatment of PAH-CTD. CCB, calcium channel blocker; DPAH, drug-induced PAH; HPAH, heritable PAH; PCA, prostacyclin analogue. [a]2015 ESC/ERS PH guidelines Table 16. [b]2015 ESC/ERS PH guidelines Table 17. [c]2015 ESC/ERS PH guidelines Table 18. [d]2015 ESC/ERS PH guidelines Table 13. [e]2015 ESC/ERS PH guidelines Table 19. [f]2015 ESC/ERS PH guidelines Table 20. [g]2015 ESC/ERS PH guidelines Table 14. [h]2015 ESC/ERS PH guidelines Table 21. [i]Maximal medical therapy is considered triple combination therapy, including a subcutaneous or an IV PCA (IV preferred in high-risk status). [j]2015 ESC/ERS PH guidelines Table 22. (Reproduced with permission of the © ERS 2024: European Respiratory Journal 53 (1) 1801889; https://doi.org/10.1183/13993003.01889-2018 Published 24 January 2019.)

diagnosed patients with PAH owing to SSc, Hassoun and colleagues[78] found significant improvement in symptoms, 6MWD, RV function assessed by echocardiography and cardiac MRI, and hemodynamics with initial combination therapy of tadalafil and ambrisentan. The improvements noted for some of these parameters significantly exceed the reported MCID, for example, RV ejection fraction on cardiac MRI. Taken together, these data suggest with initial combination therapy, patients with CTD-PAH experience significant improvement in symptoms, functional capacity, RV function, hemodynamics, and morbidity that is of similar magnitude to patients with IPAH.

Treatment of Pulmonary Hypertension-Interstitial Lung Disease in Connective Tissue Disease

Recently, the FDA approved inhaled treprostinil for use in patients with PH-ILD, including CTD-ILD. This recommendation was based on the results of the INCREASE

Table 2
Disease-specific considerations in connective tissue disease–associated pulmonary hypertension

Domain	Tool	Application to CTD-PAH
Hemodynamics	RHC, Echo	Group II and III disease confound assessment
Exercise testing	6MWD	Musculoskeletal disease/deconditioning
Dyspnea	Borg dyspnea	Non-PAH causes for dyspnea (ILD, anemia, and similar)
Adherence with therapy	Adverse events	Concomitant medications for CTD may interact
Pharmacodynamics	Bioavailability	Different due to gastrointestinal motility, malabsorption
Quality of life	SF-36/CAMPHOR	Extrapulmonary involvement affects quality of life
Global state	Survival	Poorer survival overall compared with IPAH

Adapted from Denton, C.P., Avouac, J., Behrens, F. et al. Systemic sclerosis-associated pulmonary hypertension: why disease-specific composite endpoints are needed. Arthritis Res Ther 13, 114 (2011).

study, a 16-week, randomized, double-masked controlled study of inhaled treprostinil versus placebo in patients with PH in the setting of ILD.[79] PH was defined as an mPAP $\geq$ 25 mm Hg with a PCWP $\leq$ 15 mm Hg and a PVR greater than 3 WU. Although patients with other forms of ILD were permitted to enroll if there was evidence of diffuse parenchymal disease on CT of the chest, patients with CTD also had to have a forced vital capacity less than 70% predicted to fulfill inclusion criteria. Of the 326 patients enrolled, 72 (22%) had CTD. At 16 weeks, the change in 6MWD between treatment and placebo was statistically significant (30.1 m, 95% confidence interval [CI] 16.8–45.4 m), and importantly, oxygenation did not significantly change with pulmonary vasodilator therapy. Interestingly, patients with CTD on average demonstrated greater improvement in 6MWD compared with other ILD groups (mean change 43.5 m, 95% CI 9.6–77.4 m). However, there were no improvements in secondary outcome measures such as quality of life.

TREATMENT OF OTHER FORMS OF PULMONARY HYPERTENSION
Pulmonary Hypertension Related to Left Heart Disease in Connective Tissue Disease

Unfortunately, there are no approved therapies for PH in the setting of left heart disease. Identifying the underlying cause of PH will be helpful and allow for directed therapy where appropriate, such as valve-related disease in SLE. Patients with SSc may be prone to more rapid progression of aortic stenosis, which can lead to PH as well.[80] Valve repair or replacement may be of use in select patients. Heart failure with either reduced or preserved ejection fraction (HFrEF vs HFpEF) can lead to PH, but HFpEF is more commonly encountered in CTD. Specific therapy should be directed at the underlying condition, as there are no data to support use of pulmonary vasodilator therapies for this indication.

Chronic Thromboembolic Pulmonary Hypertension in Connective Tissue Disease

Patients with CTEPH in the setting of CTD should be treated according to guideline-based recommendations.[81] When CTEPH is identified, treatment for at least 3 months with anticoagulation should be undertaken before initiating medical or surgical therapy for PH. Evaluation for surgical thromboendarterectomy should be pursued, as this is the definitive treatment for CTEPH. If the patient is not a surgical candidate, interventional therapy with balloon angioplasty or medical therapy with riociguat may be feasible and effective.[82,83] However, neither therapy is definitive, and as such, thromboendarterectomy remains the treatment of choice in appropriate candidates with appropriate anatomy.

Exercise-Induced Pulmonary Hypertension

Although the definition of PH is based on a resting mPAP at least 20 mm Hg, it is estimated that 50% to 70% of the pulmonary vasculature needs to be affected before resting mPAP is elevated. An abnormal pulmonary hemodynamic response to exercise, or exercise-induced pulmonary hypertension (Ex-PH), has therefore been postulated to represent early pulmonary vascular disease. There remains controversy regarding the appropriate definition of Ex-PH based on the hemodynamic criteria and exercise challenge used. Still, an mPAP more than 30 mm Hg and transpulmonary gradient more than 3 WU at maximal exercise have been proposed as the most suitable definition.[84,85] Using this definition applied to a retrospective cohort of patients with SSc, patients with Ex-PH not only had a worse outcome than if Ex-PH was not present but also had survival similar to patients with SSc with PAH.[86] A recent study by Zeder and colleagues[87] demonstrated that exercise hemodynamics, but not resting hemodynamics, predicted outcomes in a cohort of patients with SSc without resting PH (mPAP > 25 mm Hg), suggesting clinical relevance of exercise hemodynamics in patients without significantly elevated pulmonary pressures. However, there are limited data to support treatment of Ex-PH in SSc with pulmonary vasodilators.[88] One recent randomized controlled study examining the role of ambrisentan in a cohort of 38 patients with SSc with mild resting PH (mPAP 21–24 mm Hg) or Ex-PH did not find improvement in the primary outcome of mPAP, but did find improvement in other hemodynamic measures, both at rest and with exercise.[89] However, subgroup analyses by patients with Ex-PH alone were not reported.

Pulmonary Hypertension with Mildly Elevated Pressures (Mean Pulmonary Artery Pressure 21–24 mm Hg)

One of the major limitations to the 6th WSPH recommendations for lowering the mPAP threshold to fulfill the definition of PH is that there are no approved therapies for patients with pulmonary pressure elevations in this range. All currently approved therapies were evaluated in patients with mPAP $\geq$ 25 mm Hg. Furthermore, aside from the study by Pan and colleagues,[89] there are no randomized controlled trial data evaluating the role of pulmonary vasodilator therapy in this population. A small randomized clinical trial of sildenafil in patients with SSc with early pulmonary vascular disease is planned, but is not yet enrolling (NCT04797286).

Pulmonary Veno-Occlusive Disease in Connective Tissue Disease

PVOD is a severe form of PAH characterized by both pulmonary arterial and pulmonary venule remodeling. Patients with PVOD may have a more rapidly progressive decline and may be prone to developing pulmonary edema with pulmonary vasodilator therapy.[27] As such, careful initiation of low-dose monotherapy is generally recommended for patients with PVOD. Given the propensity for rapid progression and risk of pulmonary edema with dose escalation, patients with PVOD should be referred for lung transplantation evaluation if the diagnosis is considered possible based on the clinical scenario.

LUNG TRANSPLANTATION

Current International Society of Heart and Lung Transplantation guidelines recommend lung transplant for patients with CTD if no extrapulmonary contraindications to transplantation exist.[90] Typically, these criteria include uncontrolled gastroesophageal reflux disease or dysphagia, renal dysfunction, or significant LV dysfunction. Largely owing to these concerns, patients with CTD continue to comprise only a minority of transplant recipients. However, when recent short- and long-term outcomes are considered, outcomes for patients with CTD are comparable to other transplant recipients with similar indications for transplantation (ie, ILD and PAH).[91,92] Therefore, patients with PH in the setting of CTD should be referred for lung transplant evaluation.

SUMMARY

PH remains a common complication of CTD and can present in various forms, most commonly in the setting of left heart disease, lung disease, or PAH. The presence of PH in any form portends a poor outcome. Advances in screening for PAH in high-risk cohorts, such as SSc, along with increased awareness of treatment options for non-PAH forms of PH may help support efforts to identify pulmonary vascular disease earlier in this at-risk population and allow for intervention. Initial combination therapy is now recommended as standard of care for treatment-naive, intermediate-risk patients with PAH-CTD, and pulmonary vasodilator therapy is approved for both patients with CTEPH and patients with PH-ILD with CTD. Furthermore, lung transplant remains an option in the appropriate patient. Still, despite these advances, there remains an ongoing need to improve outcomes for patients with CTD with PH.

CLINICS CARE POINTS

- Routine, yearly screening for development of pulmonary hypertension in certain forms of connective tissue disease, such as scleroderma, is recommended.

- Thorough evaluation for pulmonary hypertension should be undertaken to ensure proper classification according to the World Health Organization Classification as treatment strategies vary between pulmonary hypertension types.

- New therapies for pulmonary hypertension in the setting of interstitial lung disease have been approved by the Federal Drug Agency recently and should be considered in the management of these patients.

DISCLOSURE

Consultancies: Actelion, Acceleron, Bayer, United Therapeutics. Funding to institution: Actelion, United Therapeutics. NHLBI: U01HL125175 (Co-PI); R01HL134905 (Co-I); R01HL11490 (Co-I). DOD: PR191839 (PI). The clinical trial (NCT04797286) referenced in the article is supported by DOD grant PR191839 (PI-Mathai).

REFERENCES

1. Chin KM, Kim NH, Rubin LJ. The right ventricle in pulmonary hypertension. Coron Artery Dis 2005;16(1):13–8.
2. Galiè N, Humbert M, Vachiery JL, et al, ESC Scientific Document Group. 2015 ESC/ERS guidelines for the diagnosis and treatment of pulmonary hypertension: the Joint Task Force for the Diagnosis and Treatment of Pulmonary Hypertension of the European Society of Cardiology (ESC) and the European Respiratory Society (ERS): endorsed by: Association for European Paediatric and Congenital

Cardiology (AEPC), International Society for Heart and Lung Transplantation (ISHLT). Eur Heart J 2016;37(1):67–119.

3. Mathai SC, Hassoun PM. Pulmonary arterial hypertension in connective tissue diseases. Heart Fail Clin 2012;8(3):413–25.

4. Simonneau G, Montani D, Celermajer DS, et al. Haemodynamic definitions and updated clinical classification of pulmonary hypertension. Eur Respir J 2019; 53(1):1801913.

5. Kovacs G, Berghold A, Scheidl S, et al. Pulmonary arterial pressure during rest and exercise in healthy subjects: a systematic review. Eur Respir J 2009;34: 888–94.

6. Maron BA, Hess E, Maddox TM, et al. Association of borderline pulmonary hypertension with mortality and hospitalization in a large patient cohort: insights from the Veterans Affairs Clinical Assessment, Reporting and Tracking program. Circulation 2016;133:1240–8.

7. Assad TR, Maron BA, Robbins IM, et al. Prognostic effect and longitudinal hemodynamic assessment of borderline pulmonary hypertension. JAMA Cardiol 2017. https://doi.org/10.1001/jamacardio.2017.3882.

8. Valerio CJ, Schreiber BE, Handler CE, et al. Borderline mean pulmonary artery pressure in patients with systemic sclerosis: transpulmonary gradient predicts risk of developing pulmonary hypertension. Arthritis Rheum 2013;65(4):1074–84.

9. Coghlan JG, Wolf M, Distler O, et al. Incidence of pulmonary hypertension and determining factors in patients with systemic sclerosis. Eur Respir J 2018; 51(4):1701197.

10. Xanthouli P, Jordan S, Milde N, et al. Haemodynamic phenotypes and survival in patients with systemic sclerosis: the impact of the new definition of pulmonary arterial hypertension. Ann Rheum Dis 2020;79(3):370–8.

11. Mathai SC, Hummers LK, Champion HC, et al. Survival in pulmonary hypertension associated with the scleroderma spectrum of diseases: impact of interstitial lung disease. Arthritis Rheum 2009;60(2):569–77.

12. Chung SM, Lee CK, Lee EY, et al. Clinical aspects of pulmonary hypertension in patients with systemic lupus erythematosus and in patients with idiopathic pulmonary arterial hypertension. Clin Rheumatol 2006;25(6):866–72.

13. Hatron PY, Tillie-Leblond I, Launay D, et al. Pulmonary manifestations of Sjogren's syndrome. Presse Med 2011;40(1 Pt 2):e49–64.

14. Szodoray P, Hajas A, Kardos L, et al. Distinct phenotypes in mixed connective tissue disease: subgroups and survival. Lupus 2012;21(13):1412–22.

15. Stewart S, Rassl D. Advances in the understanding and classification of pulmonary hypertension. Histopathology 2009;54(1):104–16.

16. Voelkel NF, Gomez-Arroyo J, Abbate A, et al. Pathobiology of pulmonary arterial hypertension and right ventricular failure. Eur Respir J 2012;40(6):1555–65.

17. Morrell NW, Aldred MA, Chung WK, et al. Genetics and genomics of pulmonary arterial hypertension. Eur Respir J 2019;53(1):1801899.

18. Jaafar S, Visovatti S, Young A, et al. Impact of the revised haemodynamic definition on the diagnosis of pulmonary hypertension in patients with systemic sclerosis. Eur Respir J 2019;54(2):1900586.

19. Launay D, Montani D, Hassoun PM, et al. Clinical phenotypes and survival of precapillary pulmonary hypertension in systemic sclerosis. PLoS One 2018;13(5): e0197112.

20. Fox BD, Shimony A, Langleben D, et al. High prevalence of occult left heart disease in scleroderma-pulmonary hypertension. Eur Respir J 2013;42:1083–91.

21. Farkas L, Gauldie J, Voelkel NF, et al. Pulmonary hypertension and idiopathic pulmonary fibrosis: a tale of angiogenesis, apoptosis, and growth factors. Am J Respir Cell Mol Biol 2011;45(1):1–15.
22. Lewandowska K, Ciurzynski M, Gorska E, et al. Antiendothelial cells antibodies in patients with systemic sclerosis in relation to pulmonary hypertension and lung fibrosis. Adv Exp Med Biol 2013;756:147–53.
23. Gabrielli A, Avvedimento EV, Krieg T. Scleroderma. N Engl J Med 2009;360(19):1989–2003.
24. van den Hoogen F, Khanna D, Fransen J, et al. 2013 classification criteria for systemic sclerosis: an American College of Rheumatology/European League Against Rheumatism Collaborative Initiative. Ann Rheum Dis 2013;72:1747–55.
25. Ranque B, Mouthon L. Geoepidemiology of systemic sclerosis. Autoimmun Rev 2010;9(5):A311–8.
26. Mathai SC, Sibley CT, Forfia PR, et al. Tricuspid annular plane systolic excursion is a robust outcome measure in systemic sclerosis-associated pulmonary arterial hypertension. J Rheumatol 2011;38(11):2410–8.
27. Dorfmuller P, Humbert M, Perros F, et al. Fibrous remodeling of the pulmonary venous system in pulmonary arterial hypertension associated with connective tissue diseases. Hum Pathol 2007;38(6):893–902.
28. Montani D, Lau EM, Dorfmuller P, et al. Pulmonary veno-occlusive disease. Eur Respir J 2016;47:1518–34.
29. Coghlan JG, Denton CP, Grunig E, et al. Evidence-based detection of pulmonary arterial hypertension in systemic sclerosis: the DETECT study. Ann Rheum Dis 2014;73(7):1340–9.
30. Hachulla E, Carpentier P, Gressin V, et al. Risk factors for death and the 3-year survival of patients with systemic sclerosis: the French ItinerAIR-Sclerodermie study. Rheumatology (Oxford) 2009;48(3):304–8.
31. Campo A, Mathai SC, Le PJ, et al. Hemodynamic predictors of survival in scleroderma-related pulmonary arterial hypertension. Am J Respir Crit Care Med 2010;182(2):252–60.
32. Rubenfire M, Huffman MD, Krishnan S, et al. Survival in systemic sclerosis with pulmonary arterial hypertension has not improved in the modern era. Chest 2013;144(4):1282–90.
33. Chung L, Domsic RT, Lingala B, et al. Survival and predictors of mortality in systemic sclerosis associated pulmonary arterial hypertension: outcomes from the PHAROS registry. Arthritis Care Res (Hoboken) 2013;65(3):454–63.
34. Mathai SC, Bueso M, Hummers LK, et al. Disproportionate elevation of N-terminal pro-brain natriuretic peptide in scleroderma-related pulmonary hypertension. Eur Respir J 2010;35(1):95–104.
35. Overbeek MJ, Lankhaar JW, Westerhof N, et al. Right ventricular contractility in systemic sclerosis-associated and idiopathic pulmonary arterial hypertension. Eur Respir J 2008;31(6):1160–6.
36. Tedford RJ, Mudd JO, Girgis RE, et al. Right ventricular dysfunction in systemic sclerosis associated pulmonary arterial hypertension. Circ Heart Fail 2013;6(5):953–63.
37. Hsu S, Kokkenen-Simon KM, Kirk JA, et al. Right ventricular myofilament functional differences in humans with systemic sclerosis-associated versus idiopathic pulmonary arterial hypertension. Circulation 2018;137:2360–70.
38. Bourji KI, Kelemen BW, Mathai SC, et al. Poor survival in patients with scleroderma and pulmonary hypertension due to heart failure with preserved ejection fraction. Pulm Circ 2017;7(2):409–20.

39. Sharp GC, Irvin WS, Tan EM, et al. Mixed connective tissue disease–an apparently distinct rheumatic disease syndrome associated with a specific antibody to an extractable nuclear antigen (ENA). Am J Med 1972;52(2):148–59.
40. Gunnarsson R, Andreassen AK, Molberg O, et al. Prevalence of pulmonary hypertension in an unselected, mixed connective tissue disease cohort: results of a nationwide, Norwegian cross-sectional multicentre study and review of current literature. Rheumatology (Oxford) 2013;52(7):1208–13.
41. Gunnarsson R, Aalokken TM, Molberg O, et al. Prevalence and severity of interstitial lung disease in mixed connective tissue disease: a nationwide, cross-sectional study. Ann Rheum Dis 2012;71(12):1966–72.
42. Chung L, Liu J, Parsons L, et al. Characterization of connective tissue disease-associated pulmonary arterial hypertension from REVEAL: identifying systemic sclerosis as a unique phenotype. Chest 2010;138(6):1383–94.
43. Khanna D, Gladue H, Channick R, et al. Recommendations for screening and detection of connective-tissue disease associated pulmonary arterial hypertension. Arthritis Rheum 2013;65(12):3194–201.
44. Condliffe R, Kiely DG, Peacock AJ, et al. Connective tissue disease-associated pulmonary arterial hypertension in the modern treatment era. Am J Respir Crit Care Med 2009;179(2):151–7.
45. Hannah JR, D'Cruz DP. Pulmonary complications of systemic lupus erythematosus. Semin Respir Crit Care Med 2019;40(2):227–34.
46. Hachulla E, Jais X, Cinquetti G, et al, French Collaborators Recruiting Members(*). Pulmonary arterial hypertension associated with systemic lupus erythematosus: results from the French Pulmonary Hypertension Registry. Chest 2018;153(01):143–51.
47. Johnson SR, Gladman DD, Urowitz MB, et al. Pulmonary hypertension in systemic lupus. Lupus 2004;13(7):506–9.
48. Flament T, Bigot A, Chaigne B, et al. Pulmonary manifestations of Sjögren's syndrome. Eur Respir Rev 2016;25(140):110–23.
49. Launay D, Hachulla E, Hatron PY, et al. Pulmonary arterial hypertension: a rare complication of primary Sjogren syndrome: report of 9 new cases and review of the literature. Medicine (Baltimore) 2007;86(5):299–315.
50. Crowson CS, Matteson EL, Myasoedova E, et al. The lifetime risk of adult-onset rheumatoid arthritis and other inflammatory autoimmune rheumatic diseases. Arthritis Rheum 2011;63(3):633–9.
51. Bernatsky S, Joseph L, Pineau CA, et al. Estimating the prevalence of polymyositis and dermatomyositis from administrative data: age, sex and regional differences. Ann Rheum Dis 2009;68(7):1192–6.
52. Mathai SC, Danoff SK. Management of interstitial lung disease associated with connective tissue disease. BMJ 2016;352:h6819.
53. Frost A, Badesch D, Gibbs JSR, et al. Diagnosis of pulmonary hypertension. Eur Respir J 2019;53(1):1801904.
54. Girgis RE, Frost AE, Hill NS, et al. Selective endothelin A receptor antagonism with sitaxsentan for pulmonary arterial hypertension associated with connective tissue disease. Ann Rheum Dis 2007;66(11):1467–72.
55. Oudiz RJ, Schilz RJ, Barst RJ, et al. Treprostinil, a prostacyclin analogue, in pulmonary arterial hypertension associated with connective tissue disease. Chest 2004;126(2):420–7.
56. Denton CP, Humbert M, Rubin L, et al. Bosentan treatment for pulmonary arterial hypertension related to connective tissue disease: a subgroup analysis of the

pivotal clinical trials and their open-label extensions. Ann Rheum Dis 2006; 65(10):1336–40.

57. Denton CP, Pope JE, Peter HH, et al. Long-term effects of bosentan on quality of life, survival, safety and tolerability in pulmonary arterial hypertension related to connective tissue diseases. Ann Rheum Dis 2008;67(9):1222–8.

58. Badesch DB, Hill NS, Burgess G, et al. Sildenafil for pulmonary arterial hypertension associated with connective tissue disease. J Rheumatol 2007;34(12): 2417–22.

59. Coghlan JG, Channick R, Chin K, et al. Targeting the prostacyclin pathway with selexipag in patients with pulmonary arterial hypertension receiving double combination therapy: insights from the randomized controlled GRIPHON study. Am J Cardiovasc Drugs 2018;18(1):37–47.

60. Coghlan JG, Galiè N, Barberà JA, et al, AMBITION Investigators. Initial combination therapy with ambrisentan and tadalafil in connective tissue disease-associated pulmonary arterial hypertension (CTD-PAH): subgroup analysis from the AMBITION trial. Ann Rheum Dis 2017;76(7):1219–27.

61. Continuous or nocturnal oxygen therapy in hypoxemic chronic obstructive lung disease: a clinical trial. Nocturnal Oxygen Therapy Trial Group. Ann Intern Med 1980;93(3):391–8.

62. Long term domiciliary oxygen therapy in chronic hypoxic cor pulmonale complicating chronic bronchitis and emphysema. Report of the Medical Research Council Working Party. Lancet 1981;1(8222):681–6.

63. Mereles D, Ehlken N, Kreuscher S, et al. Exercise and respiratory training improve exercise capacity and quality of life in patients with severe chronic pulmonary hypertension. Circulation 2006;114(14):1482–9.

64. Grunig E, Maier F, Ehlken N, et al. Exercise training in pulmonary arterial hypertension associated with connective tissue diseases. Arthritis Res Ther 2012; 14(3):R148.

65. Khan MS, Usman MS, Siddiqi TJ, et al. Is anticoagulation beneficial in pulmonary arterial hypertension? Circ Cardiovasc Qual Outcomes 2018;11(9):e004757.

66. Galiè N, Channick RN, Frantz RP, et al. Risk stratification and medical therapy of pulmonary arterial hypertension. Eur Respir J 2019;53(1):1801889.

67. Jais X, Launay D, Yaici A, et al. Immunosuppressive therapy in lupus- and mixed connective tissue disease-associated pulmonary arterial hypertension: a retrospective analysis of twenty-three cases. Arthritis Rheum 2008;58(2):521–31.

68. Sanchez O, Sitbon O, Jais X, et al. Immunosuppressive therapy in connective tissue diseases-associated pulmonary arterial hypertension. Chest 2006;130(1): 182–9.

69. Kato M, Kataoka H, Odani T, et al. The short-term role of corticosteroid therapy for pulmonary arterial hypertension associated with connective tissue diseases: report of five cases and a literature review. Lupus 2011;20(10):1047–56.

70. Miyamichi-Yamamoto S, Fukumoto Y, Sugimura K, et al. Intensive immunosuppressive therapy improves pulmonary hemodynamics and long-term prognosis in patients with pulmonary arterial hypertension associated with connective tissue disease. Circ J 2011;75(11):2668–74.

71. Benza RL, Gomberg-Maitland M, Elliott CG, et al. Predicting survival in patients with pulmonary arterial hypertension: the REVEAL risk score calculator 2.0 and comparison with ESC/ERS-based risk assessment strategies. Chest 2019; 156(2):323–37.

72. Mercurio V, Diab N, Peloquin G, et al. Risk assessment in scleroderma patients with newly diagnosed pulmonary arterial hypertension: application of the ESC/ERS risk prediction model. Eur Respir J 2018;52(4):1800497.
73. Mullin CJ, Khair RM, Damico RL, et al, PHAROS Investigators. Validation of the REVEAL prognostic equation and risk score calculator in incident systemic sclerosis-associated pulmonary arterial hypertension. Arthritis Rheumatol 2019; 71(10):1691–700.
74. Rhee RL, Gabler NB, Praestgaard A, et al. Adverse events in connective tissue disease-associated pulmonary arterial hypertension. Arthritis Rheum 2015; 67(09):2457–65.
75. Rhee RL, Gabler NB, Sangani S, et al. Comparison of treatment response in idiopathic and connective tissue disease-associated pulmonary arterial hypertension. Am J Respir Crit Care Med 2015;192(09):1111–7.
76. Mathai SC, Puhan MA, Lam D, et al. The minimal important difference in the 6-minute walk test for patients with pulmonary arterial hypertension. Am J Respir Crit Care Med 2012;186(5):428–33.
77. McLaughlin V, Zhao C, Coghlan JG, et al. Outcomes associated with modern treatment paradigms in connective tissue disease (CTD)-associated pulmonary arterial hypertension (PAH): a meta-analysis of randomized controlled trials (RCTs). Eur Heart J 2020;41(2). ehaa946.2282.
78. Hassoun PM, Zamanian RT, Damico R, et al. Ambrisentan and tadalafil up-front combination therapy in scleroderma-associated pulmonary arterial hypertension. Am J Respir Crit Care Med 2015;192(9):1102–10.
79. Waxman AB, Restrepo-Jarmillo R, Thenappan T, et al. Inhaled treprostinil in pulmonary hypertension due to interstitial lung disease. N Eng J Med 2021;384: 325–34.
80. e Groote P, Gressin V, Hachulla E, et al, ItinerAIR-Scleroderma Investigators. Evaluation of cardiac abnormalities by Doppler echocardiography in a large nationwide multicentric cohort of patients with systemic sclerosis. Ann Rheum Dis 2008;67(1):31–6.
81. Kim NH, Delcroix M, Jais X, et al. Chronic thromboembolic pulmonary hypertension. Eur Respir J 2019;53(1):1801915.
82. Ghofrani HA, D'Armini AM, Grimminger F, et al, CHEST-1 Study Group. Riociguat for the treatment of chronic thromboembolic pulmonary hypertension. N Engl J Med 2013;369(04):319–29.
83. Lang I, Meyer BC, Ogo T, et al. Balloon pulmonary angioplasty in chronic thromboembolic pulmonary hypertension. Eur Respir Rev 2017;26(143):160119.
84. Herve P, Lau EM, Sitbon O, et al. Criteria for diagnosis of exercise pulmonary hypertension. Eur Respir J 2015;46:728–37.
85. Kovacs G, Avian A, Olschewski H. Proposed new definition of exercise pulmonary hypertension decreases false-positive cases. Eur Respir J 2016;47:1270–3.
86. Stamm A, Saxer S, Lichtblau M, et al. Exercise pulmonary haemodynamics predict outcome in patients with systemic sclerosis. Eur Respir J 2016;48:1658–67.
87. Zeder K, Avian A, Bachmaier G, et al. Exercise pulmonary resistances predict long-term survival in systemic sclerosis. Chest 2021;159(2):781–90.
88. Ulrich S, Mathai SC. Performance under pressure: the relevance of pulmonary vascular response to exercise in scleroderma. Chest 2021;159:481–3.
89. Pan Z, Marra AM, Benjamin N, et al. Early treatment with ambrisentan of mildly elevated mean pulmonary arterial pressure associated with systemic sclerosis: a randomized, controlled, double-blind, parallel group study (EDITA study). Arthritis Res Ther 2019;21:217.

90. Yusen RD, Edwards LB, Dipchand AI, et al, International Society for Heart and Lung Transplantation. The Registry of the International Society for Heart and Lung Transplantation: thirty-third adult lung and heart-lung transplant report-2016; focus theme: primary diagnostic indications for transplant. J Heart Lung Transpl 2016;35:1170–84.
91. Bernstein EJ, Peterson ER, Sell JL, et al. Survival of adults with systemic sclerosis following lung transplantation: a nationwide cohort study. Arthritis Rheumatol 2015;67:1314–22.
92. Eberlein M, Mathai SC. Lung transplantation in scleroderma. Time for the pendulum to swing? Ann Am Thorac Soc 2016;13(6):767–9.

Systemic Diseases and Heart Block

Syed Rafay A. Sabzwari, MBBS, MD[a], Wendy S. Tzou, MD, FHRS[b,*]

KEYWORDS

- Heart block • Atrioventricular node • Amyloidosis • Sarcoidosis
- Systemic lupus erythematosus • Rheumatologic disorders • Thyroid disorders
- Muscular dystrophies

KEY POINTS

- Several systemic disorders can cause atrioventricular block largely because of infiltration, inflammation, or fibrosis of the conduction system owing to underlying disease process.
- Systemic disorders causing heart block can be broadly classified into infiltrative, rheumatologic, endocrine, and hereditary neuromuscular degenerative diseases.
- Infiltrative diseases like granulomas in sarcoidosis and amyloid fibrils in amyloidosis infiltrate the interstitial space including the atrioventricular nodal region causing heart block.
- Accelerated atherosclerosis leading to ischemia, vasculitis, myocarditis, and inflammatory infiltrates in rheumatologic disorders can lead to heart block.
- Myotonic, Becker, and Duchenne muscular dystrophies are inherited neuromuscular diseases that involve the myocardium in addition to the skeletal muscles and can cause progressive heart block.

INTRODUCTION

Several systemic disorders can cause atrioventricular (AV) block largely because of involvement of the myocardium and thereby the conduction system by infiltration, inflammation, or fibrosis owing to underlying disease processes (**Fig. 1**; **Table 1**). Conduction system disturbances may be permanent or transient, with conduction that is, intermittent or delayed. The underlying systemic disorder tends to govern overall presentation, as well as prognosis and management.

This article previously appeared in *Cardiology Clinics* volume 41 issue 3 August 2023.
This article originally appeared in *Cardiac Electrophysiology Clinics*, Volume 13 Issue 4, December 2021.
[a] University of Colorado Anschutz Medical Campus, 12631 East 17th Avenue, Mail Stop B130, Aurora, CO 80045, USA; [b] Cardiac Electrophysiology, University of Colorado Anschutz Medical Campus, 12401 E 17th Avenue, MS B-136, Aurora, CO 80045, USA
* Corresponding author.
E-mail address: Wendy.Tzou@cuanschutz.edu

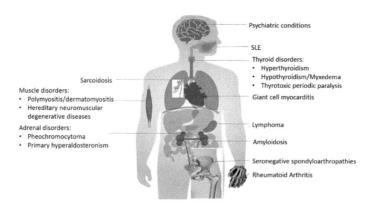

Fig. 1. Systemic diseases contributing to heart block.

CLASSIFICATION
Infiltrative Disorders

Amyloidosis
Amyloidosis can result from a spectrum of diseases characterized by extracellular deposition of amyloid within various organs and tissues. Amyloid is formed from of a number of fibrillar proteinaceous components that misfold into abnormal cross β-sheet oligomers. This conformation results in characteristic gross pathologic and histologic features. The oligomers combine with proteoglycans to form amyloid infiltrates, which may be toxic. The heart is one of the organs that can be affected, and multiple clinical manifestations may result, including cardiomyopathy, arrhythmias, and conduction system disease. The majority of cardiac amyloidosis (CA) is caused by 1 of 2 proteins: transthyretin (ATTR) or light chain. Light chains are produced as a result of a proliferative hematologic disorder where plasma cells clone and produce excessive amounts of lambda and, less commonly, kappa light chains. Light chain amyloid deposition (AL or primary amyloidosis) underlies a significant proportion of amyloidosis presentations and is generally associated with worse prognosis compared with amyloidosis resulting from ATTR deposition, whether hereditary or nonhereditary (senile or wild type).

Mechanism of heart block in cardiac amyloidosis. Unlike other inflammatory and infiltrative disorders, CA does not lead to myocardial scar formation. Amyloid fibrils deposit extracellularly throughout the heart, including in the valves and cardiac conduction system, thereby creating discontinuity and disarray between myocyte gap junctions that are critical for myocardial conduction. Additionally, amyloid deposition thickens the ventricle, producing restrictive physiology and marked diastolic dysfunction, and increased filling pressures that in turn lead to atrial dilation and atrial myopathy. Moreover, amyloid fibrils have direct toxic effect on myocardial cells, including increased calcium release owing to oxidative stress,[1] as demonstrated by impaired myocardial function and cell death in zebrafish resulting from exposure to AL light chains obtained from a patient with AL CA.[2] Also, perivascular amyloid infiltration leads to impaired vasodilation that causes continued ischemia to the myocardium, which can also affect the conduction system.[3]

Heart block in cardiac amyloidosis. AV conduction block is more often seen than sinus node dysfunction, despite the extensive atrial involvement seen in CA. Traditionally,

Table 1		
Classification of systemic diseases causing heart block		
A.	Infiltrative disorders	
	a.	Amyloidosis
	b.	Sarcoidosis
	c.	Tumors
	i.	Primary tumors
	ii.	Metastatic tumors
B.	Rheumatologic disorders	
	a.	Dermatomyositis
	b.	Polymyositis
	c.	Systemic lupus erythematosus
	d.	Systemic sclerosis
	e.	Rheumatoid arthritis
	f.	Giant cell myocarditis
	g.	HLA B27 associated seronegative spondyloarthropathies
C.	Endocrine disorders	
	a.	Thyroid gland
	i.	Hyperthyroidism
	ii.	Hypothyroidism/myxedema
	iii.	Thyrotoxic periodic paralysis
	b.	Adrenal gland
	i.	Pheochromocytoma
	ii.	Hypoaldosteronism
D.	Hereditary neuromuscular degenerative diseases	
	a.	Myotonic dystrophy
	b.	Becker muscular dystrophy
	c.	Duchenne muscular dystrophy
	d.	Kearns–Sayre syndrome
	e.	Rare muscular dystrophies
	i.	Scapuloperoneal dystrophy
	ii.	Erb's dystrophy
	iii.	Oculocraniosomatic syndrome
E.	Others	
	a.	Psychiatric conditions

the electrocardiographic features associated with high-grade AV block include prolonged PR interval, and right and left bundle branch block. However, the pathology is mostly noted in the His–Purkinje system, even in the case of first-degree AV block with preserved conduction at the nodal level. Therefore, most studies have reported a prolonged HV interval in both ATTR and AL patients with CA.[4,5] The incidence of symptomatic AV block may be higher in ATTR CA owing to older age of presentation, particularly for those with senile ATTR, who also historically have had better overall survival compared with AL CA. No difference has been found in rates of high-grade AV block between patients with wild-type and hereditary ATTR CA overall.[6] However, differences may exist based on the specific mutation among patients with hereditary TTR CA. For instance, Val122Ile compared with Thr60Ala mutation was associated with a lower prevalence of high-grade AV block at diagnosis ($P = 0.002$), although the incidence of high-grade AV block at follow-up was not different between the 2 mutations ($P = 0.15$).[6] Notably, the QRS duration tends to be normal, despite often diffuse amyloid infiltration of the bundle branches, and the mechanism is felt to be due to equal conduction delay in both bundle branches. This characteristic contrasts with other infiltrative diseases, where HV prolongation, usually more than 80 ms, is almost always associated with a widened QRS, and likely owing to a less homogenous involvement of the bundle branches.[4] For instance, in 1 series of 18 patients with advanced CA, the mean HV interval was 87 ± 27 ms.[7] In another study, the HV was prolonged (>55 ms) in all patients with CA, including 44% with a normal QRS duration (<100 ms). Reisinger and colleagues[4] also found, among 25% of patients with CA and first-degree heart block, that the His bundle deflection was greater than 30 ms, often with a notched or fragmented deflection. Importantly, the HV interval was prolonged (77 ± 18 ms) in 20 patients with a QRS of less than 120 ms, and even longer (88 ± 17 ms) in 5 patients with a QRS of greater than120 ms. Hence it is important to note that a relatively narrow QRS does not exclude patients from having infranodal disease. Therefore, when evaluating patients with high-risk syncope even in the absence of conduction abnormalities on an electrocardiogram (EKG) (normal PR interval and QRS duration), further evaluation by an electrophysiologic study should be done to exclude the possibility of infra-Hisian disease.

Sarcoidosis

Sarcoidosis is a rare but increasingly recognized disease with a reported prevalence between 0.10% and 0.16% in the United States.[8,9] It is characterized by the deposition of noncaseating granulomas with associated inflammation and fibrosis that primarily affect not only the lungs, but can also involve all other organs. Cardiac sarcoidosis is under-recognized, because it can have a variety of manifestations, including absence of symptoms, cardiomyopathy, sudden cardiac death owing to ventricular arrhythmia, and high-grade AV block.[10] An evaluation of death certificates suggests that cardiac involvement is the leading cause of death in sarcoidosis.[11]

Mechanism of heart block in cardiac sarcoidosis. The exact etiology of CS is unclear; however, it seems to result from an interplay between genetic, environmental, infectious, and immunologic factors. Polymorphism of HLA class II molecules, particularly HLA DQB*0601, and tumor necrosis factor (alpha), and particularly the TNFA2 allele, have been thought to form a potential genetic basis for CS.[12] The eventual immune response occurs owing to an interaction between immune-modulatory cells and various cytokines that lead to the characteristic noncaseating granuloma formation, which contains lymphocytes, macrophages, and epithelioid cells that fuse to form a multinucleated giant cell (**Fig. 2**). Cytokines involved include transforming growth factor beta, insulin-like growth factor 1, IL-4 and IL-5 that are subsequently responsible for fibrotic changes in the granuloma, leading to scarring.[13] CS can involve any cardiac structure, including the myocardium, valves, papillary muscles, coronary arteries, and pericardium. The inflammatory process often involves the interventricular septum and therefore can affect the AV node and His–Purkinje system, leading to heart block. Additionally, the inflammatory process and scar can involve the nodal artery causing ischemia to the AV node.[14]

Salient features and screening approach. Complete AV block is one of the most common manifestations of CS, occurring at a younger age compared with AV block from other causes. The prevalence of complete AV block in diagnosed CS is 23% to 30%.[14] Rosenthal and colleagues reported that 34% of patients aged less than

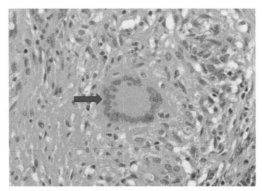

Fig. 2. Characteristic noncaseating granuloma with multinucleated giant cell (*arrow*) in cardiac sarcoidosis (hematoxylin-eosin stain, original magnification x 10). (*Adapted from* Patel B, Shah M, Gelaye A, Dusaj R. A complete heart block in a young male: a case report and review of literature of cardiac sarcoidosis. Heart Fail Rev. 2017;22(1):55-64; with permission)

60 years presenting with AV block had underlying CS.[15] This incidence is higher than reported previously, likely owing to the use of advanced imaging modalities, including a PET scan with fluorodeoxyglucose and cardiac MRI (**Fig. 3**). Similar findings have been described in a retrospective study by Kandolin and colleagues who found that in patients less than 55 years of age, 19% (14/72) had CS as the cause of new, unexplained AV block. Notably, two-thirds of these patients had only cardiac

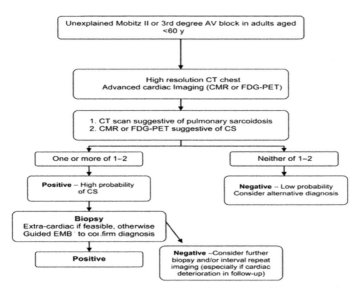

Fig. 3. Suggested algorithm for the investigation of patients with unexplained Mobitz II or third-degree AV block who are younger than 60 years. CMR, cardiovascular magnetic resonance; CS, cardiac sarcoidosis; CT, computed tomographic; ECG, electrocardiogram; EMB, endomyocardial biopsy; FDG-PET, ^{18}F-fluorodeoxyglucose–positron emission tomography. (*From* Birnie DH, Sauer WH, Bogun F, et al. HRS expert consensus statement on the diagnosis and management of arrhythmias associated with cardiac sarcoidosis. Heart Rhythm. 2014;11(7):1305-1323; with permission.)

involvement of sarcoidosis. No change in heart block was observed at 6 months of follow-up.[16]

CS should be considered in the differential diagnosis for younger patients (<60 years) with second-degree Mobitz II or third-degree AV block (class IIa).[17] Similarly, patients with biopsy-proven extracardiac sarcoidosis should be evaluated longitudinally for the development of cardiac involvement, including AV nodal conduction disease, by follow-up cardiac history (class I), EKG (class I), and echocardiogram (class IIa).[17] Subsequently, such patients who develop concerning symptoms (syncope/presyncope or palpitations) or abnormal EKG changes (pathologic Q waves, high-degree AV block, or bundle branch block) or an abnormal echocardiogram (regional wall motion abnormalities, wall aneurysm, basal septal thinning, left ventricular ejection fraction of <40%) should then undergo further evaluation with cardiac MRI or a PET scan with fluorodeoxyglucose (Class IIa).[17]

Diagnosis. In 2014, the first international consensus recommendation for diagnosis of CS was released.[17] This consensus had 2 pathways to diagnosis. The first one is through histologic diagnosis from endomyocardial biopsy. The second pathway makes CS probable if there is histologically confirmed extracardiac sarcoidosis and 1 or more typical findings of CS are present, including high-grade AV block or nonischemic left ventricular systolic dysfunction unexplained by other causes (see **Fig. 3**).[17] With advancements in imaging techniques, the diagnosis of CS has improved. Echocardiography can show evidence of increased myocardial wall thickness, basal septal thinning, aneurysms, and wall motion abnormalities in a noncoronary distribution pattern. However, echocardiography can miss early stages or "silent CS". Cardiac MRI can identify areas of late gadolinium enhancement (LGE), which in the case of CS is patchy, midmyocardial or epicardial, and commonly involves the basal septum or lateral wall. Although cardiac magnetic resonance identifies mostly the presence of fibrosis, a PET scan with fluorodeoxyglucose can pick up regions with active inflammation owing to the presence of active proinflammatory macrophages that show a higher metabolic rate and glucose use (**Fig. 4**).[12,18]

Treatment of heart block. In the inflammatory phase, Mobitz type II or third-degree heart block resulting from CS can potentially be reversed with immunosuppression, and treatment with corticosteroids is a Class IIa indication in the setting of newly diagnosed high-grade AV block and confirmed or probable CS.[17] Although there are no randomized trials to support this practice, a systematic review by Sadek and colleagues,[19] which included 10 articles in which 27 of 57 patients (47.4%) with AV block improved with corticosteroids to mostly normal AV conduction. Owing to lack of durable and reliable success in heart block recovery and unpredictable disease course, device implantation is still recommended as a Class IIa indication.[17] It is also worth mentioning that, owing to the risk of ventricular arrhythmias in CS, implantable cardioverter-defibrillator implantation is recommended in patients who require permanent pacing (class IIa recommendation), even in the absence of significant left ventricular systolic dysfunction.[17]

Tumors
Primary cardiac tumors are extremely rare, with a prevalence 0.02%, with the primary cardiac lymphomas comprising 1% to 2%. Secondary cardiac tumors owing to metastasis are more common, with a prevalence of 2.3% to 18.3% and represent 16% to 28% of extracardiac lymphomas.[20–24] AV block has accounted for up to 27% of clinical manifestations of primary cardiac lymphomas.[25–27] Metastatic tumors contributing to AV block include squamous cell cancers of the oral cavity, thyroid and

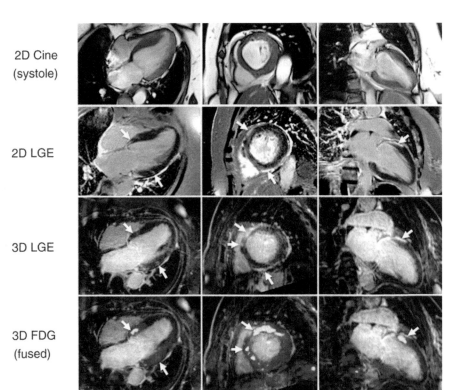

Fig. 4. Cardiac magnetic resonance images for respective 4-chamber, short-axis, and 2-chamber orientations showing systolic frame cine imaging and corresponding 2-dimensional (2D) late gadolinium enhancement (LGE) and 3-dimensional (3D) LGE scar imaging. White arrows indicate regions of abnormal LGE, consistent with mature scar. *Bottom* row shows 3D LGE images with fusion of 18F-labeled fluro-2-deoxyglucose (18F-FDG) positron emission tomography signal suggestive of active inflammation surrounding regions of established scar. (*From* White JA, Rajchl M, Butler J, et al. Active cardiac sarcoidosis: first clinical experience of simultaneous positron emission tomography–magnetic resonance imaging for the diagnosis of cardiac disease. Circulation.2013;127(22):e639-641; with permission.)

uterus. Other reported metastatic tumors that may lead to AV block include bladder cancer, Merkel cell cancer, bronchogenic carcinoma (squamous cell and adenocarcinoma), and leiomyosarcoma.[28]

Mechanism of heart block. Most tumors, and specifically metastatic tumors, involve the pericardium and myocardium; fewer than 5% involve the endocardium.[24,28] Because hematogenous spread is one of the modalities of metastases, the right atrium and right ventricle are commonly involved. Therefore, AV block has been attributed either to compression from mass effect or owing to direct infiltration of the AV node or the His–Purkinje system itself. Other mechanisms include those owing to metabolic derangements from renal involvement or directly through endocrine mechanisms leading to electrolyte abnormalities, particularly hypercalcemia. Moreover, many antineoplastic drugs can have adverse effects in the form of direct AV nodal blocking effect or from overall cardiotoxicity. These mechanisms have been discussed in Chiara Pavone and Gemma Pelargonio's article, "Reversible Causes of Atrioventricular Block," in this issue.

Rheumatologic Disorders

Mixed connective tissue disease

Mixed connective tissue disease is an autoimmune process with the combined features of multiple rheumatologic diseases, including systemic lupus erythematosus, systemic sclerosis, polymyositis, and rheumatoid arthritis (RA). It is associated with a high titer of anti-U1 ribonucleoprotein antibodies. Cardiac involvement in mixed connective tissue disease has been reported in 13% to 65% and can involve all components of the heart.[29] However, only one-fourth to one-third of the patients have symptomatic disease. Conduction disturbances have been noted in as many as 20% of patients in one of the largest series.[30]

Mechanism of heart block. Although the pathophysiology of conduction disease in mixed connective tissue disease is not completely understood, 2 post mortem series suggest myocarditis as a mechanism, similar to what has been identified in other connective tissue diseases,[31,32] with pathologic changes noted in the myocardium mimicking those found in skeletal muscle in patients with polymyositis or dermatomyositis.

Dermatomyositis and polymyositis

Polymyositis and dermatomyositis are chronic muscle inflammatory disorders clinically characterized by muscle weakness and fatigue.[33,34] Cardiac involvement, including heart failure and conduction system abnormalities, has been seen in more than 70% of patients with polymyositis and confers an increased mortality risk.[35]

Mechanism of heart block. Polymyositis and dermatomyositis are characterized by chronic inflammatory infiltrates (primarily CD4$^+$/CD8$^+$ T cells), macrophages, and dendritic cells that infiltrate muscle fascicles and perivascular regions. This inflammatory pattern, although most studied in skeletal muscles, has also been identified in those with myocardial involvement. Inflammatory changes eventually produce cardiac myocyte degeneration and fibrosis.[36,37] Similar inflammatory changes and eventual contraction-band necrosis have been observed involving the cardiac conduction system on autopsy studies.[37,38] In other post mortem studies of patients with heart block, extensive fibrous replacement of the AV node, His bundle, and bundle branches have been reported.[38–40]

Salient features. Cardiac involvement is often subclinical, and presentation delayed to a few years after the initial diagnosis of the rheumatologic condition. Most case reports describe a progressive course, evidenced by first-degree heart block, then subsequent development of hemi blocks and left bundle branch block.[41]

Giant cell myocarditis

Giant cell myocarditis (GCM) is a rare but aggressive and devastating disease characterized by rapidly progressing heart failure, ventricular arrhythmias, and conduction disease. In the 2 largest series of patients with GCM, complete heart block was noted in 5% to 31%.[42,43] The rate of death or transplant approximates 70% at 1 year after diagnosis.[44]

Mechanism of heart block. GCM is an autoimmune, virus-negative myocarditis attributed to T-lymphocyte–mediated inflammation and is associated with systemic autoimmune disorder in approximately 20% of cases. Infiltration tends to diffusely involve the myocardium, including the AV node and His–Purkinje system, leading to heart block. Histologically, multinucleated giant cells with surrounding mononuclear inflammatory cells (predominantly T-cells) are observed. Acute inflammation eventually produces necrosis of cardiac myocytes. Although certain features are similar to cardiac sarcoidosis, including the identification of granulomas in a minority of patients with advanced disease, the overall disease course and presentation are usually more fulminant.[42]

Salient features and treatment. Interestingly, more indolent presentations of AV block in GCM have been reported. Kandolin and colleagues[45] found that 6% of patients had biopsy-proven GCM when they studied 72 patients aged 18 to 55 years who had undergone pacemaker implantation for third-degree heart block. However, GCM individuals had worse 4-year outcomes, with 39% experiencing malignant ventricular arrhythmias, cardiac death, or transplantation. When compared with lymphocytic myocarditis, Davidoff and colleagues[46] reported AV block to be more common in GCM (60.0% vs 8.3%, respectively).

GCM is diagnosed by endomyocardial biopsy. Unlike sarcoidosis, the diagnostic yield of endomyocardial biopsy in GCM is relatively high owing to more widespread infiltration, ranging from 56% to 93%, depending on the biopsy protocol.[42,43]

The diagnosis of GCM along with CS should be strongly considered for adults less than 55 years of age presenting with high-degree AV block; unlike other myocarditis, expedient immunosuppressive treatment for GCM can alter the disease course by slowing or limiting its progression.[47,48] Continued immunosuppression is important as withdrawal of treatment can lead to fatal treatment relapse.[49]

Systemic lupus erythematosus, anti-RO/SSA, and anti-LA/SSB antibody

Adult complete heart block. Although atrial fibrillation, sinus tachycardia, and atrial ectopic beats are the major arrhythmias noted in systemic lupus erythematosus, progressive AV conduction abnormalities can also be seen. High-grade AV block has been shown to be the presenting symptom in a few reported cases. Tselios and colleagues[50] reported a complete heart block incidence of 1% (out of 1366 patients) from a Toronto lupus clinic database.

Mechanism of heart block The exact etiology of complete heart block in systemic lupus erythematosus is not clear, but autoantibodies seem to be involved. Natsheh and colleagues[51] reported positive antinuclear antibody in all patients, anti-DNA in 84%, anti-La in 15%, and anti-Ro in 35% of patients. Evidence that these antibodies interact with the conduction system leading to complete heart block comes from studies showing that maternal anti-Ro and anti-La antibodies block L-type and T-type calcium channels in the fetal conduction system leading to congenital complete heart block. Recent data suggest that 2 types of mechanisms may exist for anti-Ro/SSA's role in adult complete heart block.[52,53]

1. Acquired: Formation of new anti-Ro antibodies is reported to account for this type, although data supporting this theory are mixed.[54–59] Regardless, 70% of adult patients with systemic lupus erythematosus and complete heart block reported to date have shown the presence of anti-Ro antibodies.[52]
2. Late progressive congenital form: More latent and subclinical immunomodulated effects caused by maternal antibodies in utero have been observed, with first- or second-degree AV block observed in 2% to 5% of study populations, and progression to complete heart block only in adulthood.[60] Transient conduction defects have also been observed. Bergman and colleagues, demonstrated a 10% incidence of progression to first-degree AV block among children with a normal electrocardiogram within 1 month of birth, after prenatal exposure to anti-SSA/Ro52 antibodies.[61] Similarly, other studies have shown complete disappearance of first-degree AV block at birth over the ongoing years.[62] A Swedish nationwide

retrospective study showed that 24.5% of 53 cases of isolated complete heart block of unknown origin had a seropositive mother for anti-Ro/SSA antibodies.[63] An infectious insult in adult life is postulated to act as the trigger for the manifestation of complete heart block in some cases.[52] This finding in turn implies that at least approximately 10% of adults with isolated complete heart block in the general population may have a seropositive mother, would not themselves be seropositive and therefore not respond to immunosuppressants.

Fig. 5 summarizes the assessment of complete heart block of unknown origin in adults with anti-Ro/SSA antibodies. However, the predominant antibody type in adult complete heart block is anti-DNA and not anti-Ro/SSA.[51] Besides, myocarditis in systemic lupus erythematosus consists of apoptosis of myocardiocytes leading to conduction system fibrosis in addition to ischemic heart disease associated nodal artery occlusive disease owing to vasculitis and accelerated atherosclerosis.[50,51,64,65] Moreover, in patients with systemic lupus erythematosus without cardiac involvement, antimalarial treatment of systemic lupus erythematosus can also contribute to cardiomyopathy as well as heart block as reviewed in Chiara Pavone and Gemma Pelargonio's article, "Reversible Causes of Atrioventricular Block," in this issue. In 1 series, 17 of 47 patients with biopsy-confirmed antimalarial cardiomyopathy had complete heart block, with majority of them requiring permanent pacemaker implantation.[66]

Salient features in adults As with systemic lupus erythematosus in general, complete heart block in systemic lupus erythematosus almost exclusively has been seen in females (94% cases) with a median age of 37 years (range, 12–63 years) at a median time of 10 years (range, 1–25 years) after systemic lupus erythematosus

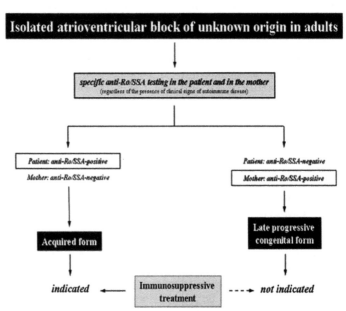

Fig. 5. Algorithm in assessment of complete heart block of unknown origin adults associated with anti-Ro/SSA antibodies. (*From* Lazzerini PE, Capecchi PL, Laghi-Pasini F. Isolated atrioventricular block of unknown origin in adults and anti-Ro/SSA antibodies: clinical evidence, putative mechanisms, and therapeutic implications. Heart Rhythm. 2015;12(2):449-454; with permission.)

diagnosis.[51] However, in only 5 reported cases, syncope owing to complete heart block was the initial manifestation leading to the diagnosis of systemic lupus erythematosus. In most of these cases, systemic manifestations of systemic lupus erythematosus usually took days to weeks to develop and in one case up to several years. An EKG before the development of complete heart block can be normal, but can also show evidence of first-degree and second-degree AV block as well as intraventricular conduction delays.[51] Owing to predominant involvement of the AV node and His–Purkinje system the QRS in these patients is usually narrow (**Fig. 6A**).

Anti-Ro/SSA–associated AV block in adults in the absence of clinical autoimmune disease can represent 20% of all cases of isolated complete heart block of unknown origin.[52] **Fig. 6A** shows the EKG of a 29-year-old woman with positive anti-Ro/SSA antibodies who was noted to have sudden onset complete heart block in the absence of any signs or symptoms of systemic lupus erythematosus.[53] Hence, the possibility of this mechanism in patients with "idiopathic" complete heart block should be considered and accordingly should prompt investigation of anti-Ro antibodies in both the patient and mother. The results of this testing can help to categorize the patient's AV block as either acquired or late progressive. The timely institution of immunosuppressants will only help to treat the acquired form (see **Fig. 6B**), whereas the remainder might require implantation of a permanent pacemaker.

Neonatal complete heart block. Since the 1980s, congenital complete heart block has been thought to be associated with maternal anti-Ro/SSA and anti-La/SSB antibodies not necessarily dependent on clinical evidence of maternal Sjogren syndrome and systemic lupus erythematosus.[67–69] Congenital complete heart block represents the most severe and representative effect of anti-Ro/SSA antibodies in the fetal heart and these antibodies account for 80% to 95% of congenital complete heart block in the absence of structural heart disease.[67,70] The risk of congenital complete heart block in first anti-Ro positive pregnancy is 1% to 2%, but it increases significantly to 12% to 20% with future pregnancies. It is thought that congenital complete heart block is a manifestation of a spectrum of progressively worsening heart block starting from first then second and eventually irreversible congenital complete heart block.[62,71]

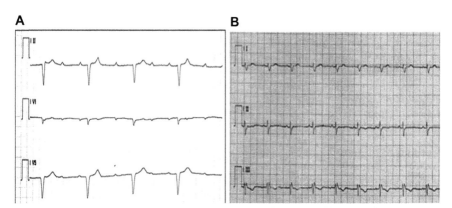

Fig. 6. (*A*) A 29-years-old woman with positive anti-Ro/SSA antibodies and no history of SLE with sudden onset complete heart block. (*B*) Normal AV conduction after 2 weeks of immunosuppressive therapy with prednisone. SLE, systemic lupus erythematosus. (*From* Lazzerini PE, Brucato A, Capecchi PL, et al. Isolated atrioventricular block of unknown origin in the adult and autoimmunity: diagnostic and therapeutic considerations exemplified by 3 anti-Ro/SSA-associated cases. HeartRhythm Case Rep. 2015;1(5):293-299; with permission.)

Mechanism of heart block In comparison with the association of complete heart block to anti-Ro antibodies, data supporting an association of complete heart block with anti-La antibodies are less robust. Two studies suggested anti-La to be more associated with neonatal cutaneous lupus erythematosus than complete heart block; however, another study suggested anti-La antibodies increasing the risk of congenital complete heart block.[72–74] Hence, the consensus remains that congenital complete heart block can develop with either of the 2 antibodies or even in their absence. Although the exact mechanism is not known, there are a few theories proposed for development of complete heart block in neonates. (1) The inflammatory theory proposes inflammation-driven injury to the AV node owing to interaction between anti-Ro/SSA and specific antigens expressed in the fetal conduction system; (2) an electrophysiology theory based on experimental models, suggesting a rapidly occurring and fully reversing electrophysiologic interference demonstrated by anti-Ro/SSA on AV conduction; and (3) calcium-channel theory incorporates a unique pathophysiologic interaction between anti-Ro/SSA and fetal calcium channels, predominantly L-type Ca channels that are more predominant in neonates than adults for AV conduction owing to underdeveloped sarcoplasmic reticula, with decreased calcium storage and therefore greater dependence on trans-sarcolemmal calcium entry through L-type calcium channels.[62,71,75,76] Moreover, experimental studies have also suggested that IgG bind to L- and T-type calcium channels, thereby significantly inhibiting their currents.

Salient features in neonates Fetal monitoring in the peripartum period is usually recommended when the antibody titer is more than 8 enzyme-linked immunosorbent assay units in commercial laboratories. Neonates are most at risk for heart block during the first 18 to 24 weeks of gestation. However, the risk is less during the 26th to 30th weeks and very rare after 30 weeks of pregnancy. Second-degree AV block, mostly Mobitz type 1 owing to impaired AV node conduction, has a better prognosis with chance of reversibility based on a meta-analysis of 4 studies in which 24% of the patients recovered normal conduction regardless of therapy.[77]

Hickstein and colleagues[78] suggested immunoadsorption as a possible treatment for pregnant women with high titers of SSA antibodies. However, infants with complete heart block and particularly those with a heart rate of less than 50 beats/min before delivery may require a permanent pacemaker.[79] This is likely due to the involvement of His–Purkinje system in infants with complete heart block. As in adults, owing to the predominant involvement of the AV node and His–Purkinje system, the QRS duration usually remains normal.

Rheumatoid arthritis

AV nodal block in RA is very rare, but is usually complete.[80] The incidence is estimated to be 1 in 1000 to 1600 patients.[81,82]

Mechanism of heart block. Patients with RA can have primary infiltration of the AV node by mononuclear cells consisting of lymphocytes, plasma cells, and histiocytes or rheumatoid granulomas. Continued inflammation in the AV node results in fibroelastosis.[83] Other mechanisms include AV nodal artery vasculitis, hemorrhage into a rheumatoid nodule, or extension of the inflammatory front from adjacent mitral or aortic valve. Villecco and colleagues noted antibodies directed against the conduction system more often than in RA patients with RBBB compared with those without (76% vs 21%).[83] It is also thought that the incidence might be higher in patients treated primarily with corticosteroids because there is a higher incidence of necrotizing arteritis in such patients.[84]

Salient features. The majority of patients with complete heart block have established erosive, nodular RA with clinical features of extra-articular RA and high titers of rheumatoid factor. The progression from normal conduction to complete heart block can be sudden and permanent, although rare reports of spontaneous recovery exist.[80]

Systemic sclerosis
Complete heart block is very rare in systemic sclerosis, although lesser degrees of AV block can be more common, with first-degree AVB in 6% to 10%, and second- and third-degree AV block in up to 2% of patients.[85–88]

Mechanism of heart block. AV block in systemic sclerosis is primarily owing to advanced fibrosis of the myocardium extending to the AV node, although selective fibrosis of the conduction system has not been established definitively.[89] Additionally, inflammatory involvement of the arterial blood supply and the conduction tissue can also play a role.[80] Volta and colleagues[90] showed that 25% of the patients with progressive systemic sclerosis had antibodies against the conduction system.

HLA B27 and seronegative ankylospondyloarthropathies
Seronegative spondyloarthropathies, which are primarily composed of ankylosing spondylitis and Reiter's syndrome, are characterized by a variable but strong association with immunogenetically important cell surface protein HLA B27, sacroiliitis, and an absence of rheumatoid factor.

Mechanism of heart block. The primary mechanism underlying complete heart block is the same for aortic regurgitation in these patients and is due to an inflammatory process in the aortic root and the adjacent myocardium, which in turn leads to varying degrees of fibrosis.[91,92]

Salient features. There has been an association of HLA B-27 and complete heart block noted even in the absence of clinical or radiographic evidence of rheumatic disease in 15% to 20% of men with complete heart block.[93] It is noteworthy that complete heart block in HLA B-27 predominantly involves the His bundle and is therefore associated with complete heart block owing to intra-His rather than infra-Hisian block, correlating with a normal PR interval. This finding is supported by a series of 12 patients with complete heart block and HLA B27 disease (8 having ankylosing spondylitis) who underwent an electrophysiologic study; only 1 patient had infra-Hisian block, whereas 10 patients had supra-Hisian second- or third-degree AV block.[94]

Another important feature is the tendency of complete heart block to occur paroxysmally. Although consequences from the disease process overall might resolve without significant clinical sequelae, complete and long-lasting remission rarely occurs.[93,95,96]

Management. Treatment is directed toward the underlying disease process and includes corticosteroids in the acute setting and eventual transition to disease-modifying antirheumatic drugs. In most rheumatologic disorders, by the time high-grade AV block is diagnosed, the disease process has advanced enough that complete or durable reversibility of AV block is unlikely. Therefore, patients often require permanent pacemaker implantation. However, those patients who are asymptomatic or without evidence of high-grade AV block can be monitored periodically in the form of either outpatient follow-up EKGs or Holter monitor. There are no specific guideline recommendations for the implantation of permanent pacemaker in rheumatologic disorders.

Endocrine disorders

Hyperthyroidism

Thyroid hormones have mechanism of action on the heart with mostly positive inotropic, chronotropic, and dromotropic responses leading to faster heart rates and improved cardiac output.[97–99] Although hyperthyroidism has been mostly known in relation to tachyarrhythmias, it has been rarely associated with heart block. Most reported cases have described other disease processes such as infectious disease, hypercalcemia, rheumatic fever or digitalis treatment concomitantly present with thyrotoxicosis; however, primary involvement with only thyrotoxicosis has also been reported.[100–102]

Mechanism of heart block. Thyroid hormones effect sodium pump density and enhance the permeability of Na^+ and K^+ permeability within myocytes.[103,104] The exact mechanism of heart block in hyperthyroidism is not well-known. Data from case reports and autopsy studies describe potential pathophysiology, although the correlation of biochemical evidence of elevated T4 and T3 levels to postmortem histopathologic evidence is challenging owing to immediate postmortem decreases in T4 and fluctuating T3 levels.[102] Interstitial inflammation and focal myocarditis around the AV node have been noted, along with myocyte necrosis and hypertrophy, myocardial edema, and interstitial and perivascular fibrosis that can lead to AV nodal conduction abnormalities through direct injury or ischemic effects.[102,105] Ortmann and colleagues[102] described microscopic evidence of degenerative changes with vacuolization with negative immunohistochemical finding excluding necrosis (**Fig. 7**). Ischemic effects are likely augmented in the setting of baseline atherosclerotic coronary artery disease, which is found in the majority of patients with thyrotoxicosis, and in whom increased work of the heart can worsen ischemia to the conduction system and AV node in general. Finally, under the influence of excessive thyroid hormone levels, the autonomic nervous system has a reciprocal action of exacerbating hypervagatonia, which might have been present before hyperthyroidism, and may precipitate AV nodal conduction abnormalities.[106,107]

Treatment. Treatment of thyroid storm involves administration of intravenous glucocorticoids, which can also help to decrease peri-AV nodal inflammation and thereby improve AV conduction. Additionally, antithyroid medication can eventually decrease

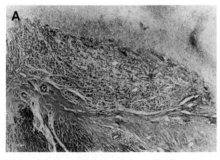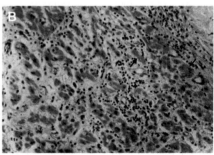

Fig. 7. (A) Penetrating His bundle shows interstitial edema and mixed infiltrate. Inflammation cells are also seen in the fibrous body close to the bundle (stain: hematoxylin and eosin; original magnification ×25). (B) Absence of necrosis of the His bundle myocytes. Degenerative changes with vacuolization (↑) and mixed interstitial inflammation. (*Adapted from* Ortmann C, Pfeiffer H, Du Chesne A, Brinkmann B. Inflammation of the cardiac conduction system in a case of hyperthyroidism. Int J Legal Med. 1999;112(4):271-274.)

circulating T4 and T3 levels, improving the constant myocardial proinflammatory state. Administration of beta-blockers such as propranolol in thyrotoxicosis, given especially when tachyarrhythmias are present, can in turn promote AV block. However, in patients with gradual and progressive perinodal fibrosis, glucocorticoids may not be effective in reversing AV block, and pacemaker implantation might be required.

Hypothyroidism and myxedema

Myxedema has been associated with AV block, as demonstrated through multiple case reports and histopathologic studies.[108–113] Given that AV block in this context can be reversible with thyroid replacement therapy, the yield of screening patients for hypothyroidism is particularly high.

Mechanism of heart block. Various histopathologic changes in the myxedema heart have been identified that may increase risk of AV block, including interstitial edema, myocardial fibrosis, and mucinous vacuolization with positive periodic acid-Schiff staining. However, because some of these changes persist after resolution of AV block after treatment with thyroid replacement therapy, their exact contribution is not completely certain.[114,115] As is true in the context of other systemic processes that lead to increased myocardial oxygen demand, ischemia to the AV node may be enhanced in the presence of underlying coronary artery disease. Significant interstitial edema may also lead to mechanical compression of the AV node. Possibly most relevant, thyroid hormones have direct and indirect stimulatory effects, the latter mediated through increased catecholamines, on AV nodal conduction; in the setting of insufficient thyroid hormone levels, bradycardia and AV block can therefore result, as well as be effectively treated with thyroid replacement therapy.[116,117]

Salient features. The clinical presentation of myxedema can be very insidious, especially in the elderly. Given the therapeutic reversibility of heart block in myxedema, the presentation of heart block of an unclear etiology should warrant screening for thyroid status particularly if clinical signs are also suggestive of thyroid dysfunction. Complete heart block in a small subset of patients might not reverse despite thyroid replacement, which may result from extensive myocardial fibrosis to prolonged thyroid deficiency.[117]

Pheochromocytoma

Pheochromocytoma is a rare but potentially life-threatening tumor of the adrenal medulla with an incidence of 1 in 100,000.[118] It is characterized by excessive secretion of norepinephrine, epinephrine, and dopamine leading to imbalances in the autonomic nervous system that, in turn, can affect cardiac conduction.[119]

Mechanism of heart block. Prolonged exposure to catecholamines in pheochromocytoma can lead to myocardial hypertrophy, ischemia, and eventually cardiomyopathy. The exact mechanism of heart block in pheochromocytoma is not known, and existing data are limited primarily to case reports; chronic ischemia leading to development of cardiomyopathy, along the lines of the inflammatory disorders discussed elsewhere in this article, may be mechanistic.[120–122] Additionally, AV block has been particularly noted during hypertensive paroxysms during which baroreceptor stimulation results in reflex vagal nerve stimulation that can lead owing to both sinus arrest as well as AV block.[120] Other mechanism include adrenergic receptor desensitization and particularly negative chronotropic effects of noradrenaline infusion.[122]

Primary Hyperaldosteronism

Primary hyperaldosteronism accounts for 5% to 15% of all hypertensive patients and is characterized by minerocorticoid (aldosterone) excess leading to hypertension and hypokalemia.[123] Patients with primary hyperaldosteronism have adverse cardiovascular effects that cannot just be explained by effects of hypertension.

Mechanism of heart block. Data on AV block in primary hyperaldosteronism are limited and therefore the mechanism is not understood entirely. Besides hypertension, excess aldosterone leads to cardiac remodeling owing to cell proliferation and deposition of collagen fibers in the myocardium including the conduction system.[123] Fibrosis leads to reduced sodium current, reduced cell-to-cell coupling with connexin (CX43) downregulation, and microfibrosis-associated decreased transfer coupling.[124] Additionally conduction velocity across the AV node and His bundle is also adversely affected by hypokalemia. Effect of electrolyte abnormalities on membrane potential is discussed in Chiara Pavone and Gemma Pelargonio's article, "Reversible Causes of Atrioventricular Block," in this issue.

Salient features and treatment. Progressive PR prolongation has been noted in patients with primary hyperaldosteronism. First-degree AV block was present in 16% of patients with primary hyperaldosteronism and correlated positively with interventricular septal wall thickness, left ventricular mass index, plasma aldosterone level, and degree of hypokalemia.[123,125] Patients with primary hyperaldosteronism with marked left ventricular hypertrophy, hypokalemia, and prominent aldosterone elevation are at risk for complete heart block when treated with beta blockers and nondyhydropyridine calcium channel blockers.[126]

With the treatment of underlying hyperaldosteronism with adrenalectomy, including judicious use of AV nodal blockers, PR interval prolongation and heart block have been noted to reverse completely in patients with primary hyperaldosteronism.[125]

Hereditary neuromuscular dystrophies

Myotonic dystrophy

Myotonic dystrophy is the most common autosomal-dominant adult-onset muscular dystrophy, particularly in adults of European ancestry. The prevalence of myotonic dystrophy ranges from 1 in 7400 to 1 in 10,700 in Europe.[127–129] It has 2 types: myotonic dystrophy type 1 and type 2. It is characterized by delayed skeletal muscle relaxation after contraction and systemic manifestations including cardiac arrhythmias, both AV block and ventricular arrhythmias that can lead to sudden cardiac death.[130] In a population-based study, the risk of cardiac conduction system disease was noted to be 60 times higher than in the general population.[131] Therefore, those meeting pacing indications are also recommended to undergo implantable cardioverter-defibrillator implantation if life expectancy exceeds a year.[132]

Mechanism of heart block. The general mechanism is related to RNA toxicity. Myotonic dystrophy type 1 results from an expansion of a cytosine–thymine–guanine trinucleotide repeat in the 3′-untranslated region of the dystrophia myotonica protein kinase gene on chromosome 19q 13.3. Myotonic dystrophy type 2 results from expanded cytosine–cytosine–thymine–guanine tetranucleotide repeat expansion located on chromosome 3q 21.3. Although the exact cause of cardiac conduction involvement is unknown, multiple potential mechanisms exist. First, impaired function of the dystrophia myotonica protein kinase gene and/or protein encoded by a gene on a nearby locus result in abnormal cellular metabolism and cell damage by progressive interstitial fibrosis, fatty and lymphocyte infiltration, and myofiber disarray. On electron microscopy, myofibrillar degeneration and prominent I-bands have been identified to involve the sinoatrial node, AV node, and His bundle.[130,133] Additionally, abnormal glucose metabolism and phosphorylation in the myocardium, controlled by MMRGlu and κ3, respectively, can result from direct effects of abnormal protein serine–threonine protein kinase produced in myotonic dystrophy patients.[130]

Salient features. Although there are limited data correlating histologic and EKG abnormalities in myotonic dystrophy, AV node fibrosis has been histologically confirmed in asymptomatic patients without EKG abnormalities, suggesting the relative inadequacy of EKG in identifying patients at risk for sudden cardiac death.[133] The risk of AV block is most significant in patients with myotonic dystrophy type 1. In a study of 406 patients, baseline EKG abnormalities including a PR interval of greater than 240 ms, second- or third-degree AV block, and a prolonged QRS interval were noted in 24%.[134] An increased PR interval has been noted in 21% to 40% of patients, and an increased HV interval in 56% of patients with myotonic dystrophy type 1.[130,135] Philips and colleagues compared studies that investigated the rate of change of conduction abnormalities and, although the data were mixed, the authors concluded that, although the rate of progression is gradual, it is occasionally rapid, and the rate of progression is not an accurate predictor of future sudden cardiac death risk.[130,136]

AV block has also been noted in myotonic dystrophy type 2, although with much less data compared with myotonic dystrophy type 1. In 2 studies, the risk of conduction abnormalities including AV block was noted to be 11% and 24%.[137,138]

Kearns–Sayre syndrome
Kearns–Sayre syndrome is a mitochondrial myopathy, with incidence of 1 in 125,000 live births, and results in a constellation of chronic progressive external ophthalmoplegia with pigmentary retinopathy and at least 1 other systemic manifestation, including AV block, usually before the age of 20 years.[139] Chronic progressive external ophthalmoplegia, which can also exist in isolation, is characterized by paresis of extraocular muscles and bilateral ptosis. Kearns–Sayre syndrome can be sporadic, autosomal dominant, autosomal recessive, or maternal owing to the involvement of either nuclear or mitochondrial DNA.[140]

Mechanism of heart block. The exact reason for abnormal cardiac conduction is unknown. Cardiac biopsy of Kearns–Sayre syndrome patients have shown an absolute increase in the number and size of mitochondria in the cardiomyocytes owing to progressive mtDNA depletion leading to decreased mitochondrial enzyme activity that can, in turn, lead to cell death and conduction system fibrosis.[139,141,142] The involvement of the His–Purkinje system compared with the rest of the myocardium is specifically thought to result from differences in its dedicated vascular supply and electrophysiologic characteristic of increased spontaneous (phase 4) depolarization that requires increased mitochondrial enzymatic activity.

Salient features. Incident AV block was noted in 20 of 33 (61%) of patients with Kearns–Sayre syndrome and 8 of 78 (10%) of patients with chronic progressive external ophthalmoplegia in 1 study.[143] Another study reported the incidence of complete heart block to be 40%, and all patients progressed from left anterior fascicular block to bifascicular block.[139] Therefore, fascicular blocks in Kearns–Sayre syndrome carry a high, sudden, and often fatal risk of progression to complete heart block.[144]

Indications for permanent pacemaker implantation. The 2018 American College of Cardiology/American Heart Association Task Force on Clinical Practice Guidelines, and the Heart Rhythm Society guideline recommendations for permanent pacing are summarized in **Fig. 8**. Notably, pacemaker implantation is recommended (Class I) among patients with myotonic dystrophy or Kearns–Sayre syndrome with second

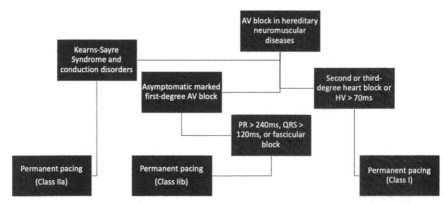

Fig. 8. Pacing indications for AV block in neuromuscular diseases. (*Data from* Kusumoto FM, Schoenfeld MH, Barrett C, et al. 2018 ACC/AHA/HRS Guideline on the Evaluation and Management of Patients With Bradycardia and Cardiac Conduction Delay: Executive Summary: A Report of the American College of Cardiology/American Heart Association Task Force on Clinical Practice Guidelines, and the Heart Rhythm Society. J Am Coll Cardiol. 2019;74(7):932-987)

or third-degree AV block or an HV of more than 70 ms on electrophysiologic study.[132] Additionally, pacemaker implantation should be considered (Class IIa) among patients with Kearns–Sayre syndrome with other conduction abnormalities or among patients with myotonic dystrophy with a PR of greater than 240 ms and a left bundle branch block.[132] Patients with asymptomatic myotonic dystrophy or Kearns–Sayre syndrome without conduction abnormalities should be evaluated at least annually with an EKG,

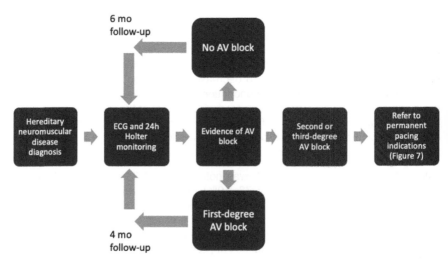

Fig. 9. Monitoring algorithm for AV block in neuromuscular diseases. ECG, electrocardiogram. (*Data from* Kusumoto FM, Schoenfeld MH, Barrett C, et al. 2018 ACC/AHA/HRS Guideline on the Evaluation and Management of Patients With Bradycardia and Cardiac Conduction Delay: Executive Summary: A Report of the American College of Cardiology/ American Heart Association Task Force on Clinical Practice Guidelines, and the Heart Rhythm Society. J Am Coll Cardiol. 2019;74(7):932-987)

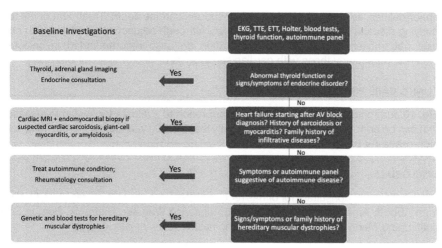

Fig. 10. Diagnostic algorithm for investigating high-grade AV block in young adults. ETT, exercise tolerance test; TTE, transthoracic echocardiogram. (*Data from* Barra SN, Providencia R, Paiva L, Nascimento J, Marques AL. A review on advanced atrioventricular block in young or middle-aged adults. Pacing Clin Electrophysiol. 2012;35(11):1395-1405)

with consideration of electrophysiologic study for further risk stratification to identify patients with AV nodal disease and need for permanent pacing (**Fig. 9**).

There is also an increased risk of sudden cardiac death owing to ventricular arrhythmias in patients with myotonic dystrophy and Kearns–Sayre syndrome. In a prospective study, the overall sudden cardiac death risk was 33%.[134] Therefore, the guidelines also recommend implantable cardioverter-defibrillator implantation for any pacing indication in these patients if there is more than 1 year of meaningful expected survival.[132]

Duchenne and Becker muscular dystrophies
Duchenne muscular dystrophy (DMD) and Becker muscular dystrophy are X-linked disorders causing myopathy owing to dystrophin gene mutations on chromosome Xp21.1 and primarily result in weakness of affected skeletal muscles. DMD is associated with earlier onset and most severe clinical symptoms, although cardiac involvement is a more predominant feature in Becker muscular dystrophy. AV block in DMD has been noted in a few case reports, particularly after the development of cardiomyopathy, although it can be the first manifestation of cardiac involvement.[145,146] First-degree AV block is reported in 2% of patients with Becker muscular dystrophy, with complete AV block in both early and later decades of life reported as the initial manifestation of cardiac involvement.[147–149]

Mechanism of heart block. Dystrophin is a sarcolemmal protein that binds actin to extracellular matrix and is localized to the membrane surface of the His–Purkinje fibers.[150] The absence of dystrophin in His–Purkinje tissue, particularly in DMD, not only leads to abnormal conduction, but also to progressive replacement of cardiomyocytes by connective tissue or fat.[146,151] Electrophysiologic studies have shown conduction disturbance at the His and infra-Hisian levels.[145]

SUMMARY

Multiple systemic disease processes of widely varying etiology and clinical characteristics can result in cardiac infiltration that produces significant conduction system abnormalities, as well as increased risk of sudden cardiac death. Treatment of the underlying disease should be of primary focus, although adjunctive treatment with cardiac pacemaker or defibrillator implantation are also recommended in selected patients, particularly those with cardiac sarcoidosis or neuromuscular disorders.

CLINICS CARE POINTS

Fig. 10 summarizes a general diagnostic approach to evaluate for systemic diseases that can be adopted for young adults, mostly less than 60 years of age, presenting with high-grade AV block.

DISCLOSURE

Dr W.Z. Tzou is a consultant for or has received speaker honoraria, or research funding from Abbott, American Heart Association, Biosense Webster, Biotronik, Boston Scientific, and Medtronic. Dr S.R.A. Sabzwari has no relevant disclosures.

REFERENCES

1. Brenner DA, Jain M, Pimentel DR, et al. Human amyloidogenic light chains directly impair cardiomyocyte function through an increase in cellular oxidant stress. Circ Res 2004;94(8):1008–10.
2. Mishra S, Guan J, Plovie E, et al. Human amyloidogenic light chain proteins result in cardiac dysfunction, cell death, and early mortality in zebrafish. Am J Physiol Heart Circ Physiol 2013;305(1):H95–103.
3. Coelho T, Maurer MS, Suhr OB. THAOS - the Transthyretin Amyloidosis Outcomes Survey: initial report on clinical manifestations in patients with hereditary and wild-type transthyretin amyloidosis. Curr Med Res Opin 2013;29(1):63–76.
4. Reisinger J, Dubrey SW, Lavalley M, et al. Electrophysiologic abnormalities in AL (primary) amyloidosis with cardiac involvement. J Am Coll Cardiol 1997;30(4):1046–51.
5. Barbhaiya CR, Kumar S, Baldinger SH, et al. Electrophysiologic assessment of conduction abnormalities and atrial arrhythmias associated with amyloid cardiomyopathy. Heart Rhythm 2016;13(2):383–90.
6. Donnellan E, Wazni OM, Saliba WI, et al. Prevalence, incidence, and impact on mortality of conduction system disease in transthyretin cardiac amyloidosis. Am J Cardiol 2020;128:140–6.
7. John RM. Arrhythmias in cardiac amyloidosis. J Innov Card Rhythm Manag 2018;9(3):3051–7.
8. Arkema EV, Cozier YC. Epidemiology of sarcoidosis: current findings and future directions. Ther Adv Chronic Dis 2018;9(11):227–40.
9. Patel N, Kalra R, Doshi R, et al. Hospitalization rates, prevalence of cardiovascular manifestations, and outcomes associated with sarcoidosis in the United States. J Am Heart Assoc 2018;7(2):e007844.
10. Swigris JJ, Olson AL, Huie TJ, et al. Sarcoidosis-related mortality in the United States from 1988 to 2007. Am J Respir Crit Care Med 2011;183(11):1524–30.
11. Birnie DH, Kandolin R, Nery PB, et al. Cardiac manifestations of sarcoidosis: diagnosis and management. Eur Heart J 2017;38(35):2663–70.
12. Birnie DH, Nery PB, Ha AC, et al. Cardiac sarcoidosis. J Am Coll Cardiol 2016;68(4):411–21.

13. Patel B, Shah M, Gelaye A, et al. A complete heart block in a young male: a case report and review of literature of cardiac sarcoidosis. Heart Fail Rev 2017;22(1): 55–64.
14. Sekhri V, Sanal S, Delorenzo LJ, et al. Cardiac sarcoidosis: a comprehensive review. Arch Med Sci 2011;7(4):546–54.
15. Rosenthal DG, Fang CD, Groh CA, et al. Heart failure, atrioventricular block, and ventricular tachycardia in sarcoidosis. J Am Heart Assoc 2021;10(5):e017692.
16. Kandolin R, Lehtonen J, Airaksinen J, et al. Cardiac sarcoidosis: epidemiology, characteristics, and outcome over 25 years in a nationwide study. Circulation 2015;131(7):624–32. https://doi.org/10.1161/CIRCULATIONAHA.114.011522.
17. Birnie DH, Sauer WH, Bogun F, et al. HRS expert consensus statement on the diagnosis and management of arrhythmias associated with cardiac sarcoidosis. Heart Rhythm 2014;11(7):1305–23.
18. White JA, Rajchl M, Butler J, et al. Active cardiac sarcoidosis: first clinical experience of simultaneous positron emission tomography–magnetic resonance imaging for the diagnosis of cardiac disease. Circulation 2013;127(22):e639–41.
19. Sadek MM, Yung D, Birnie DH, et al. Corticosteroid therapy for cardiac sarcoidosis: a systematic review. Can J Cardiol 2013;29(9):1034–41.
20. Chim CS, Chan AC, Kwong YL, et al. Primary cardiac lymphoma. Am J Hematol 1997;54(1):79–83.
21. Reynen K. Frequency of primary tumors of the heart. Am J Cardiol 1996; 77(1):107.
22. Tai CJ, Wang WS, Chung MT, et al. Complete atrio-ventricular block as a major clinical presentation of the primary cardiac lymphoma: a case report. Jpn J Clin Oncol 2001;31(5):217–20.
23. Curtsinger CR, Wilson MJ, Yoneda K. Primary cardiac lymphoma. Cancer 1989; 64(2):521–5.
24. Montiel V, Maziers N, Dereme T. Primary cardiac lymphoma and complete atrio-ventricular block: case report and review of the literature. Acta Cardiol 2007; 62(1):55–8.
25. Miguel CE, Bestetti RB. Primary cardiac lymphoma. Int J Cardiol 2011;149(3): 358–63.
26. Shapiro LM. Cardiac tumours: diagnosis and management. Heart 2001;85(2): 218–22.
27. Faganello G, Belham M, Thaman R, et al. A case of primary cardiac lymphoma: analysis of the role of echocardiography in early diagnosis. Echocardiography 2007;24(8):889–92.
28. Andrianto A, Mulia EPB, Suwanto D, et al. Case report: complete heart block as a manifestation of cardiac metastasis of oral cancer. F1000Res 2020;9:1243.
29. Ungprasert P, Wannarong T, Panichsillapakit T, et al. Cardiac involvement in mixed connective tissue disease: a systematic review. Int J Cardiol 2014; 171(3):326–30.
30. Rebollar-Gonzalez V, Torre-Delgadillo A, Orea-Tejeda A, et al. Cardiac conduction disturbances in mixed connective tissue disease. Rev Invest Clin 2001; 53(4):330–4.
31. Hajas A, Szodoray P, Nakken B, et al. Clinical course, prognosis, and causes of death in mixed connective tissue disease. J Rheumatol 2013;40(7):1134–42.
32. Lash AD, Wittman AL, Quismorio FP Jr. Myocarditis in mixed connective tissue disease: clinical and pathologic study of three cases and review of the literature. Semin Arthritis Rheum 1986;15(4):288–96.

33. Love LA, Leff RL, Fraser DD, et al. A new approach to the classification of idiopathic inflammatory myopathy: myositis-specific autoantibodies define useful homogeneous patient groups. Medicine (Baltimore) 1991;70(6):360–74.

34. Brouwer R, Hengstman GJ, Vree Egberts W, et al. Autoantibody profiles in the sera of European patients with myositis. Ann Rheum Dis 2001;60(2):116–23.

35. Alyan O, Ozdemir O, Geyik B, et al. Polymyositis complicated with complete atrioventricular block–a case report and review of the literature. Angiology 2003;54(6):729–31.

36. Denbow CE, Lie JT, Tancredi RG, et al. Cardiac involvement in polymyositis: a clinicopathologic study of 20 autopsied patients. Arthritis Rheum 1979;22(10):1088–92.

37. Haupt HM, Hutchins GM. The heart and cardiac conduction system in polymyositis-dermatomyositis: a clinicopathologic study of 16 autopsied patients. Am J Cardiol 1982;50(5):998–1006.

38. Lightfoot PR, Bharati S, Lev M. Chronic dermatomyositis with intermittent trifascicular block. An electrophysiologic-conduction system correlation. Chest 1977;71(3):413–6.

39. Lynch PG. Cardiac involvement in chronic polymyositis. Br Heart J 1971;33(3):416–9.

40. Schaumburg HH, Nielsen SL, Yurchak PM. Heart block in polymyositis. N Engl J Med 1971;284(9):480–1.

41. Reid JM, Murdoch R. Polymyositis and complete heart block. Br Heart J 1979;41(5):628–9.

42. Kandolin R, Lehtonen J, Salmenkivi K, et al. Diagnosis, treatment, and outcome of giant-cell myocarditis in the era of combined immunosuppression. Circ Heart Fail 2013;6(1):15–22.

43. Cooper LT Jr, Berry GJ, Shabetai R. Idiopathic giant-cell myocarditis–natural history and treatment. Multicenter giant cell myocarditis study Group investigators. N Engl J Med 1997;336(26):1860–6.

44. Barra SN, Providencia R, Paiva L, et al. A review on advanced atrioventricular block in young or middle-aged adults. Pacing Clin Electrophysiol 2012;35(11):1395–405.

45. Kandolin R, Lehtonen J, Kupari M. Cardiac sarcoidosis and giant cell myocarditis as causes of atrioventricular block in young and middle-aged adults. Circ Arrhythm Electrophysiol 2011;4(3):303–9.

46. Davidoff R, Palacios I, Southern J, et al. Giant cell versus lymphocytic myocarditis. A comparison of their clinical features and long-term outcomes. Circulation 1991;83(3):953–61.

47. Ren H, Poston RS Jr, Hruban RH, et al. Long survival with giant cell myocarditis. Mod Pathol 1993;6(4):402–7.

48. Davies RA, Veinot JP, Smith S, et al. Giant cell myocarditis: clinical presentation, bridge to transplantation with mechanical circulatory support, and long-term outcome. J Heart Lung Transpl 2002;21(6):674–9.

49. Menghini VV, Savcenko V, Olson LJ, et al. Combined immunosuppression for the treatment of idiopathic giant cell myocarditis. Mayo Clin Proc 1999;74(12):1221–6.

50. Tselios K, Gladman DD, Harvey P, et al. Severe brady-arrhythmias in systemic lupus erythematosus: prevalence, etiology and associated factors. Lupus 2018;27(9):1415–23.

51. Natsheh A, Shimony D, Bogot N, et al. Complete heart block in lupus. Lupus 2019;28(13):1589–93.

52. Lazzerini PE, Capecchi PL, Laghi-Pasini F. Isolated atrioventricular block of unknown origin in adults and anti-Ro/SSA antibodies: clinical evidence, putative mechanisms, and therapeutic implications. Heart Rhythm 2015;12(2):449–54.
53. Lazzerini PE, Brucato A, Capecchi PL, et al. Isolated atrioventricular block of unknown origin in the adult and autoimmunity: diagnostic and therapeutic considerations exemplified by 3 anti-Ro/SSA-associated cases. HeartRhythm Case Rep 2015;1(5):293–9.
54. Behan WM, Behan PO, Gairns J. Cardiac damage in polymyositis associated with antibodies to tissue ribonucleoproteins. Br Heart J 1987;57(2):176–80.
55. Logar D, Kveder T, Rozman B, et al. Possible association between anti-Ro antibodies and myocarditis or cardiac conduction defects in adults with systemic lupus erythematosus. Ann Rheum Dis 1990;49(8):627–9.
56. O'Neill TW, Mahmoud A, Tooke A, et al. Is there a relationship between subclinical myocardial abnormalities, conduction defects and Ro/La antibodies in adults with systemic lupus erythematosus? Clin Exp Rheumatol 1993;11(4):409–12.
57. Gordon PA, Rosenthal E, Khamashta MA, et al. Absence of conduction defects in the electrocardiograms [correction of echocardiograms] of mothers with children with congenital complete heart block. J Rheumatol 2001;28(2):366–9.
58. Lodde BM, Sankar V, Kok MR, et al. Adult heart block is associated with disease activity in primary Sjogren's syndrome. Scand J Rheumatol 2005;34(5):383–6.
59. Costa M, Gameiro Silva MB, Silva JA, et al. Anti-RO anti-LA anti-RNP antibodies and eletrocardiogram's PR interval in adult patients with systemic lupus erythematosus. Acta Reumatol Port 2008;33(2):173–6.
60. Askanase AD, Friedman DM, Copel J, et al. Spectrum and progression of conduction abnormalities in infants born to mothers with anti-SSA/Ro-SSB/La antibodies. Lupus 2002;11(3):145–51.
61. Bergman G, Eliasson H, Mohlkert LA, et al. Progression to first-degree heart block in preschool children exposed in utero to maternal anti-SSA/Ro52 autoantibodies. Acta Paediatr 2012;101(5):488–93.
62. Ambrosi A, Wahren-Herlenius M. Congenital heart block: evidence for a pathogenic role of maternal autoantibodies. Arthritis Res Ther 2012;14(2):208.
63. Bergman G, Skog A, Tingstrom J, et al. Late development of complete atrioventricular block may be immune mediated and congenital in origin. Acta Paediatr 2014;103(3):275–81.
64. Lo CH, Wei JCC, Tsai CF, et al. Syncope caused by complete heart block and ventricular arrhythmia as early manifestation of systemic lupus erythematosus in a pregnant patient: a case report. Lupus 2018;27(10):1729–31.
65. Prochaska MT, Bergl PA, Patel AR, et al. Atrioventricular heart block and syncope coincident with diagnosis of systemic lupus erythematosus. Can J Cardiol 2013;29(10):1330.e5–7.
66. Tselios K, Deeb M, Gladman DD, et al. Antimalarial-induced cardiomyopathy: a systematic review of the literature. Lupus 2018;27(4):591–9.
67. Jaeggi ET, Hamilton RM, Silverman ED, et al. Outcome of children with fetal, neonatal or childhood diagnosis of isolated congenital atrioventricular block. A single institution's experience of 30 years. J Am Coll Cardiol 2002;39(1):130–7.
68. Llanos C, Izmirly PM, Katholi M, et al. Recurrence rates of cardiac manifestations associated with neonatal lupus and maternal/fetal risk factors. Arthritis Rheum 2009;60(10):3091–7.

69. Waltuck J, Buyon JP. Autoantibody-associated congenital heart block: outcome in mothers and children. Ann Intern Med 1994;120(7):544–51.

70. Buyon JP, Clancy RM, Friedman DM. Cardiac manifestations of neonatal lupus erythematosus: guidelines to management, integrating clues from the bench and bedside. Nat Clin Pract Rheumatol 2009;5(3):139–48.

71. Brucato A, Cimaz R, Caporali R, et al. Pregnancy outcomes in patients with autoimmune diseases and anti-Ro/SSA antibodies. Clin Rev Allergy Immunol 2011;40(1):27–41.

72. Silverman ED, Buyon J, Laxer RM, et al. Autoantibody response to the Ro/La particle may predict outcome in neonatal lupus erythematosus. Clin Exp Immunol 1995;100(3):499–505.

73. Jaeggi E, Laskin C, Hamilton R, et al. The importance of the level of maternal anti-Ro/SSA antibodies as a prognostic marker of the development of cardiac neonatal lupus erythematosus a prospective study of 186 antibody-exposed fetuses and infants. J Am Coll Cardiol 2010;55(24):2778–84.

74. Gordon P, Khamashta MA, Rosenthal E, et al. Anti-52 kDa Ro, anti-60 kDa Ro, and anti-La antibody profiles in neonatal lupus. J Rheumatol 2004;31(12): 2480–7.

75. Karnabi E, Boutjdir M. Role of calcium channels in congenital heart block. Scand J Immunol 2010;72(3):226–34.

76. Itzhaki I, Schiller J, Beyar R, et al. Calcium handling in embryonic stem cell-derived cardiac myocytes: of mice and men. Ann N Y Acad Sci 2006;1080: 207–15.

77. Ciardulli A, D'Antonio F, Magro-Malosso ER, et al. Maternal steroid therapy for fetuses with second-degree immune-mediated congenital atrioventricular block: a systematic review and meta-analysis. Acta Obstet Gynecol Scand 2018;97(7): 787–94.

78. Hickstein H, Kulz T, Claus R, et al. Autoimmune-associated congenital heart block: treatment of the mother with immunoadsorption. Ther Apher Dial 2005; 9(2):148–53.

79. Maisch B, Ristic AD. Immunological basis of the cardiac conduction and rhythm disorders. Eur Heart J 2001;22(10):813–24.

80. Seferovic PM, Ristic AD, Maksimovic R, et al. Cardiac arrhythmias and conduction disturbances in autoimmune rheumatic diseases. Rheumatology (Oxford) 2006;45(Suppl 4):iv39–42.

81. Ahern M, Lever JV, Cosh J. Complete heart block in rheumatoid arthritis. Ann Rheum Dis 1983;42(4):389–97.

82. Rasker JJ, Cosh JA. Cause and age at death in a prospective study of 100 patients with rheumatoid arthritis. Ann Rheum Dis 1981;40(2):115–20.

83. Villecco AS, de Liberali E, Bianchi FB, et al. Antibodies to cardiac conducting tissue and abnormalities of cardiac conduction in rheumatoid arthritis. Clin Exp Immunol 1983;53(3):536–40.

84. Kemper JW, Baggenstoss AH, Slocumb CH. The relationship of therapy with cortisone to the incidence of vascular lesions in rheumatoid arthritis. Ann Intern Med 1957;46(5):831–51.

85. Janosik DL, Osborn TG, Moore TL, et al. Heart disease in systemic sclerosis. Semin Arthritis Rheum 1989;19(3):191–200.

86. Escudero J, Mc DE. The electrocardiogram in scleroderma: analysis of 60 cases and review of the literature. Am Heart J 1958;56(6):846–55.

87. Follansbee WP, Curtiss EI, Rahko PS, et al. The electrocardiogram in systemic sclerosis (scleroderma). Study of 102 consecutive cases with functional correlations and review of the literature. Am J Med 1985;79(2):183–92.
88. Roberts NK, Cabeen WR Jr, Moss J, et al. The prevalence of conduction defects and cardiac arrhythmias in progressive systemic sclerosis. Ann Intern Med 1981;94(1):38–40.
89. Ridolfi RL, Bulkley BH, Hutchins GM. The cardiac conduction system in progressive systemic sclerosis. Clinical and pathologic features of 35 patients. Am J Med 1976;61(3):361–6.
90. Volta U, Villecco AS, Bianchi FB, et al. Antibodies to cardiac conducting tissue in progressive systemic sclerosis. Clin Exp Rheumatol 1985;3(2):131–5.
91. Bulkley BH, Roberts WC. Ankylosing spondylitis and aortic regurgitation. Description of the characteristic cardiovascular lesion from study of eight necropsy patients. Circulation 1973;48(5):1014–27.
92. Davidson P, Baggenstoss AH, Slocumb CH, et al. Cardiac and aortic lesions in rheumatoid spondylitis. Proc Staff Meet Mayo Clin 1963;38:427–35.
93. Bergfeldt L, Moller E. Complete heart block–another HLA B27 associated disease manifestation. Tissue Antigens 1983;21(5):385–90.
94. Bergfeldt L, Vallin H, Edhag O. Complete heart block in HLA B27 associated disease. Electrophysiological and clinical characteristics. Br Heart J 1984; 51(2):184–8.
95. Kinsella TD, Johnson LG, Ian R. Cardiovascular manifestations of ankylosing spondylitis. Can Med Assoc J 1974;111(12):1309–11.
96. Bergfeldt L, Edhag O, Vallin H. Cardiac conduction disturbances, an underestimated manifestation in ankylosing spondylitis. A 25-year follow-up study of 68 patients. Acta Med Scand 1982;212(4):217–23.
97. Eom YS, Oh PC. Graves' disease presenting with complete atrioventricular block. Case Rep Endocrinol 2020;2020:6656875.
98. Kramer MR, Shilo S, Hershko C. Atrioventricular and sinoatrial block in thyrotoxic crisis. Br Heart J 1985;54(6):600–2.
99. Eraker SA, Wickamasekaran R, Goldman S. Complete heart block with hyperthyroidism. JAMA 1978;239(16):1644–6.
100. Stern MP, Jacobs RL, Duncan GW. Complete heart block complicating hyperthyroidism. JAMA 1970;212(12):2117–9.
101. Sataline L, Donaghue G. Hypercalcemia, heart-block, and hyperthyroidism. JAMA 1970;213(8):1342.
102. Ortmann C, Du Chesne A, Brinkmann B. Inflammation of the cardiac conduction system in a case of hyperthyroidism. Int J Leg Med 1999;112(4):271–4.
103. Kim D, Smith TW. Effects of thyroid hormone on sodium pump sites, sodium content, and contractile responses to cardiac glycosides in cultured chick ventricular cells. J Clin Invest 1984;74(4):1481–8.
104. Haber RS, Loeb JN. Stimulation of potassium efflux in rat liver by a low dose of thyroid hormone: evidence for enhanced cation permeability in the absence of Na,K-ATPase induction. Endocrinology 1986;118(1):207–11.
105. Shirani J, Barron MM, Pierre-Louis ML, et al. Congestive heart failure, dilated cardiac ventricles, and sudden death in hyperthyroidism. Am J Cardiol 1993; 72(3):365–8.
106. Toloune F, Boukili A, Ghafir D, et al. [Hyperthyroidism and atrioventricular block. Pathogenic hypothesis. Apropos of a case and review of the literature]. Arch Mal Coeur Vaiss 1988;81(9):1131–5.

107. Topaloglu S, Topaloglu OY, Ozdemir O, et al. Hyperthyroidism and complete atrioventricular block–a report of 2 cases with electrophysiologic assessment. Angiology 2005;56(2):217–20.
108. Schantz ET, Dubbs AW. Complete auriculoventricular block in myxedema with reversion to normal sinus rhythm on thyroid therapy. Am Heart J 1951;41(4): 613–9.
109. Lee JK, Lewis JA. Myxoedema with complete A-V block and Adams-Stokes disease abolished with thyroid medication. Br Heart J 1962;24:253–6.
110. Ohler WR. The heart in myxedema. Arch Intern Med 1934;53:165–87.
111. Davis JC. Myxedema heart with report of one case. Ann Intern Med 1930;4: 733–41.
112. Luten D. Myxedema with partial heart block and severe anemia both of which disappeared under thyroid therapy. Mo Med 1929;26:73–7.
113. Aub JC, Stern SN. The influence of large doses of thyroid extract on the total metabolism and heart in a case of heart-block. Arch Intern Med 1918;21:130–8.
114. Brewer DB. Myxoedema: an autopsy report with histochemical observations on the nature of the mucoid infiltrations. J Pathol Bacteriol 1951;63(3):503–12.
115. Hamilton JD, Greenwood WF. Myxedema heart disease. Circulation 1957;15(3): 442–7.
116. Zoll PM, Linenthal AJ, Gibson W, et al. Intravenous drug therapy of Stokes-Adams disease; effects of sympathomimetic amines on ventricular rhythmicity and atrioventricular conduction. Circulation 1958;17(3):325–39.
117. Singh JB, Starobin OE, Guerrant RL, et al. Reversible atrioventricular block in myxedema. Chest 1973;63(4):582–5.
118. Beard CM, Sheps SG, Kurland LT, et al. Occurrence of pheochromocytoma in Rochester, Minnesota, 1950 through 1979. Mayo Clin Proc 1983;58(12):802–4.
119. Zweiker R, Tiemann M, Eber B, et al. Bradydysrhythmia-related presyncope secondary to pheochromocytoma. J Intern Med 1997;242(3):249–53.
120. Paschalis-Purtak K, Pucilowska B, Prejbisz A, et al. Cardiac arrests, atrioventricular block, and pheochromocytoma. Am J Hypertens 2004;17(6):544–5.
121. McHirgui N, Rojbi I, Oueslati I, et al. Atrioventricular dissociation due to pheochromocytoma: a case report. Tunis Med 2014;92(10):645–6.
122. Haine SE, Miljoen HP, Blankoff I, et al. Atrioventricular dissociation due to pheochromocytoma in a young adult. Clin Cardiol 2010;33(12):E65–7.
123. Curione M, Petramala L, Savoriti C, et al. Electrical and myocardial remodeling in primary aldosteronism. Front Cardiovasc Med 2014;1:7.
124. de Jong S, van Veen TA, van Rijen HV, et al. Fibrosis and cardiac arrhythmias. J Cardiovasc Pharmacol 2011;57(6):630–8.
125. Rossi GP, Sacchetto A, Pavan E, et al. Remodeling of the left ventricle in primary aldosteronism due to Conn's adenoma. Circulation 1997;95(6):1471–8.
126. Rossi GP. Cardiac consequences of aldosterone excess in human hypertension. Am J Hypertens 2006;19(1):10–2.
127. Magee A, Nevin NC. The epidemiology of myotonic dystrophy in Northern Ireland. Community Genet 1999;2(4):179–83.
128. Siciliano G, Manca M, Gennarelli M, et al. Epidemiology of myotonic dystrophy in Italy: re-apprisal after genetic diagnosis. Clin Genet 2001;59(5):344–9.
129. Norwood FL, Harling C, Chinnery PF, et al. Prevalence of genetic muscle disease in Northern England: in-depth analysis of a muscle clinic population. Brain 2009;132(Pt 11):3175–86.
130. Phillips MF, Harper PS. Cardiac disease in myotonic dystrophy. Cardiovasc Res 1997;33(1):13–22.

131. Johnson NE, Abbott D, Cannon-Albright LA. Relative risks for comorbidities associated with myotonic dystrophy: a population-based analysis. Muscle Nerve 2015;52(4):659–61.

132. Kusumoto FM, Schoenfeld MH, Barrett C, et al. 2018 ACC/AHA/HRS guideline on the evaluation and management of patients with bradycardia and cardiac conduction delay: executive summary: a report of the American College of Cardiology/American Heart Association Task Force on clinical practice guidelines, and the Heart Rhythm Society. J Am Coll Cardiol 2019;74(7): 932–87.

133. Nguyen HH, Wolfe JT 3rd, Holmes DR Jr, et al. Pathology of the cardiac conduction system in myotonic dystrophy: a study of 12 cases. J Am Coll Cardiol 1988; 11(3):662–71.

134. Groh WJ, Groh MR, Saha C, et al. Electrocardiographic abnormalities and sudden death in myotonic dystrophy type 1. N Engl J Med 2008;358(25):2688–97.

135. Olofsson BO, Forsberg H, Andersson S, et al. Electrocardiographic findings in myotonic dystrophy. Br Heart J 1988;59(1):47–52.

136. Prystowsky EN, Pritchett LC, Smith WM, et al. Electrophysiologic assessment of the atrioventricular conduction system after surgical correction of ventricular preexcitation. Circulation 1979;59(4):789–96.

137. Wahbi K, Meune C, Becane HM, et al. Left ventricular dysfunction and cardiac arrhythmias are frequent in type 2 myotonic dystrophy: a case control study. Neuromuscul Disord 2009;19(7):468–72.

138. Day JW, Ricker K, Jacobsen JF, et al. Myotonic dystrophy type 2: molecular, diagnostic and clinical spectrum. Neurology 2003;60(4):657–64.

139. Di Mambro C, Tamborrino PP, Silvetti MS, et al. Progressive involvement of cardiac conduction system in paediatric patients with Kearns-Sayre syndrome: how to predict occurrence of complete heart block and sudden cardiac death? Europace 2021;23(6):948–57.

140. DiMauro S, Schon EA, Carelli V, et al. The clinical maze of mitochondrial neurology. Nat Rev Neurol 2013;9(8):429–44.

141. Larsson NG, Holme E, Kristiansson B, et al. Progressive increase of the mutated mitochondrial DNA fraction in Kearns-Sayre syndrome. Pediatr Res 1990;28(2): 131–6.

142. Polak PE, Zijlstra F, Roelandt JR. Indications for pacemaker implantation in the Kearns-Sayre syndrome. Eur Heart J 1989;10(3):281–2.

143. Yamashita S, Nishino I, Nonaka I, et al. Genotype and phenotype analyses in 136 patients with single large-scale mitochondrial DNA deletions. J Hum Genet 2008;53(7):598.

144. Welzing L, von Kleist-Retzow JC, Kribs A, et al. Rapid development of life-threatening complete atrioventricular block in Kearns-Sayre syndrome. Eur J Pediatr 2009;168(6):757–9.

145. Altekin RE, Yanikoglu A, Ucar M, et al. Complete AV block and cardiac syncope in a patient with Duchenne muscular dystrophy. J Cardiol Cases 2011;3(2): e68–70.

146. Fayssoil A, Orlikowski D, Nardi O, et al. Complete atrioventricular block in Duchenne muscular dystrophy. Europace 2008;10(11):1351–2.

147. Akdemir R, Ozhan H, Gunduz H, et al. Complete atrioventricular block in Becker muscular dystrophy. N Z Med J 2004;117(1194):U895.

148. Quinlivan R, Ball J, Dunckley M, et al. Becker muscular dystrophy presenting with complete heart block in the sixth decade. J Neurol 1995;242(6):398–400.

149. Angelini C, Fanin M, Freda MP, et al. Prognostic factors in mild dystrophinopathies. J Neurol Sci 1996;142(1–2):70–8.

150. Bies RD, Friedman D, Roberts R, et al. Expression and localization of dystrophin in human cardiac Purkinje fibers. Circulation 1992;86(1):147–53.

151. Finsterer J, Stollberger C. The heart in human dystrophinopathies. Cardiology 2003;99(1):1–19.

Imaging of Pulmonary Manifestations of Connective Tissue Disease

Kimberly Kallianos, MD

KEYWORDS

- Connective tissue disease • Interstitial lung disease
- Nonspecific interstitial pneumonia • Organizing pneumonia
- Lymphoid interstitial pneumonia • Usual interstitial pneumonia
- Interstitial pneumonia with autoimmune features

KEY POINTS

- The diagnosis of connective tissue disease-related interstitial lung disease is a multidisciplinary process, integrating clinical findings, serologic data, and imaging patterns.
- Although connective tissue disease-associated interstitial lung disease connective tissue disease-related usual interstitial pneumonia (CTD-ILD) can present with any pattern, the most commonly seen patterns are nonspecific interstitial pneumonia (NSIP), organizing pneumonia (OP), NSIP/OP overlap, and lymphoid interstitial pneumonia. CTD-UIP is also seen, most commonly in patients with rheumatoid arthritis.
- Multicompartmental disease, when seen, supports a diagnosis of CTD-ILD. These features include airways disease, pleural/pericardial effusions, and pulmonary hypertension.

CLINICAL DIAGNOSIS OF CONNECTIVE TISSUES DISEASE

The majority of connective tissue diseases (CTDs) are multisystem disorders that are often heterogeneous in their presentation and do not have a single laboratory, histologic, or radiologic feature that is defined as the gold standard to support a specific diagnosis.[1] Given this challenging situation, the diagnosis of CTD is a process that requires the synthesis of multidisciplinary data which may include patient clinical symptoms, serologic evaluation, laboratory testing, histology from tissue biopsy, and imaging (**Table 1**).[2–6]

Thus, the goals of a radiologist in the workup of a patient with suspected CTD are several. Image interpretation and identification of pulmonary and extrapulmonary

This article previously appeared in *Radiologic Clinics* volume 60 issue 6 November 2022.
The author has nothing to disclose.
Department of Radiology and Biomedical Imaging, UCSF, 505 Parnassus Avenue, M391, San Francisco, CA 94143, USA
E-mail address: Kimberly.Kallianos@ucsf.edu

Rheum Dis Clin N Am 50 (2024) 409–422
https://doi.org/10.1016/j.rdc.2024.03.002
rheumatic.theclinics.com

Table 1
Classification criteria for connective tissue diseases

Lupus	Scleroderma	Rheumatoid Arthritis	Myositis	Sjogren
Skin rash/photosensitivity	Sclerodactyly	Joint symptoms	Proximal muscle weakness	Ocular symptoms
Oral ulcers	Fingertip lesions	Duration > 6 wk	Dysphagia	Oral symptoms
Arthritis	Telangiectasia	Rheumatoid nodules	Muscle biopsy	Salivary gland biopsy
Serositis	Pulmonary hypertension and/or interstitial lung disease	Rheumatoid factor	Elevated skeletal muscle enzymes	Sjogren-related autoantibodies
Systemic disorders—renal, neurologic, hematologic, immunologic	Raynaud phenomenon	Radiographic erosions	EMG findings	
Antinuclear antibody	SSc-related autoantibodies		Skin rash	

manifestations that would suggest an underlying CTD is a primary goal; however, the radiologist also must be comfortable with the multidisciplinary data supplied by the other arms of the patient's workup so as to place the imaging findings in the appropriate clinical context. In fact, a radiologist with broad knowledge of the features and presentation of CTD is a great asset in the diagnosis of CTD patients, as imaging findings are not infrequently the initial presenting symptom. In a series of 114 patients evaluated in an interstitial lung disease program, 34 (30%) satisfied criteria American College of Rheumatology criteria for a CTD, 17 (15%) of which were newly diagnosed with CTD as a direct result of their evaluation by the interstitial lung disease program.[7] In addition, a subset of patients with presumed idiopathic interstitial pneumonia such as idiopathic pulmonary fibrosis followed longitudinally will subsequently be diagnosed with a CTD at follow-up. In one series of 68 patients diagnosed with idiopathic interstitial lung disease, 13 patients (19%) developed a CTD over the 1 to 11 year follow-up period.[8]

SEROLOGIC ANALYSIS

Evaluation for the presence of autoantibodies is a key feature in the workup of patients with presumed CTD. Although a comprehensive understanding of the breath of autoantibodies evaluated in the practice of rheumatology is beyond the scope of practice for radiologists, a general familiarity with the common autoantibodies associated with CTDs allows radiologists involved in the diagnosis of patients with interstitial lung disease to engage fully in the multidisciplinary conversation that takes place to distinguish patients with idiopathic ILD from those with an underlying connective tissue disorder. Multidisciplinary assessment of patients with interstitial lung disease has been shown in the literature to improve dialogistic certainty, resulting in a change in diagnosis from IPF to CTD-ILD in 28% of patients.[9]

The ATS/ERS/JRS/ALAT Clinical Practice Guidelines for patients with newly diagnosed interstitial lung disease who are clinically suspected of having IPF recommend serologic testing to aid in the exclusion CTD as a cause of the patient's lung disease.[10,11] Guidelines recommend testing for antinuclear antibody (ANA), anti-cyclic citrullinated peptide (anti-CCP), and rheumatoid factor (RF) in all patients with suspected ILD. More focused antibody tests such as Scl70, SSA/Ro, SSB/La, RNP, and myositis–related antibodies can be performed in specific cases, as discussed below.

ANA titers are very commonly tested in patients with presumed CTD. Low-level titers (for example 1:40 dilution) can be seen in up to 32% of normal individuals, and thus a higher cut-off of 1:160 or 1:320 dilution improves the identification of a clinically significant positive ANA result.[12] Positive ANA is sensitive for the diagnosis of lupus (93%) and scleroderma (85%); however, it can be less helpful in the diagnosis of other connective tissue disorders. For example, myositis or anti-synthetase syndrome is classically ANA negative.[13] In addition to the presence of a positive ANA, the pattern of staining is also a relevant feature—with options including nuclear, nucleolar, and centromeric patterns. Anti-centromeric pattern is strongly associated with scleroderma.[14]

Rheumatoid factor positivity has a high sensitivity and specificity for the diagnosis of rheumatoid arthritis (both near 70%), whereas anti-CCP has an even higher specificity (95%–99%).[12] Anti-topoisomerase I, also known as anti-Scl70 has a very high specificity for scleroderma (90%–100%). Other highly specific autoantibodies for a defined CTD include anti-ds-DNA and anti-Smith antibodies which have a specificity for SLE of 97% and 96% respectively. A positive anti-RNP in isolation is both highly sensitive and specific for mixed CTD. The combination of positive anti-SSA/Ro and anti-SSB/La antibodies is suggestive of Sjogren's disease, although positive SSA in isolation can also be seen with a variety of other CTDs, particularly scleroderma.[15] Finally, a variety of autoantibodies can be detected in patients with myositis (either polymyositis or dermatomyositis) and are associated with an increased risk of interstitial lung disease. Anti-tRNA synthetase antibodies (Jo-1, PL-7, PL-12, EJ, OJ, KS, Ha, Zo) are specific for the diagnosis of myositis, of which anti Jo-1 is the most common (seen in 20%–30%), followed by anti PL-7 and PL-12 (seen in 3%–4%).[15] Anti-Jo1 antibody positivity is seen in 30% to 75% of myositis patients with ILD.[16]

CT FINDINGS IN CONNECTIVE TISSUE DISEASE PATIENTS

Nearly all patterns of interstitial lung disease can be seen in patients with CTD, although the four most common patterns of interstitial lung disease seen in patients with CTD are nonspecific interstitial pneumonia (NSIP), organizing pneumonia (OP), NSIP/OP overlap, and lymphoid interstitial pneumonia (LIP). Surgical biopsy to confirm a particular pattern of interstitial lung disease is rarely performed, and therefore high-resolution computed tomography (CT) is very frequently used to determine the primary pattern of lung pathology.

The most common pattern of interstitial lung disease seen in patients with CTD is NSIP (**Fig. 1**). CT findings in NSIP include (1) symmetric bilateral ground-glass opacity, (2) irregular reticulation, and (3) traction bronchiectasis.[17] The combination of ground-glass opacity with reticulation and relatively minimal honeycombing has a 96% sensitivity for NSIP versus UIP; however, only a moderate specificity (41%).[18] Histologically, these findings correspond to varying degrees of fibrosis and interstitial inflammation uniformly involving the peripheral and basilar lung.[19] Relative subpleural sparing, although not a sensitive finding, is highly specific for distinguishing NSIP from UIP pattern (96%).[20]

Organizing pneumonia seen in patients with CTD has a similar CT appearance to organizing pneumonia due to other causes (**Fig. 2**). Common findings include symmetric, peripheral, or peribronchovascular ground-glass opacity and consolidation.[21] The atoll or reverse halo sign characterized by rounded or crescentic regions of consolidation with central clearing or ground-glass opacity may also be seen in 20% of patients

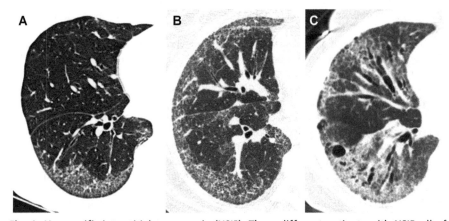

Fig. 1. Nonspecific interstitial pneumonia (NSIP). Three different patients with NSIP, all of which show basilar predominant findings with subpleural sparing. The spectrum of findings seen in NSIP include ground-glass opacity (A), irregular reticulation (B), and traction bronchiectasis (C).

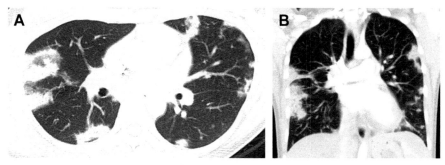

Fig. 2. Organizing pneumonia. Axial (A) and coronal reformatted (B) images show typical findings of organizing pneumonia in a patient with systemic lupus erythematosus. Patchy basilar predominant subpleural and peribronchovascular regions of consolidation with the reversed halo sign are typical findings.

with OP.[22] Combined features of NSIP and OP, also called "NSIP/OP overlap", include the greater extent of consolidation and greater frequency of combined peripheral plus peribronchovascular distribution than is seen in patients with isolated NSIP pattern[23] (**Fig. 3**).

LIP/follicular bronchiolitis is characterized by interstitial infiltration by lymphocytes and plasma cells; however, these are polyclonal in origin, which helps to distinguish from these findings from low-grade lymphoma. The major CT findings corresponding to this histology include ground-glass opacity, small ill-defined nodules, and perivascular cysts[24] (**Fig. 4**).

Usual interstitial pneumonia (UIP) pattern is also seen in patients with CTD. CTD-UIP patients tend to be younger and more likely to be female compared with patients with UIP pattern due to idiopathic pulmonary fibrosis (IPF).[25] UIP pattern is defined by basilar and peripheral predominate fibrosis with reticulation, traction bronchiectasis, and honeycombing[11] (**Fig. 5**). Several CT findings have been reported as useful in distinguishing UIP pattern due to CTD versus UIP pattern in patients with IPF. These include the "anterior upper lobe sign", with concentration of fibrosis in the anterior lung and relative sparing of other regions; the "straight edge sign", with a sharp line of demarcation in the craniocaudal plane between normal lung and regions involved

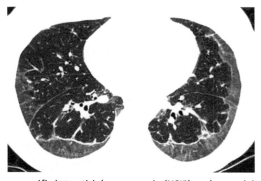

Fig. 3. Overlap of nonspecific interstitial pneumonia (NSIP) and organizing pneumonia (OP). Subpleural and basilar predominant ground-glass opacity is present in a patient with polymyositis. Note the rim of consolidation at the interface between the ground glass opacity and normal lung. This appearance is typical of an overlap of NSIP and OP.

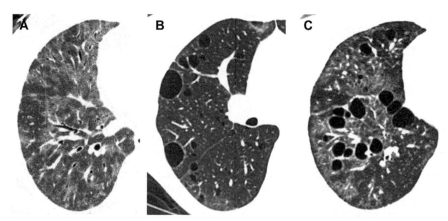

Fig. 4. Lymphoid interstitial pneumonia. Three separate patients with connective tissue disease and lymphoid interstitial pneumonia. Typical findings include ground-glass opacity (*A*), isolated cysts (*B*), and a combination of ground glass and cysts (*C*).

by fibrosis; and the "exuberant honeycombing sign", with exuberant honeycomb cysts occupying 70% of the fibrotic involvement of the lung. The specificities of each of these signs alone exceed 87% for CTD-UIP, and the presence of two of the three signs has a sensitivity for CTD-UIP of 95%.[26] It is important to acknowledge that CT findings may evolve over time. Over 3 years of longitudinal follow-up in a series of 48 patients with biopsy-proven NSIP, 28% of patients with NSIP pattern on initial CT progressed to findings of UIP pattern[27] (**Fig. 6**).

In addition to pulmonary parenchymal involvement by interstitial lung disease, there are associated "multicompartmental" findings which also support a diagnosis of connective tissue-related ILD. These include intrinsic airway disease (such as bronchiolitis obliterans as manifested by mosaic perfusion on inspiratory imaging and air trapping on expiratory imaging), pleural or pericardial effusions, and pulmonary vascular disease such as pulmonary hypertension[28] (**Fig. 7**).

Pulmonary hypertension is defined as elevated pulmonary artery pressures greater than 25 mm Hg at rest of greater than 30 mm Hg during exercise. A variety of size thresholds of the pulmonary artery have been described in the literature; however, pulmonary artery size has only moderate sensitivity (range 47%–87%) and specificity

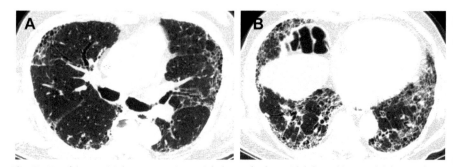

Fig. 5. Usual interstitial pneumonia. Axial through the mid (*A*) and lower (*B*) lungs shows typical findings of fibrosis and honeycombing (*arrow*) with a patchy subpleural and basilar predominance.

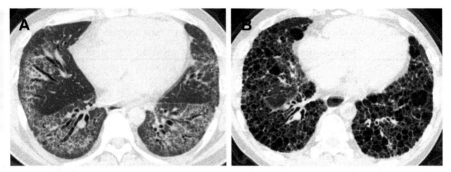

Fig. 6. Nonspecific interstitial pneumonia, evolution over time. Baseline CT (A) shows typical findings of nonspecific interstitial pneumonia with basilar predominant reticulation and traction bronchiectasis with subpleural sparing. Six years later (B), the same patient shows findings typical of usual interstitial pneumonia with extensive honeycombing.

(range 41%–100%) for the detection of pulmonary hypertension. Pulmonary artery to aorta ratio greater than 1 is a stronger predictor for pulmonary hypertension than pulmonary artery diameter alone, with a positive predictive value of 92% to 95%.[29,30]

SPECIFIC CONNECTIVE TISSUE DISEASES

There is no one pattern of interstitial lung disease that is diagnostic of a particular CTD, and all patterns have been seen across the spectrum of patients with CTD. However, certain patterns are seen more commonly or are more strongly associated with particular CTD diagnoses. These trends are summarized in **Table 2** and discussed in further detail below.

Scleroderma (**Figs. 8** and **9**)—Interstitial lung disease occurs most commonly in scleroderma compared with the other CTDs, occurring in up to 90% of patients with both limited and diffuse forms of the disease. Interstitial lung disease and pulmonary

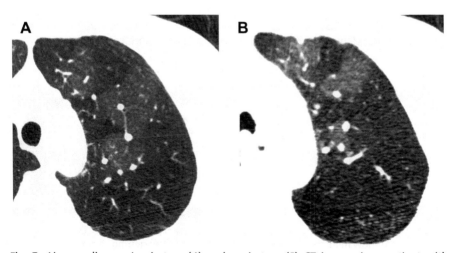

Fig. 7. Airways disease. Inspiratory (A) and expiratory (B) CT images in a patient with constrictive bronchiolitis showing mosaic perfusion, geographic regions of decreased lung density, and corresponding air trapping on the expiratory phase.

Table 2
Common and less common manifestations of connective tissue diseases by diagnosis

	Scleroderma	Rheumatoid Arthritis	Myositis	Sjogrens	Lupus
Common	NSIP PAH	UIP NSIP	NSIP OP	LIP	Edema Hemorrhage DAD
Less common	UIP	Airways disease OP	DAD	Airways disease	Fibrosis

hypertension contribute to the majority (60%) of deaths in this patient population.[31] The most common pattern of ILD seen in scleroderma patients is NSIP (77%), although UIP pattern can be seen less commonly. At biopsy, fibrotic NSIP is more common than cellular NSIP.[32]

Rheumatoid arthritis (**Fig. 10**)—Interstitial lung disease is reported in up to 40% of patients with rheumatoid arthritis. Although both UIP and NSIP patterns are seen in this population, with UIP pattern reported more frequently (41%–56% vs 30%–33%).[33,34] The presence of UIP pattern in patients with RA-ILD is also associated with more rapid disease progression and increased mortality compared with NSIP pattern, although there is mixed data regarding the prognosis of patients with UIP in the setting of RA-ILD versus IPF.[35] Rheumatoid arthritis is also associated with airways disease such as bronchiolitis obliterans as well as organizing pneumonia.[36]

Myositis (**Fig. 11**)—Anti-synthetase syndrome occurs in a subset of patients with inflammatory myositis (dermatomyositis/polymyositis) who have myositis-related antibodies, including antibodies to the aminoacyl-tRNA synthetase enzymes. A substantial proportion of patients with the anti-synthetase syndrome (70%–90%) have interstitial lung disease, with the most common CT patterns in this patient population including NSIP (45%), OP (21%), or NSIP/OP overlap (24%).[37] The natural history of ILD in this patient population is a decrease of resolution of consolidation over time in the majority of patients following treatment with corticosteroids and immunosuppression; however, fibrosis develops in a subset (38%), and the minority of patients evolve to UIP pattern of fibrosis.[38] Patients with anti-synthetase syndrome and anti-MDA-5 antibodies may also present with fulminant respiratory failure and diffuse alveolar damage, with a particularly high risk of mortality (84%).[39]

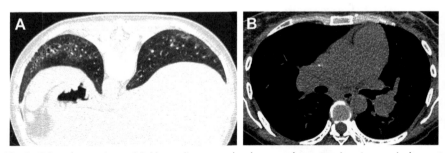

Fig. 8. Scleroderma, interstitial lung disease and pulmonary hypertension. Lung windows at the bases (*A*) show mild ground-glass opacity with subpleural sparing compatible with early nonspecific interstitial pneumonia in a patient with marked dyspnea. Soft tissue windows (see *B*) shows a markedly enlarged pulmonary artery, measuring 4.1 cm, compatible with pulmonary hypertension.

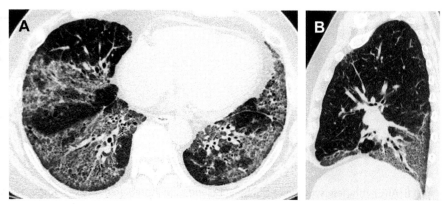

Fig. 9. Scleroderma. Axial (A) and sagittal reformatted (B) images show basilar predominant reticulation and traction bronchiectasis with subpleural sparing. Nonspecific interstitial pneumonia is the most common pattern seen in scleroderma patients.

Sjogren syndrome **(Fig. 12)**—LIP is the most common interstitial lung disease seen in patients with Sjogren syndrome, seen in 50%. Airways diseases such as follicular bronchiolitis, bronchiolitis, and bronchiectasis less commonly occur.[40]

Systemic lupus erythematosus **(Fig. 13)**—The most common CT abnormality seen in up to 50% to 60% of patients with lupus is serositis including pleuritis and pleural/pericardial effusions, with lung parenchymal involvement such as pulmonary hemorrhage, pulmonary edema, and lupus pneumonitis/diffuse alveolar damage occurring in a smaller subset (3%–7%).[41,42] Pulmonary fibrosis is seen much less commonly in lupus patients than in those with other CTDs.[36]

Mixed Connective Tissue Disease (MCTD)—The CT features of mixed connective tissue disease (MCTD) most closely mimic those of scleroderma (NSIP) and myositis (OP), as well as an overlap of these features.[43]

Idiopathic Pneumonia with Autoimmune Features—Patients with clinical features suggesting a diagnosis of CTD but not meeting established criteria for any disorder may present with interstitial lung disease. Several different terms have been used to

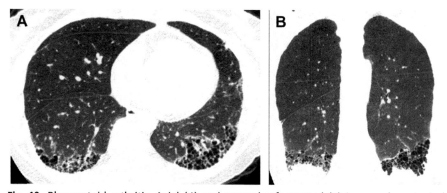

Fig. 10. Rheumatoid arthritis. Axial (A) and coronal reformatted (B) images show typical findings of usual interstitial pneumonia with peripheral and basilar fibrosis with honeycombing. In the setting of connective tissue disease, usual interstitial pneumonia is most closely associated with rheumatoid arthritis.

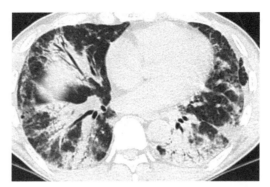

Fig. 11. Antisynthetase syndrome. A subpleural and basilar predominance of consolidation is typical of an overlap of nonspecific interstitial pneumonia and organizing pneumonia. This pattern is often seen with myositis and antisynthetase syndrome.

describe these patients including "idiopathic pneumonia with autoimmune features (IPAF)", "undifferentiated CTD", "lung-dominant CTD", and "autoimmune-featured diffuse lung disease".

To establish a diagnosis of IPAF, patients must (1) have an interstitial pneumonia by HRCT or lung biopsy, (2) not meet diagnostic criteria for a defined CTD, (3) not have another explanation for their lung disease, and (4) meet at least one feature from two of three domains—clinical, serologic, and morphologic.[44]

Imaging findings fall under the morphologic domain, with suggestive HRCT patterns including NSIP, OP, NSIP/OP overlap, and LIP or the presence of multicompartment involvement (as described above) in addition to ILD. Other patterns of ILD have been described in patients diagnosed with IPAF (for example UIP); however, this pattern of ILD does not fulfill one of the necessary domains, and as such, features from two other domains such as clinical and serologic must also be present.[45–47]

EXACERBATION OF INTERSTITIAL LUNG DISEASE

In addition to the utility of imaging for the diagnosis of CTD, CT is also useful for the evaluation of acute symptoms in CTD patients, which may be due to worsening/

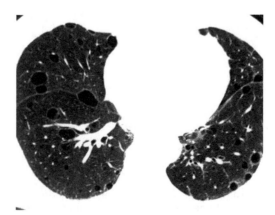

Fig. 12. Sjogren syndrome. Axial image shows thin-walled pulmonary cysts and mild ground-glass opacity in a patient with Sjogren syndrome.

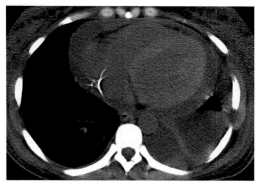

Fig. 13. Systemic lupus erythematosus (SLE). Serositis is a common finding in patients with SLE. In this patient with SLE, pericardial effusion/thickening and left-sided pleural effusion is indicative of a serositis.

exacerbation of ILD versus infection. Exacerbation of interstitial lung disease manifests with worsening fibrosis, organizing pneumonia, and/or diffuse alveolar damage—which will appear as increased diffuse ground glass and/or consolidation. Overall prognosis of ILD exacerbation is poor, with a 66% mortality rate in one series of 24 biopsy-proven ILD patients, which included patients with CTD-NSIP (3/24) and CTD-UIP (8/24).[48]

SUMMARY

Although any pattern of interstitial lung disease can be seen in patients with CTD, NSIP, OP, NSIP/OP overlap, LIP, and less commonly UIP are classically associated with CTD as described above. Familiarity with these common imaging patterns, as well as the clinical and serologic manifestations of CTD, will allow the radiologist to contribute fully in the multidisciplinary diagnosis of patients with CTD.

CLINICS CARE POINTS

- Common CT patterns in CTD-ILD include NSIP, OP, NSIP/OP overlap, LIP, and UIP

- Multicompartmental disease including pulmonary hypertension and airways disease also support a diagnosis of CTD-ILD

REFERENCES

1. Aggarwal R, Ringold S, Khanna D, et al. Distinctions between diagnostic and classification criteria? Arthritis Care Res 2015;67(7):891–7.
2. van den Hoogen F, Khanna D, Fransen J, et al. 2013 classification criteria for systemic sclerosis: an American college of rheumatology/European league against rheumatism collaborative initiative. Ann Rheum Dis 2013;72(11): 1747–55.
3. Vitali C, Bombardieri S, Jonsson R, et al. Classification criteria for Sjögren's syndrome: a revised version of the European criteria proposed by the American-European Consensus Group. Ann Rheum Dis 2002;61(6):554–8.

4. Arnett FC, Edworthy SM, Bloch DA, et al. The American Rheumatism Association 1987 revised criteria for the classification of rheumatoid arthritis. Arthritis Rheum 1988;31(3):315–24.
5. Dalakas MC, Hohlfeld R. Polymyositis and dermatomyositis. Lancet 2003; 362(9388):971–82.
6. Tan EM, Cohen AS, Fries JF, et al. The 1982 revised criteria for the classification of systemic lupus erythematosus. Arthritis Rheum 1982;25(11):1271–7.
7. Mittoo S, Gelber AC, Christopher-Stine L, et al. Ascertainment of collagen vascular disease in patients presenting with interstitial lung disease. Respir Med 2009;103(8):1152–8.
8. Homma Y, Ohtsuka Y, Tanimura K, et al. Can interstitial pneumonia as the sole presentation of collagen vascular diseases be differentiated from idiopathic interstitial pneumonia? Respiration 1995;62(5):248–51.
9. Castelino FV, Goldberg H, Dellaripa PF. The impact of rheumatological evaluation in the management of patients with interstitial lung disease. Rheumatology 2010; 50(3):489–93.
10. Raghu G, Rochwerg B, Zhang Y, et al. An Official ATS/ERS/JRS/ALAT Clinical Practice Guideline: Treatment of Idiopathic Pulmonary Fibrosis. An Update of the 2011 Clinical Practice Guideline. Am J Respir Crit Care Med 2015;192(2): e3–19.
11. Raghu G, Remy-Jardin M, Myers JL, et al. Diagnosis of Idiopathic Pulmonary Fibrosis. An Official ATS/ERS/JRS/ALAT Clinical Practice Guideline. Am J Respir Crit Care Med 2018;198(5):e44–68.
12. Satoh M, Vázquez-Del Mercado M, Chan EKL. Clinical interpretation of antinuclear antibody tests in systemic rheumatic diseases. Mod Rheumatol 2009; 19(3):219–28.
13. Solomon DH, Kavanaugh AJ, Schur PH. Evidence-based guidelines for the use of immunologic tests: antinuclear antibody testing. Arthritis Rheum 2002;47(4): 434–44.
14. Ho KT, Reveille JD. The clinical relevance of autoantibodies in scleroderma. Arthritis Res Ther 2003;5(2):80–93.
15. Jee AS, Adelstein S, Bleasel J, et al. Role of autoantibodies in the diagnosis of connective-tissue disease ILD (CTD-ILD) and interstitial pneumonia with autoimmune features (IPAF). J Clin Med 2017;6(5):51.
16. Fischer A, Swigris JJ, du Bois RM, et al. Anti-synthetase syndrome in ANA and anti-Jo-1 negative patients presenting with idiopathic interstitial pneumonia. Respir Med 2009;103(11):1719–24.
17. Travis WD, Costabel U, Hansell DM, et al. An official American Thoracic Society/ European Respiratory Society statement: Update of the international multidisciplinary classification of the idiopathic interstitial pneumonias. Am J Respir Crit Care Med 2013;188(6):733–48.
18. Elliot TL, Lynch DA, Newell JD Jr, et al. High-resolution computed tomography features of nonspecific interstitial pneumonia and usual interstitial pneumonia. J Comput Assist Tomogr 2005;29(3):339–45.
19. Johkoh T, Müller NL, Colby TV, et al. Nonspecific interstitial pneumonia: correlation between thin-section CT findings and pathologic subgroups in 55 patients. Radiology 2002;225(1):199–204.
20. Silva CIS, Müller NL, Lynch DA, et al. Chronic hypersensitivity pneumonitis: differentiation from idiopathic pulmonary fibrosis and nonspecific interstitial pneumonia by using thin-section CT. Radiology 2008;246(1):288–97.

21. Zare Mehrjardi M, Kahkouee S, Pourabdollah M. Radio-pathological correlation of organizing pneumonia (OP): a pictorial review. Br J Radiol 2017;90(1071): 20160723.
22. Kim SJ, Lee KS, Ryu YH, et al. Reversed halo sign on high-resolution CT of cryptogenic organizing pneumonia: diagnostic implications. AJR Am J Roentgenol 2003;180(5):1251–4.
23. Enomoto N, Sumikawa H, Sugiura H, et al. Clinical, radiological, and pathological evaluation of "NSIP with OP overlap" pattern compared with NSIP in patients with idiopathic interstitial pneumonias. Respir Med 2020;174:106201.
24. Lynch DA, Travis WD, Müller NL, et al. Idiopathic interstitial pneumonias: CT features. Radiology 2005;236(1):10–21.
25. Park JH, Kim DS, Park IN, et al. Prognosis of fibrotic interstitial pneumonia: idiopathic versus collagen vascular disease-related subtypes. Am J Respir Crit Care Med 2007;175(7):705–11.
26. Chung JH, Cox CW, Montner SM, et al. CT features of the usual interstitial pneumonia pattern: differentiating connective tissue disease-associated interstitial lung disease from idiopathic pulmonary fibrosis. AJR Am J Roentgenol 2018; 210(2):307–13.
27. Silva CI, Müller NL, Hansell DM, et al. Nonspecific interstitial pneumonia and idiopathic pulmonary fibrosis: changes in pattern and distribution of disease over time. Radiology 2008;247(1):251–9.
28. Oldham JM, Adegunsoye A, Valenzi E, et al. Characterisation of patients with interstitial pneumonia with autoimmune features. Eur Respir J 2016;47(6):1767–75.
29. Peña E, Dennie C, Veinot J, et al. Pulmonary hypertension: how the radiologist can help. Radiographics 2012;32(1):9–32.
30. Mohamed Hoesein FA, Besselink T, Pompe E, et al. Accuracy of CT Pulmonary Artery Diameter for Pulmonary Hypertension in End-Stage COPD. Lung 2016; 194(5):813–9.
31. Solomon JJ, Olson AL, Fischer A, et al. Scleroderma lung disease. Eur Respir Rev 2013;22(127):6–19.
32. Bouros D, Wells AU, Nicholson AG, et al. Histopathologic subsets of fibrosing alveolitis in patients with systemic sclerosis and their relationship to outcome. Am J Respir Crit Care Med 2002;165(12):1581–6.
33. Lee HK, Kim DS, Yoo B, et al. Histopathologic pattern and clinical features of rheumatoid arthritis-associated interstitial lung disease. Chest 2005;127(6): 2019–27.
34. Tanaka N, Kim JS, Newell JD, et al. Rheumatoid arthritis-related lung diseases: CT findings. Radiology 2004;232(1):81–91.
35. Kim EJ, Collard HR, King TE Jr. Rheumatoid arthritis-associated interstitial lung disease: the relevance of histopathologic and radiographic pattern. Chest 2009;136(5):1397–405.
36. Mayberry JP, Primack SL, Müller NL. Thoracic Manifestations of Systemic Autoimmune Diseases: Radiographic and High-Resolution CT Findings. RadioGraphics 2000;20(6):1623–35.
37. Debray MP, Borie R, Revel MP, et al. Interstitial lung disease in anti-synthetase syndrome: initial and follow-up CT findings. Eur J Radiol 2015;84(3):516–23.
38. Tillie-Leblond I, Wislez M, Valeyre D, et al. Interstitial lung disease and anti-Jo-1 antibodies: difference between acute and gradual onset. Thorax 2008;63(1):53–9.
39. Vuillard C, Pineton de Chambrun M, de Prost N, et al. Clinical features and outcome of patients with acute respiratory failure revealing anti-synthetase or

anti-MDA-5 dermato-pulmonary syndrome: a French multicenter retrospective study. Ann Intensive Care 2018;8(1):87.

40. Kim EA, Lee KS, Johkoh T, et al. Interstitial Lung Diseases Associated with Collagen Vascular Diseases: Radiologic and Histopathologic Findings. Radio-Graphics 2002;22(suppl_1):S151–65.

41. Murin S, Wiedemann HP, Matthay RA. Pulmonary manifestations of systemic lupus erythematosus. Clin Chest Med 1998;19(4):641–65, viii.

42. Cervera R, Khamashta MA, Font J, et al. Systemic lupus erythematosus: clinical and immunologic patterns of disease expression in a cohort of 1,000 patients. Eur Working Party Systemic Lupus Erythematosus. Med (Baltimore) 1993;72(2):113–24.

43. Yamanaka Y, Baba T, Hagiwara E, et al. Radiological images of interstitial pneumonia in mixed connective tissue disease compared with scleroderma and polymyositis/dermatomyositis. Eur J Radiol 2018;107:26–32.

44. Fischer A, Antoniou KM, Brown KK, et al. An official European Respiratory Society/American Thoracic Society research statement: interstitial pneumonia with autoimmune features. Eur Respir J 2015;46(4):976–87.

45. Fischer A, Collard HR, Cottin V. Interstitial pneumonia with autoimmune features: the new consensus-based definition for this cohort of patients should be broadened. Eur Respir J 2016;47(4):1295.

46. Dai J, Wang L, Yan X, et al. Clinical features, risk factors, and outcomes of patients with interstitial pneumonia with autoimmune features: a population-based study. Clin Rheumatol 2018;37(8):2125–32.

47. Ahmad K, Barba T, Gamondes D, et al. Interstitial pneumonia with autoimmune features: Clinical, radiologic, and histological characteristics and outcome in a series of 57 patients. Respir Med 2017;123:56–62.

48. Silva CIS, Müller NL, Fujimoto K, et al. Acute exacerbation of chronic interstitial pneumonia: high-resolution computed tomography and pathologic findings. J Thorac Imaging 2007;22(3):221–9.

Connective Tissue Disease Associated Interstitial Lung Disease

Scott M. Matson, MD[a], M. Kristen Demoruelle, MD, PhD[b],*

KEYWORDS

- Autoimmunity • Interstitial lung disease • Connective tissue disease
- Immunosuppression • Subclinical interstitial lung disease • Antifibrotic

KEY POINTS

- Connective tissue disease associated interstitial lung disease (CTD-ILD) is a heterogenous collection of autoimmune and CTDs with myriad manifestations of interstitial lung disease (ILD) including cellular, inflammatory lung disease and progressive, fibrotic manifestations.
- Subclinical CTD-ILD may offer an important treatment window; however, with the lack of clinical data to guide clinicians, there are currently only expert consensus guidelines within SSc to guide screening for ILD in CTD populations, and it remains unclear how early intervention will impact these conditions.
- Immunosuppression in CTD-ILD is supported by several randomized, placebo-controlled trials (RCTs) in patients with scleroderma and several observational, retrospective studies in other autoimmune conditions.
- There is increasing data and clinical interest in the addition of antifibrotic therapy for patients with CTD-ILD.
- There are urgent needs for RCTs, which test the efficacy of immunosuppression and antifibrotic agents, including in combination and the sequence of use, in fibrotic CTD-ILD populations as well as study of intervention in subclinical CTD-ILD populations.

INTRODUCTION

Interstitial lung disease (ILD) occurs in a portion of patients with underlying connective tissue disease (CTD), most commonly effecting patients with rheumatoid arthritis (RA), systemic sclerosis (SSc), and idiopathic inflammatory myositis (IIM). The field of

This article previously appeared in *Immunology and Allergy Clinics* volume 43 issue 2 May 2023.
[a] Division of Pulmonary, Critical Care and Sleep Medicine, University of Kansas School of Medicine, 3901 Rainbow boulevard, Mailstop 3007, Kansas City, KS 66160, USA; [b] Division of Rheumatology, University of Colorado School of Medicine, 1775 Aurora Court, Mail Stop B-115, Aurora, CO 80045, USA
* Corresponding author.
E-mail address: kristen.demoruelle@cuanschutz.edu

Rheum Dis Clin N Am 50 (2024) 423–438
https://doi.org/10.1016/j.rdc.2024.03.001
0889-857X/24/© 2024 Elsevier Inc. All rights reserved.

424	Matson & Demoruelle

connective tissue disease associated interstitial lung disease (CTD-ILD) has seen major advances in the past several years. However, there remain many unanswered questions for which further study is critically needed. In this review, we will discuss recent advances in treatment options that have had a major influence on the clinical approach to patients with CTD-ILD. We will also review what is known about pathogenic pathways in different CTD-ILDs and the entity of subclinical CTD-ILD, both areas in which further research is likely to change the current paradigm of CTD-ILD management.

EPIDEMIOLOGY AND CLINICAL OUTCOMES

ILD is one of the more severe forms of pulmonary involvement in patients with CTD. It involves varying degrees of inflammation and fibrosis in the interstitial compartment of the lung. For effected patients, it is a common cause of poor quality of life and early mortality. ILD can affect any patient with any CTD but the prevalence is higher in certain types of CTD and in patients with certain risk factors. Clinically diagnosed CTD-ILD is most common in patients with RA, SSc, and IIM, ranging from 5% to 10% in RA to 20% to 60% in SSc and 20% to 80% in IIM.[1–3] It is of note, that despite the lower rates of ILD in patients with RA, the number of patients affected by RA-ILD is similar or higher compared with the number of patients affected by SSc-ILD and IIM-ILD, given the overall higher prevalence of RA in the population. Moreover, it is notable that studies report a wide range of CTD-ILD prevalence, often differing based on the population studied, mode of detection, retrospective versus prospective data collection, clinical cohort versus claims-based cohort, and whether subclinical ILD was included along with clinically diagnosed ILD.

It is well established that different CTD-ILDs have different patterns of lung involvement. For example, SSc and IIM commonly display a pattern of nonspecific interstitial pneumonia (NSIP) with or without organizing pneumonia, whereas patients with RA are more likely to have a pattern of usual interstitial pneumonia (UIP). Overall, patients with CTD-ILD have a more favorable outcome compared with those with idiopathic disease,[4] although patients with RA with a UIP pattern are a notable exception and can progress at rates similar to those seen in idiopathic pulmonary fibrosis (IPF).[5] Different predictors of prognosis have been reported in the different CTD-ILDs but significant impairment in physiology at baseline or worsening in physiology over time as measured by percent predicted forced vital capacity (FVC) is associated with a poor prognosis across CTD-ILDs.[6–8]

More clarity is needed to understand the exact prevalence of CTD-ILDs, and a major gap in the field continues to be a lack of standardized screening guidelines, which can lead to delays in diagnosis or diagnosis at late-stage disease when treatment options are less effective. As therapeutic options for CTD-ILD increase (discussed further below), prompt identification of CTD-ILD will become increasing necessary for optimal patient care, and consensus guidelines on who and how to screen as well as what constitutes clinically significant disease will be critical. Of note, consensus statements for SSc-ILD have been published[9] and support screening with high-resolution computed tomography (HRCT), pulmonary function tests (PFTs), and chest auscultation in all patients with SSc. However, given the much higher prevalence of RA, HRCT, and PFT, screening of all patients with RA presents logistical and financial challenges. As such, the use of HRCT or PFTs for ILD screening in patients with RA is often reserved for patients with respiratory symptoms, although screening may also be appropriate in asymptomatic patients with RA with multiple ILD risk factors (eg, male sex, older age, smoking history). In addition to a lack of screening guidelines, there are also no standardized guidelines for monitoring ILD progression once CTD-

ILD has been identified, a gap in the field made more critical with the approval of treatments for patients with CTD-ILD with progressive pulmonary fibrosis (PPF).[10] A common clinical approach is to repeat PFTs every 3 months and HRCT annually but evidence-based guidelines are needed. Given the uncertainties highlighted, a multidisciplinary approach between pulmonologists, rheumatologists, radiologists, pathologists, and other health-care providers can be beneficial in the clinical management of patients with CTD-ILD.[10]

THERAPEUTIC OPTIONS AND ADVANCES

Clinicians approaching treatment options for CTD-ILD face several important decision points and currently many of these questions lack high-quality data to answer. It is important to highlight that nearly all randomized, controlled trials for CTD-ILD are derived from scleroderma ILD (SSc-ILD) and subsequently extrapolated to other autoimmune lung diseases. However, many questions remain about the applicability of SSc-ILD broadly across all types of CTD-ILDs and patterns, that is, do more fibrotic ILDs represent the same conditions as more cellular, inflammatory ILD patterns commonly encountered in SSc-ILD? There is increasingly more interest in the expanded use of antifibrotic therapy to non-IPF conditions including CTD-ILD, and many questions remain regarding sequencing of therapies in these patients.

This field is dynamic and evolving but for the purposes of this review, the authors have chosen to highlight 3 important stages of CTD-ILD treatment considerations: (1) considerations of medication-induced lung injury in the baseline autoimmune regimen, (2) role of added "ILD-specific" immunosuppression, and (3) the role of antifibrotic therapy in CTD-ILD.

Considerations of Medication-Induced Lung Injury in Baseline Autoimmune Regimens

Retrospective, observational data in CTD-ILD led to a persistent and common vagary that has driven many of the considerations in this field for decades. For instance, methotrexate is a first-line disease modifying anti-rheumatic drug (DMARD) for patients with RA.[11] It is typically continued for many years, either as monotherapy or as a foundation to which other conventional or biologic DMARDs are added. As such, methotrexate is broadly applied to the most severe patients with the condition during times of most significant disease progression. Therefore, it was difficult to differentiate this temporal relationship in historical records, that is, did these patients with RA who developed RA-ILD do so because of the risk from methotrexate or because those patients with RA on methotrexate represented a progressive phenotype of patients with RA and thus the most likely to develop ILD as an extra-articular manifestation.[12] For decades, the clinical management of patients with CTD-ILD was influenced by this observation and clinicians were faced with a difficult decision, that is, do you remove an effective DMARD when patients develop ILD given this concern for its role in ILD risk. However, recent evidence has absolved methotrexate from its previous putative role in causing or contributing to progressive fibrotic ILDs in patients with RA, indicating that the relationship was correlative and not causative.[13]

This pursuit of high-quality evidence in CTD-ILD has led to a paradigm shift in newly diagnosed fibrotic ILDs where there is no longer concern for continuing methotrexate. Subsequently, clinicians can safely continue methotrexate as an effective DMARD in patients with ILD who were achieving adequate articular disease control.[14] However, important caveats remain, including the rare potential for methotrexate to cause a cellular, acute hypersensitivity pneumonitis, which is clinically distinct from fibrotic

ILDs and can typically be differentiated based on cellular analysis of bronchoalveolar lavage if indicated for diagnostic uncertainty.[15]

Methotrexate is illustrative in CTD-ILD treatment where it is often difficult to separate the temporal relationship between DMARD use and the underlying autoimmune disease progression. For instance, a similar controversy still surrounds the use of biologic anti-tumor necrosis factor (TNF) therapy in patients with CTD-ILD given observational associations with ILD exacerbations and potential harm in a meta-analysis of retrospective studies[16–18] despite several initial reports of improved ILD-specific outcomes with these agents.[19]

Table 1 highlights several known toxicities of medications used in the baseline treatment of autoimmune diseases, which may complicate ILD diagnosis and treatment in CTD-ILD.

Finally, there is an important observed association between autoimmune disease activity and ILD prognosis, which is important to consider for baseline autoimmune therapy in patients with ILD. For instance, RA disease activity is associated with both incidence of ILD and severity/prognosis of ILD in 2 recent studies.[20,21] This evidence supports the role of optimizing typical DMARD therapy in patients with ILD aside from ILD-specific immunosuppression given the association with disease activity and ILD outcomes. As mentioned above, for these complex clinical decisions, the authors of this review strongly endorse the use of multidisciplinary discussions to place the patient's baseline therapy in context, which requires the balance of autoimmune disease activity with the potential impact of current therapies on ILD exacerbation such as the use of anti-TNF therapy in patients with previous difficult-to-control autoimmune disease.

Interstitial Lung Disease-Specific Immunosuppression

There are 3 randomized, placebo-controlled trials (RCTs) that address the important question of the impact of immunosuppression in CTD-ILD (Fig. 1).[22–24] As mentioned

Table 1
Baseline autoimmune therapies with potential for lung toxicity

Drug	Toxicity
Methotrexate	Most commonly presents with acute hypersensitivity pneumonitis, up to 50% will have peripheral eosinophilia and associated with broncho-alveolar lymphocytosis[15]
Leflunomide	Associated with low risk of alveolar pneumonitis, especially in those patients with underlying ILD or history of methotrexate-induced lung toxicity[69]
Biologic agents	Direct inflammatory pneumonitis resulting from treatment with biologic agents in RA is reported. However, a direct pathogenic link between the agent and the pneumonitis has not been shown. Given the clinical efficacy of these agents in treating the synovial manifestations of RA, their use in patients with autoimmune-ILD remains controversial[16,19,70]
Gold	Although no longer commonly used, a typical but rare pulmonary toxicity was known to be associated with gold administration. Patients with gold-induced pulmonary toxicity have a fever and develop an NSIP pattern with lymphocytes in the lung[71]
Sulfasalazine and non-steroidal anti-inflammatory drugs (NSAIDs)	Associated with an eosinophilic alveolar infiltrate with fever which is steroid-responsive[72,73]

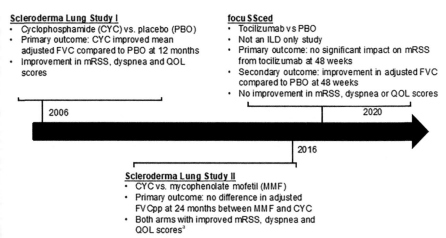

Scleroderma Lung Study I
- Cyclophosphamide (CYC) vs. placebo (PBO)
- Primary outcome: CYC improved mean adjusted FVC compared to PBO at 12 months
- Improvement in mRSS, dyspnea and QOL scores

focuSSced
- Tocilizumab vs PBO
- Not an ILD only study
- Primary outcome: no significant impact on mRSS from tocilizumab at 48 weeks
- Secondary outcome: improvement in adjusted FVC compared to PBO at 48 weeks
- No improvement in mRSS, dyspnea or QOL scores

2006

2020

2016

Scleroderma Lung Study II
- CYC vs. mycophenolate mofetil (MMF)
- Primary outcome: no difference in adjusted FVCpp at 24 months between MMF and CYC
- Both arms with improved mRSS, dyspnea and QOL scores[a]

Fig. 1. *Timeline of randomized, controlled trials for immunosuppression in SSc-ILD* with primary efficacy results highlighted in each study. [a]Quality of life evaluation from SLSII was published in a second article, separate from the main article.[80] CYC, cyclophosphamide; FVC, forced vital capacity; FVCpp, forced vital capacity percent predicted; ILD, Interstitial lung disease; MMF, mycophenolate mofetil; mRSS, modified Rodnan skin score; PBO, placebo; QOL, quality of life. (*Adapted from* Volkmann ER, Tashkin DP, LeClair H, et al. Treatment with mycophenolate and cyclophosphamide leads to clinically meaningful improvements in patientreported outcomes in scleroderma lung disease: results of scleroderma lung study II. ACR Open Rheumatol 2020;2:362-70.)

previously, all 3 of these seminal RCTs were performed in patients with SSc-ILD. However, there are important lessons learned from these data and each study can inform current clinical practice in CTD-ILD.

The first RCT in CTD-ILD was the initial Scleroderma Lung Study (SLS), which compared cyclophosphamide with placebo. SLS found that cyclophosphamide preserved decline in FVC compared with placebo and had important improvements in skin thickening scores and health-related quality of life metrics.[23] Given the toxicity profile of cyclophosphamide, investigators performed SLS II where mycophenolate mofetil (MMF) was compared with cyclophosphamide. SLS II demonstrated an improvement in FVC during the intervention period from both therapies.[24] More recently, tocilizumab was studied in SSc-ILD in the focuSSced trial (which included patients with SSc with ILD and was enriched for a progressive phenotype including patients with elevated interleukin-6).[22] In this 48-week, placebo-controlled, randomized, double-blind study, the primary endpoint (change in modified Rodnan skin fibrosis score [mRSS]) was not significant between groups.[22] However, the investigators report a prespecified secondary endpoint which showed preservation in FVC % predicted with tocilizumab compared with placebo at 48 weeks (−0.4 vs −4.6 change in % predicted FVC).[22]

These 3 studies and their therapies make up the primary backbone of immunosuppression used in clinical practice in CTD-ILD given their data, which confirms efficacy when compared with placebo. All other clinical agents used in CTD-ILD lack confirmatory efficacy trials. However, various levels of evidence exist in CTD-ILD from prospective studies of therapy without control arms to multisite observational studies to single-site retrospective study design (**Table 2**). Further specific discussion of individual choice of immunosuppressive agent for each specific CTD-ILD is beyond the scope of this review; however, it is worth addressing one important question that remains in CTD-ILD

Table 2
Immunosuppression therapy in autoimmune interstitial lung diseases and level of evidence

Therapy	Highest Level of Evidence	Outcome	Study
Glucocorticoids	Observational in multiple autoimmune ILDs	Lung function stability	Cassone et al,[74] 2020
Cyclophosphamide	Randomized, placebo-controlled	Improves lung function, QOL	Tashkin et al,[23] 2006
Mycophenolate	Randomized, noninferiority to CYC	Improves lung function, QOL	Tashkin et al,[24] 2016
Azathioprine	Multisite observational (fibrotic autoimmune ILD)	Lung function stability	Oldham et al,[75] 2016
Rituximab	Observational	Lung function stability	Md Yusof et al,[76] 2017
Anti-TNF biologics	Observational	Mixed outcomes	16–18
Abatacept	Prospective, observational (RA)	Lung function stability, steroid-sparing effect	Mena-Vázquez et al,[77] 2022
Tocilizumab	Randomized, placebo controlled (SSc)	Lung function with less decline compared with placebo	Khanna et al,[22] 2020
IVIG	Observational (Myositis)	Lung function stability	Huapaya et al,[78] 2019
Tacrolimus	Observational	Lung function improvement	Witt et al,[79] 2016

Abbreviations: CYC, cyclophosphamide; ILD, interstitial lung disease; IVIG, intravenous immunoglobulin; QOL, quality of life; RA, rheumatoid arthritis; SSc, systemic scleroderma; TNF, tumor necrosis factor.

treatment: the impact of immunosuppression on outcomes for patients with CTD-ILD with the UIP pattern ILD.

In 2012, investigators revealed the results of Prednisone, Azathioprine, and N-Acetylcysteine: A Study That Evaluates Response in Idiopathic Pulmonary Fibrosis (PANTHER-IPF), an RCT comparing the effect of combined azathioprine, prednisone, and N-acetylcysteine to placebo for patients with IPF. In this study, there was harm associated with the treatment arm with worse survival from the immunosuppression-based strategy.[25] Although IPF is not thought to be an autoimmune disease, there was significant observational data before the PANTHER study to support an anti-inflammatory strategy, and these results highlight the limitations of retrospective treatment data. However, there are potentially important implications of the PANTHER outcomes considering the clinical, genetic, and radiographic overlaps between IPF and several autoimmune conditions, most notably RA-ILD.[26]

The observed similarities between CTD-ILDs with the UIP pattern and IPF lead to an important clinical quandary in CTD-ILD: how do clinicians safely approach immunosuppression in patients with CTD-ILD in UIP patterns? The current state of the literature offers only expert opinion as guidance for now, with observational level evidence to guide these decisions. It is the opinion of the authors of this review that UIP represents a pathologic, end-stage fibrotic pattern, which is corollary to "cirrhosis" in hepatic disease, and that treatment should be directed at the underlying cause of the pattern and not the pattern itself including, when appropriate, immunosuppression to improve autoimmune disease activity.[27] However, we continue to stress the need for prospective, randomized data to address this important question.

Antifibrotics in Autoimmune Interstitial Lung Disease

Antifibrotics are a broad "class" of therapies that include 2 Federal Drug Administration (FDA)-approved therapies (nintedanib and pirfenidone) that have been shown to reduce the decline of FVC in patients with IPF in 3 RCTs published in 2014.[28,29] Given the overlaps of CTD-ILD and IPF as mentioned previously, there has been interest in expanding the use of these novel therapies beyond only IPF.

In the SENSCIS trial, nintedanib was found to slow the decline in FVC over time compared with placebo in a study that allowed for the background immunosuppression in SSc-ILD.[30] Additionally, in 2022, the results of the Safety, tolerability, and efficacy of pirfenidone in patients with rheumatoid arthritis-associated interstitial lung disease: a randomised, double-blind, placebo-controlled, phase 2 study (TRAIL-1) were published, the first-ever RCT in RA-ILD, which found no statistically significant difference between pirfenidone and placebo in their primary endpoint (proportion of RA-ILD subjects with more than 10% or more FVC decline from baseline or death).[31] It is important to point out that FVC decline as a secondary endpoint in TRAIL-1 was similar to the trends seen in all other RCTs of antifibrotic therapy and reached statistical significance but the study was underpowered and underrecruited for multiple reasons including the coronavirus disease 2019 pandemic. It is also important to point out that patients with autoimmune ILD made-up 24.7% of the treatment arm of an RCT of nintedanib versus placebo that explored the role of nintedanib in a subset of patients with PPF, which met its primary end-point.[32]

Considered in totality, these studies highlight primarily one major takeaway: for patients with CTD-ILD with fibrotic features who have progressive loss of lung function, the addition of an antifibrotic agent is associated with slower lung function decline compared with placebo. However, these data fail to address the impact of these therapies on survival or quality of life; they also are unable to properly guide clinicians on choice or sequence of therapy when several other immunosuppressive agents would be available to a clinician when a patient with CTD-ILD experiences progression.

There is a reasonably renewed interest and excitement regarding this era of treatment afforded by this novel modality of treatment in CTD-ILD. However, we currently lack data regarding many of the important questions that these therapies raise in CTD-ILD. For instance, are there particular features of CTD-ILD that should guide treatment approaches such as earlier antifibrotic use for those patients with the UIP featured ILD?

Multidisciplinary discussion between rheumatologists and pulmonologists with experience treating these conditions and familiarity with these therapies remains the gold-standard for clinical decision-making in the absence of the level of data required to fully guide these complex decisions. However, there is hope that adaptive randomized trial platforms and global collaborative initiatives will fill these large clinical gaps in knowledge for patients with CTD-ILD in the coming decade.

PATHOGENIC PATHWAYS IN CONNECTIVE TISSUE DISEASE ASSOCIATED INTERSTITIAL LUNG DISEASE

As discussed above, CTD-ILD can be challenging to treat. The treatment approach may differ based on the ILD subtype (ie, UIP vs NSIP) but the treatment approach is not often specific for the underlying CTD despite marked differences in the clinical phenotypes associated with each CTD. These differences raise the question of whether the pathogenesis of ILD is also markedly different among different CTDs, in such a way that should be considered when investigating new treatment targets. Understanding more about the overlapping and distinct pathogenic pathways across CTD-ILDs could lead to improved screening and potentially more effective treatment approaches in CTD-ILD.

The pathogenesis of all CTD-ILDs includes interactions among genetic, environmental, and immunologic risk factors. In general, ILDs develop following repetitive alveolar epithelial and endothelial damage and activation of lung fibroblasts that transform into profibrotic myofibroblasts.[33,34] However, the initiating and propagating factors that ultimately lead to ILD in a patient with CTD likely have both shared and distinct features based on the underlying CTD. For the purposes of this review, we will highlight 4 areas that are of interest in considering whether CTD-ILDs develop through distinct pathways based on the underlying CTD: (1) genetics, (2) environmental risk factors, (3) autoantibodies, and (4) neutrophil extracellular traps (NETs).

Genetic Risk Alleles in Autoimmune Interstitial Lung Disease

As with autoimmune diseases, in general, genetics clearly play a role in CTD-ILD development. One of the strongest genetic links in CTD-ILD has been demonstrated between the gain-of-function polymorphism in the promoter of the mucin 5b (*MUC5B*) gene and RA-ILD, particularly the UIP pattern of RA-ILD.[35,36] The same polymorphism has also been strongly linked to risk of IPF,[37] suggesting shared pathways of disease development between RA-ILD and IPF. However, in SSc-ILD and IIM-ILD, other genetic variants have been identified, and the MUC5B genetic risk variant has not been associated with these forms of ILD (reviewed in ref[38]). Overall suggesting the likelihood that distinct pathogenic pathways contribute to the development of RA-ILD compared with other NSIP-predominant CTD-ILDs such as SSc-ILD and IIM-ILD.

Environmental Risk Factors and Autoimmune Interstitial Lung Disease

A number of environmental factors have been identified that are associated with increased CTD-ILD risk. However, they often vary depending on the underlying CTD. For example, cigarette smoking is consistently associated with increased RA-ILD risk but not with risk of ILD in SSc or IIM.[39–42] Longer disease duration is often associated with ILD risk in RA, whereas shorter disease duration is associated with ILD risk in SSc. These differences are likely informative regarding distinct pathways of ILD development across CTD-ILDs. However, there are also risk factors shared across CTD-ILDs, such as older age,[39,41] and shared risk factors likely inform overlapping pathways of ILD development. A deeper understanding of the mechanisms by which each risk factor leads to ILD development, including immunologic responses in the lung associated with each risk factor, will likely be informative to an improved understanding of the distinct and shared pathways in CTD-ILDs.

Autoantibodies and Autoimmune Interstitial Lung Disease

Autoantibodies play a critical role in the clinical diagnosis of most CTDs because they are often distinguishing between different CTDs. When considering how autoantibodies may be informative of CTD-ILD pathogenesis, it is of interest that there are typically a small subset of autoantibodies within a larger group of CTD-specific autoantibodies that are associated with ILD. For example, there are 3 common SSc-associated autoantibodies but antitopoisomerase I is consistently associated with SSc-ILD.[43,44] Similarly, there are multiple myositis-associated and myositis-specific autoantibodies but antisynthetase antibodies and antimelanoma differentiation-associated gene 5 carry the strongest association with IIM-ILD.[45] In RA-ILD, rheumatoid factor, anticyclic citrullinated peptide, and antipeptidylarginine deiminase-4 antibodies have been associated with RA-ILD.[39,40,46] The strong association of specific autoantibodies with CTD-ILD suggest a potential role in pathogenesis but more research is needed to understand whether these autoantibodies are directly pathogenic or an epiphenomenon arising from a separate pathogenic process. It is of note that each CTD-ILD has its own ILD-associated autoantibodies, perhaps suggesting distinct pathways by which ILD develops but it may also be that different autoantibodies trigger similar pathways that culminate in a similar downstream pathway of ILD development.

Neutrophil Extracellular Traps and Autoimmune Interstitial Lung Disease

NET formation (termed NETosis) is an innate immune response to infection or inflammation that is distinct from neutrophil apoptosis or necrosis.[47] During NETosis, neutrophils decondense and expel their DNA in complex with intracellular proteins. Proteins contained within NET remnants have antimicrobial properties but can also induce inflammation, damage surrounding tissues, and enhanced NETosis has been associated with multiple autoimmune diseases, including RA, SSc, and IIM.[48–50] Relevant to this review, NETs have also been associated with several forms of chronic lung disease, including ILD.[51,52] Several key pathways implicated in ILD pathogenesis can be influenced by NETs including that several NET-bound proteins are cytotoxic to alveolar epithelial cells,[51] NETs can activate human lung fibroblasts to differentiate into myofibroblasts,[52,53] and NETs can be a source of matrix-metalloproteinase-9 (MMP-9).[54] Moreover, in animal models, NET inhibition has been associated with a reduction in lung fibrosis.[55]

NETs in the lung have not been well studied in CTD-ILD. Our group has reported that neutrophils isolated from the sputum of patients with RA demonstrate enhanced NET formation[56] but it is unknown if this phenomenon is further exaggerated in patients with RA with ILD. It is notable that lung neutrophilia has been associated with increased mortality in IPF,[57] and based on unpublished data from our group, we suspect that this association is mediated through increased NET formation in the lung. Given these data in aggregate, it will be highly informative to better understand the function of neutrophils in the lung in different CTD-ILDs, particularly lung neutrophil predilection for NET formation. It is of note that distinct protein cargo is expressed in the NETs generated in patients with RA compared with osteoarthritis controls.[49] It will therefore be of particular interest to identify the protein content of NETs generated in the lung in different CTDs because differences could potentially inform distinct pathways of CTD-ILD development, whereas similarities could potentially identify common pathways of CTD-ILD pathogenesis.

SUBCLINICAL DISEASE

Disease modification in autoimmune conditions such as RA highlights the positive impact that translational biomedical research can have on human disease. For instance, the identification of highly sensitive biomarkers in RA and research-based screening in the first-degree family members has led to identification of a "preclinical" state in which an individual does not meet classification for RA but has demonstrated features that strongly increase that individual's risk for developing RA in the future. In RA, the identification of this preclinical state has provided valuable lessons regarding pathogenesis and has also led to several clinical trials aimed at an early intervention with the goal of prevention.[58,59] In the preclinical state of RA, joint disease has not yet developed but similar concepts can be applied to a "subclinical" state of ILD during which lung fibrosis is present on imaging but pulmonary function testing and symptoms do not indicate a clinically significant level of ILD.

There are 2 primary principles of fibrotic ILD that make the identification of a subclinical fibrotic ILD state important: (1) pulmonary fibrosis is devastating and irreversible for patients and (2) treatment exists but often patients present in late stages of disease severity when therapy only offers to reduce the rate of progression. The long-range goal of pulmonary fibrosis research is the development of reliable clinical or molecular-based prediction systems to facilitate reliable, early identification of subclinical ILD states. Autoimmune conditions at risk for ILD could allow for novel insights into subclinical ILD states, including the identification of factors associated with the progression to clinically meaningful disease and, in time, could facilitate early intervention trials to alter the natural history of ILD.

Rates of Subclinical Interstitial Lung Disease in Autoimmune Disease States

Recently, 2 large RA cohorts were screened, prospectively, for the presence of subclinical ILD via high-resolution cross-sectional chest imaging.[60,61] These 2 studies identified subclinical ILD in 21% and 18% of the screened patients with RA, respectively. Both studies found associations between subclinical ILD and the previously discussed *MUC5B* promoter polymorphism that is a primary genetic risk factor for IPF and clinical RA-ILD.[37,62] Estimates of lifetime risk for the development of clinical ILD within RA cohorts vary but typically they are thought to be between 5% and 10%.[1,63]

SSc cohorts without known lung disease have also undergone prospective evaluation for subclinical ILD via high-resolution cross-sectional computed tomography (CT) chest imaging.[64–66] Although the methods differ in these 3 studies, the primary takeaway is that SSc cohorts have high rates of subclinical ILD when screened (as high as 197/305 with 1 to >20% fibrosis on CT chest from Hoffman-Vold and colleagues[64]).

Additionally, a large, pooled analysis of a national cohort of patients with many autoimmune diseases including SSc, antisynthetase syndrome, mixed-CTD was screened for the presence of subclinical ILD and found that 67/525 (13%) of patients with autoimmune diseases had radiographic evidence of subclinical ILD.[67] Recent expert consensus statements were published regarding screening for ILD and early intervention within SSc populations, which will be an important step toward understanding these important questions.[9,68]

A more exhaustive discussion of all observational data in subclinical CTD-ILD is beyond the scope of this review; however, these prospective studies highlight one very important principle: subclinical ILD is common in autoimmune disease states and is readily identifiable via HRCT scans of the chest.

Screening in Autoimmune Disease

Although data have been presented in this review of subclinical ILD rates in autoimmune disease, there remains no clear data to guide the *clinical* utility of screening in autoimmune disease, that is to say, there remains no clear proven benefit to identifying subclinical ILD in this population. One might surmise that an early intervention in these states would be beneficial; however, this remains only a hypothesis without clinical data to support this decision. As highlighted in the treatment section of this review, there are only 4 RCTs of therapy in CTD-ILD and none of those 4 are focused on a subclinical state. The same is true in the field of pulmonary fibrosis or ILD writ large, where no interventional trials have been undertaken in preclinical or subclinical states.

Therefore, for now, the primary utility of approaching subclinical states of ILD in autoimmunity remains within the realm of translational and clinical research. However, there are several reasons highlighted in this review, which point out the potential benefits of ongoing research in this field, which could even translate beyond autoimmune disease into all realms of subclinical ILD.

RESEARCH AGENDA

In recent years, there have been many important advances in our understanding of CTD-ILD pathogenesis and clinical management but there remain many gaps in this area that need further study. The authors of this review think that the following areas of research focus during the coming years are likely to have the biggest impact on the field and the biggest impact on patient outcomes.

- Establish clinical screening and monitoring guidelines for CTD-ILD such that patients can be identified at the earliest stage of disease.
- Understand the pathogenesis of subclinical ILD such that patients can be identified who are most likely to benefit from earlier treatment.
- Identify shared and distinct pathogenic pathways across CTD-ILDs such that therapeutics targeting disease-specific pathways can improve the efficacy of CTD-ILD treatments.

SUMMARY

ILD is a common manifestation of several autoimmune diseases, and its association with poor quality of life and mortality warrant further study that can lead to more effective screening and treatment. There have been advances in the treatment of CTD-ILD in recent years but many unanswered questions remain. The pathogenesis of CTD-ILDs likely have both shared and distinct pathways, and understanding how genetics, environmental factors, and immune responses in each CTD contribute to ILD development will likely improve our understanding of pathogenesis and the effectiveness of our treatments for patients with CTD-ILD.

CLINICS CARE POINTS

- Prevalent ILD and ILD prognosis are associated with disease activity scores in CTD; therefore, a pillar of effective CTD-ILD treatment management remains adequate baseline DMARD treatment to control primary CTD manifestations.

- Methotrexate neither causes fibrotic ILD nor does it exacerbate the underlying ILD in RA; therefore, it is safe to continue as an effective DMARD in patients with adequate disease control.

- Added immunosuppression or alterations of the immunosuppression regimen for new ILD manifestations (or ILD progression) in patients with underlying autoimmune disease should be carefully considered between pulmonary and rheumatology physicians with experience balancing these entities.

- Three therapies have randomized, placebo-controlled level evidence in SSc-ILD, which supports their safety, improvement in lung function over placebo, and, in the case of mycophenolate and cyclophosphamide, improvement in health-related quality of life (mycophenolate, cyclophosphamide, and tocilizumab).

- Antifibrotic therapy seems to have a role as adjunctive therapy for patients with CTD-ILD with progressive fibrotic features in patients with adequate CTD disease activity control.

- There are high rates of subclinical ILD in autoimmune disease populations but there remains unclear clinical benefit to early intervention in screened populations.
- Randomized, placebo-controlled studies are urgently needed in both subclinical and clinical CTD-ILD with fibrotic features to determine the safety of added immunosuppression and to determine the clinical efficacy of early intervention in subclinical ILD states.

DECLARATION OF INTERESTS

S.M. Matson is supported by P20GM130423 and the Joseph A. Cates Pulmonary Fibrosis Research fund at the University of Kansas Medical Center. M.K. Demoruelle has investigator-initiated research funding from Pfizer, United States and Boehringer Ingelheim, United States.

REFERENCES

1. Bongartz T, Nannini C, Medina-Velasquez YF, et al. Incidence and mortality of interstitial lung disease in rheumatoid arthritis: a population-based study. Arthritis Rheum 2010;62:1583–91.
2. Hoffmann-Vold AM, Fretheim H, Halse AK, et al. Tracking impact of interstitial lung disease in systemic sclerosis in a complete nationwide cohort. Am J Respir Crit Care Med 2019;200:1258–66.
3. Marie I, Hachulla E, Cherin P, et al. Interstitial lung disease in polymyositis and dermatomyositis. Arthritis Rheum 2002;47:614–22.
4. Park JH, Kim DS, Park IN, et al. Prognosis of fibrotic interstitial pneumonia: idiopathic versus collagen vascular disease-related subtypes. Am J Respir Crit Care Med 2007;175:705–11.
5. Solomon JJ, Ryu JH, Tazelaar HD, et al. Fibrosing interstitial pneumonia predicts survival in patients with rheumatoid arthritis-associated interstitial lung disease (RA-ILD). Respir Med 2013;107:1247–52.
6. Solomon JJ, Chung JH, Cosgrove GP, et al. Predictors of mortality in rheumatoid arthritis-associated interstitial lung disease. Eur Respir J 2016;47:588–96.
7. Fujisawa T, Hozumi H, Kono M, et al. Prognostic factors for myositis-associated interstitial lung disease. PLoS One 2014;9:e98824.
8. Volkmann ER, Tashkin DP, Sim M, et al. Short-term progression of interstitial lung disease in systemic sclerosis predicts long-term survival in two independent clinical trial cohorts. Ann Rheum Dis 2019;78:122–30.
9. Hoffmann-Vold A-M, Maher TM, Philpot EE, et al. The identification and management of interstitial lung disease in systemic sclerosis: evidence-based European consensus statements. The Lancet Rheumatology 2020;2:e71–83.
10. Raghu G, Remy-Jardin M, Richeldi L, et al. Idiopathic pulmonary fibrosis (an update) and progressive pulmonary fibrosis in adults: an official ATS/ERS/JRS/ALAT clinical practice guideline. Am J Respir Crit Care Med 2022;205:e18–47.
11. Fraenkel L, Bathon JM, England BR, et al. 2021 American college of rheumatology guideline for the treatment of rheumatoid arthritis. Arthritis Rheumatol 2021;73:1108–23.
12. Cannon GW, Ward JR, Clegg DO, et al. Acute lung disease associated with low-dose pulse methotrexate therapy in patients with rheumatoid arthritis. Arthritis Rheum 1983;26:1269–74.
13. Juge P-A, Lee JS, Lau J, et al. Methotrexate and rheumatoid arthritis associated interstitial lung disease. Eur Respir J 2020;57(2):2000337.

14. Mehta P, Redhead G, Nair A, et al. Can we finally exonerate methotrexate as a factor in causing or exacerbating fibrotic interstitial lung disease in patients with rheumatoid arthritis? Clin Rheumatol 2022;41:2925–8.
15. Schnabel A, Richter C, Bauerfeind S, et al. Bronchoalveolar lavage cell profile in methotrexate induced pneumonitis. Thorax 1997;52:377–9.
16. Nakashita T, Ando K, Kaneko N, et al. Potential risk of TNF inhibitors on the progression of interstitial lung disease in patients with rheumatoid arthritis. BMJ Open 2014;4:e005615.
17. Wolfe F, Caplan L, Michaud K. Rheumatoid arthritis treatment and the risk of severe interstitial lung disease. Scand J Rheumatol 2007;36:172–8.
18. Huang Y, Lin W, Chen Z, et al. Effect of tumor necrosis factor inhibitors on interstitial lung disease in rheumatoid arthritis: angel or demon? Drug Des Dev Ther 2019;13:2111–25.
19. Panopoulos ST, Sfikakis PP. Biological treatments and connective tissue disease associated interstitial lung disease. Curr Opin Pulm Med 2011;17:362–7.
20. Rojas-Serrano J, Mejía M, Rivera-Matias PA, et al. Rheumatoid arthritis-related interstitial lung disease (RA-ILD): a possible association between disease activity and prognosis. Clin Rheumatol 2022;41:1741–7.
21. Sparks JA, He X, Huang J, et al. Rheumatoid arthritis disease activity predicting incident clinically apparent rheumatoid arthritis-associated interstitial lung disease: a prospective cohort study. Arthritis Rheumatol 2019;71:1472–82.
22. Khanna D, Lin CJF, Furst DE, et al. Tocilizumab in systemic sclerosis: a randomised, double-blind, placebo-controlled, phase 3 trial. Lancet Respir Med 2020;8:963–74.
23. Tashkin DP, Elashoff R, Clements PJ, et al. Cyclophosphamide versus placebo in scleroderma lung disease. N Engl J Med 2006;354:2655–66.
24. Tashkin DP, Roth MD, Clements PJ, et al. Mycophenolate mofetil versus oral cyclophosphamide in scleroderma-related interstitial lung disease (SLS II): a randomised controlled, double-blind, parallel group trial. Lancet Respir Med 2016;4:708–19.
25. Raghu G, Anstrom KJ, King TE Jr, et al. Prednisone, azathioprine, and N-acetylcysteine for pulmonary fibrosis. N Engl J Med 2012;366:1968–77.
26. Matson S, Lee J, Eickelberg O. Two sides of the same coin? A review of the similarities and differences between idiopathic pulmonary fibrosis and rheumatoid arthritis associated interstitial lung disease. Eur Respir J 2021;57(5):2002533.
27. Mukhopadhyay S. Usual interstitial pneumonia (UIP): a clinically significant pathologic diagnosis. Mod Pathol 2022;35:580–8.
28. Richeldi L, du Bois RM, Raghu G, et al. Efficacy and safety of nintedanib in idiopathic pulmonary fibrosis. N Engl J Med 2014;370:2071–82.
29. King TE Jr, Bradford WZ, Castro-Bernardini S, et al. A phase 3 trial of pirfenidone in patients with idiopathic pulmonary fibrosis. N Engl J Med 2014;370:2083–92.
30. Distler O, Highland KB, Gahlemann M, et al. Nintedanib for systemic sclerosis-associated interstitial lung disease. N Engl J Med 2019;380:2518–28.
31. Solomon JJ, Danoff SK, Woodhead FA, et al. Safety, tolerability, and efficacy of pirfenidone in patients with rheumatoid arthritis-associated interstitial lung disease: a randomised, double-blind, placebo-controlled, phase 2 study. Lancet Respir Med 2023;11(1):87–96.
32. Flaherty KR, Wells AU, Cottin V, et al. Nintedanib in progressive fibrosing interstitial lung diseases. N Engl J Med 2019;381:1718–27.
33. Wuyts WA, Agostini C, Antoniou KM, et al. The pathogenesis of pulmonary fibrosis: a moving target. Eur Respir J 2013;41:1207–18.

34. Laurent GJ, McAnulty RJ, Hill M, et al. Escape from the matrix: multiple mechanisms for fibroblast activation in pulmonary fibrosis. Proc Am Thorac Soc 2008; 5:311–5.
35. Juge PA, Lee JS, Ebstein E, et al. MUC5B promoter variant and rheumatoid arthritis with interstitial lung disease. N Engl J Med 2018;379:2209–19.
36. Palomaki A, FinnGen Rheumatology Clinical Expert G, Palotie A, et al. Lifetime risk of rheumatoid arthritis-associated interstitial lung disease in MUC5B mutation carriers. Ann Rheum Dis 2021;80:1530–6.
37. Seibold MA, Wise AL, Speer MC, et al. A common MUC5B promoter polymorphism and pulmonary fibrosis. N Engl J Med 2011;364:1503–12.
38. Shao T, Shi X, Yang S, et al. Interstitial lung disease in connective tissue disease: a common lesion with heterogeneous mechanisms and treatment considerations. Front Immunol 2021;12:684699.
39. Doyle TJ, Patel AS, Hatabu H, et al. Detection of Rheumatoid Arthritis-Interstitial Lung Disease Is Enhanced by Serum Biomarkers. Am J Respir Crit Care Med 2015;191:1403–12.
40. Kelly CA, Saravanan V, Nisar M, et al. British Rheumatoid Interstitial Lung N. Rheumatoid arthritis-related interstitial lung disease: associations, prognostic factors and physiological and radiological characteristics–a large multicentre UK study. Rheumatology 2014;53:1676–82.
41. Nihtyanova SI, Schreiber BE, Ong VH, et al. Prediction of pulmonary complications and long-term survival in systemic sclerosis. Arthritis Rheumatol 2014;66: 1625–35.
42. Zhang L, Wu G, Gao D, et al. Factors associated with interstitial lung disease in patients with polymyositis and dermatomyositis: a systematic review and meta-analysis. PLoS One 2016;11:e0155381.
43. Nihtyanova SI, Sari A, Harvey JC, et al. Using Autoantibodies and Cutaneous Subset to Develop Outcome-Based Disease Classification in Systemic Sclerosis. Arthritis Rheumatol 2020;72:465–76.
44. Khanna D, Tashkin DP, Denton CP, et al. Etiology, risk factors, and biomarkers in systemic sclerosis with interstitial lung disease. Am J Respir Crit Care Med 2020; 201:650–60.
45. Teel A, Lu J, Park J, et al. The role of myositis-specific autoantibodies and the management of interstitial lung disease in idiopathic inflammatory myopathies: a systematic review. Semin Arthritis Rheum 2022;57:152088.
46. Giles JT, Darrah E, Danoff S, et al. Association of cross-reactive antibodies targeting peptidyl-arginine deiminase 3 and 4 with rheumatoid arthritis-associated interstitial lung disease. PLoS One 2014;9:e98794.
47. Brinkmann V, Reichard U, Goosmann C, et al. Neutrophil extracellular traps kill bacteria. Science 2004;303:1532–5.
48. Kuley R, Stultz RD, Duvvuri B, et al. N-Formyl methionine peptide-mediated neutrophil activation in systemic sclerosis. Front Immunol 2021;12:785275.
49. Khandpur R, Carmona-Rivera C, Vivekanandan-Giri A, et al. NETs are a source of citrullinated autoantigens and stimulate inflammatory responses in rheumatoid arthritis. Sci Transl Med 2013;5:178ra140.
50. Seto N, Torres-Ruiz JJ, Carmona-Rivera C, et al. Neutrophil dysregulation is pathogenic in idiopathic inflammatory myopathies. JCI Insight 2020;5(3):e134189.
51. Saffarzadeh M, Juenemann C, Queisser MA, et al. Neutrophil extracellular traps directly induce epithelial and endothelial cell death: a predominant role of histones. PLoS One 2012;7:e32366.

52. Chrysanthopoulou A, Mitroulis I, Apostolidou E, et al. Neutrophil extracellular traps promote differentiation and function of fibroblasts. J Pathol 2014;233: 294–307.
53. Zhang S, Jia X, Zhang Q, et al. Neutrophil extracellular traps activate lung fibroblast to induce polymyositis-related interstitial lung diseases via TLR9-miR-7-Smad2 pathway. J Cell Mol Med 2020;24(2):1658–69.
54. Carmona-Rivera C, Zhao W, Yalavarthi S, et al. Neutrophil extracellular traps induce endothelial dysfunction in systemic lupus erythematosus through the activation of matrix metalloproteinase-2. Ann Rheum Dis 2015;74:1417–24.
55. Takemasa A, Ishii Y, Fukuda T. A neutrophil elastase inhibitor prevents bleomycin-induced pulmonary fibrosis in mice. Eur Respir J 2012;40:1475–82.
56. Okamoto Y, Devoe S, Seto N, et al. Association of Sputum Neutrophil Extracellular Trap Subsets With IgA Anti-Citrullinated Protein Antibodies in Subjects at Risk for Rheumatoid Arthritis. Arthritis Rheumatol 2022;74:38–48.
57. Kinder BW, Brown KK, Schwarz MI, et al. Baseline BAL neutrophilia predicts early mortality in idiopathic pulmonary fibrosis. Chest 2008;133:226–32.
58. Gerlag DM, Safy M, Maijer KI, et al. Effects of B-cell directed therapy on the preclinical stage of rheumatoid arthritis: the PRAIRI study. Ann Rheum Dis 2019;78: 179–85.
59. Krijbolder DI, Verstappen M, van Dijk BT, et al. Intervention with methotrexate in patients with arthralgia at risk of rheumatoid arthritis to reduce the development of persistent arthritis and its disease burden (TREAT EARLIER): a randomised, double-blind, placebo-controlled, proof-of-concept trial. Lancet (London, England) 2022;400:283–94.
60. Matson SM, Deane KD, Peljto AL, et al. Prospective Identification of Subclinical Interstitial Lung Disease in Rheumatoid Arthritis Cohort is Associated with the MUC5B Promoter Variant. Am J Respir Crit Care Med 2022;205(4):473–6.
61. Juge PA, Granger B, Debray MP, et al. A risk score to detect subclinical rheumatoid arthritis-associated interstitial lung disease. Arthritis Rheumatol 2022;74(11): 1755–65.
62. Juge PA, Borie R, Kannengiesser C, et al. Shared genetic predisposition in rheumatoid arthritis-interstitial lung disease and familial pulmonary fibrosis. Eur Respir J 2017;49(5):1602314.
63. Turesson C, O'Fallon WM, Crowson CS, et al. Extra-articular disease manifestations in rheumatoid arthritis: incidence trends and risk factors over 46 years. Ann Rheum Dis 2003;62:722–7.
64. Hoffmann-Vold AM, Aaløkken TM, Lund MB, et al. Predictive value of serial high-resolution computed tomography analyses and concurrent lung function tests in systemic sclerosis. Arthritis Rheumatol 2015;67:2205–12.
65. Launay D, Remy-Jardin M, Michon-Pasturel U, et al. High resolution computed tomography in fibrosing alveolitis associated with systemic sclerosis. J Rheumatol 2006;33:1789–801.
66. Reyes-Long S, Gutierrez M, Clavijo-Cornejo D, et al. Subclinical interstitial lung disease in patients with systemic sclerosis. A pilot study on the role of ultrasound. Reumatol Clínica 2021;17:144–9.
67. Hoffmann-Vold AM, Andersson H, Reiseter S, et al. Subclinical ILD is frequent and progresses across different connective tissue diseases. Eur Respir J 2021; 58:OA2973.
68. Rahaghi FF, Hsu VM, Kaner RJ, et al. Expert consensus on the management of systemic sclerosis-associated interstitial lung disease. Respir Res 2023;24:6.

69. Suissa S, Hudson M, Ernst P. Leflunomide use and the risk of interstitial lung disease in rheumatoid arthritis. Arthritis Rheum 2006;54:1435–9.
70. Perez-Alvarez R, Perez-de-Lis M, Diaz-Lagares C, et al. Interstitial lung disease induced or exacerbated by TNF-targeted therapies: analysis of 122 cases. Semin Arthritis Rheum 2011;41:256–64.
71. Tomioka R, King TE Jr. Gold-induced pulmonary disease: clinical features, outcome, and differentiation from rheumatoid lung disease. Am J Respir Crit Care Med 1997;155:1011–20.
72. Goodwin SD, Glenny RW. Nonsteroidal anti-inflammatory drug-associated pulmonary infiltrates with eosinophilia. Review of the literature and Food and Drug Administration adverse drug reaction reports. Arch Intern Med 1992;152:1521–4.
73. Parry SD, Barbatzas C, Peel ET, et al. Sulphasalazine and lung toxicity. Eur Respir J 2002;19:756–64.
74. Cassone G, Manfredi A, Vacchi C, et al. Treatment of rheumatoid arthritis-associated interstitial lung disease: lights and shadows. J Clin Med 2020;9:1082.
75. Oldham JM, Lee C, Valenzi E, et al. Azathioprine response in patients with fibrotic connective tissue disease-associated interstitial lung disease. Respir Med 2016; 121:117–22.
76. Md Yusof MY, Kabia A, Darby M, et al. Effect of rituximab on the progression of rheumatoid arthritis-related interstitial lung disease: 10 years' experience at a single centre. Rheumatology 2017;56:1348–57.
77. Mena-Vázquez N, Rojas-Gimenez M, Fuego-Varela C, et al. Safety and effectiveness of abatacept in a prospective cohort of patients with rheumatoid arthritis-associated interstitial lung disease. Respir Med 2019;154:6–11.
78. Huapaya JA, Hallowell R, Silhan L, et al. Long-term treatment with human immunoglobulin for antisynthetase syndrome-associated interstitial lung disease. Respir Med 2019;154:6–11.
79. Witt LJ, Demchuk C, Curran JJ, et al. Benefit of adjunctive tacrolimus in connective tissue disease-interstitial lung disease. Pulm Pharmacol Ther 2016;36:46–52.
80. Volkmann ER, Tashkin DP, LeClair H, et al. Treatment with mycophenolate and cyclophosphamide leads to clinically meaningful improvements in patient-reported outcomes in scleroderma lung disease: results of scleroderma lung study II. ACR Open Rheumatol 2020;2:362–70.

Clinically Relevant Biomarkers in Connective Tissue Disease-Associated Interstitial Lung Disease

Janelle Vu Pugashetti, MD, MS[a],*, Dinesh Khanna, MD, MS[b],
Ella A. Kazerooni, MD, MS[a,c], Justin Oldham, MD, MS[a,d]

KEYWORDS

• Connective tissue disease • Interstitial lung disease • Computed tomography
• Biomarkers

KEY POINTS

• Blood-based biomarkers that reflect lung epithelial cell dysfunction, aberrant immunity, and abnormal lung remodeling may discriminate the presence of interstitial lung disease in patients with connective tissue diseases.
• High-resolution computed tomography (HRCT) is the current best diagnostic tool for ILD and may have prognostic value in CTD-ILD.
• Texture-based and volumetric HRCT analysis show promise as prognostic biomarkers in CTD-ILD.
• Composite biomarkers improve risk prediction compared with stand-alone biomarkers, showing high promise in the diagnosis and prognosis of patients with connective tissue-associated interstitial lung disease.
• The combination of large blood-based platforms, radiomic algorithms, and use of machine learning is expected to advance the study of CTD-ILD in coming years.

INTRODUCTION

Interstitial lung disease (ILD) is a common manifestation of connective tissue disease (CTD), most often affecting patients with rheumatoid arthritis (RA), systemic sclerosis

This article previously appeared in *Anesthesiology Clinics* volume 42 issue 1 March 2024.
[a] Division of Pulmonary and Critical Care Medicine, Department of Internal Medicine, University of Michigan; [b] Scleroderma Program, Division of Rheumatology, Department of Internal Medicine, University of Michigan; [c] Division of Cardiothoracic Radiology, Department of Radiology, University of Michigan; [d] Department of Epidemiology, University of Michigan
* Corresponding author. 1150 West Medical Center Drive, 6220 MSRB III / SPC 5642, Ann Arbor, MI 48109.
E-mail address: vupugash@med.umich.edu

(SSc), idiopathic inflammatory myopathy (IIM), and mixed CTD.[1–5] ILD can also develop in patients with Sjögren syndrome (SS) and systemic lupus erythematosus, but is less common with these disorders.[6,7] Among patients who do develop CTD-ILD, a subset will develop a progressive phenotype, leading to parenchymal destruction, lung function decline, and early mortality.[8–21] Early and accurate diagnosis is essential for effectively managing patients with CTD-ILD, particularly because effective treatments exist to stabilize disease and sometimes improve lung function.[13–15,22–24] Diagnosing ILD is often nuanced and difficult, as many patients with CTD-ILD have no respiratory symptoms, and symptoms are nonspecific when they do develop.[25,26] Pulmonary function testing (PFT) can help raise suspicion for ILD in patients with CTD, but test performance characteristics are modest.[25,27] Once ILD is diagnosed, the inability to discriminate patients likely to progress remains elusive. Clinical prediction models have been developed to predict ILD progression in patients with CTD, but many are CTD specific, reducing generalizability to the larger CTD-ILD population. The ability to predict CTD-ILD progression would empower patients and clinicians to make better informed decisions about treatment, lung transplantation, and goals of care.

Biomarkers, defined as indicators of normal biological processes and pathogenic processes, hold promise for improving our ability to accurately diagnose ILD and predict disease trajectory.[28] The ideal biomarker should be noninvasive or minimally invasive, with high accuracy for predicting the end point of interest. Biomarkers most likely to inform clinical decision making in patients with CTD are those that predict early disease before the development of respiratory symptoms and a progressive phenotype. In the past decade, numerous studies have identified candidate blood-based and high-resolution computed tomography (HRCT) biomarkers, and recent -omics investigations have added composite biomarkers to the list of potentially clinically relevant biomarkers in the CTD-ILD population. However, barriers to clinical implementation remain. This review provides an overview of recent advances in CTD-ILD biomarker investigation, focusing on blood-based and HRCT biomarkers, and highlights strategies to advance these biomarkers toward clinical implementation in patients with CTD-ILD.

BLOOD-BASED DIAGNOSTIC BIOMARKERS

Blood-based biomarkers carry high promise for diagnosing ILD in patients with CTD and providing prognostic information for these patients, because many reflect molecular pathways involved in fibrogenesis and can signal early disease before the development of overt fibrosis and respiratory symptoms. Furthermore, the minimally invasive nature of peripheral blood acquisition better positions this class of biomarkers for clinical implementation when compared with more invasive procedures such as bronchoalveolar lavage and surgical lung biopsy. Blood-based biomarkers include clinically approved autoantibodies and inflammatory markers, and research biomarkers identified through targeted and unbiased analysis. The major challenge remaining with blood-based biomarkers, however, is achieving adequate test performance to justify clinical implementation; this is particularly difficult in patients with CTD, because many blood-based biomarkers may reflect systemic and extrapulmonary processes.

The detection of autoantibodies serves a critical role in the diagnosis of CTD-ILD, and autoantibodies are the only blood biomarkers available for clinical use. There are a number of autoantibodies found in patients with CTD that are associated with higher risk of ILD. In patients with SSc, antitopoisomerase I antibody (anti-Scl70) has repeatedly been associated with ILD across cohorts.[29–33] Anti-Th/To ribonucleo-protein antibodies and anti-PM/Scl have also been shown to be associated with ILD, although they are more rarely detected in patients with SSc.[34,35] In addition, in 2 large SSc cohorts, the presence of anti-SSA/Ro was found to be associated with at least a 2-fold increased odds of SSc-ILD.[36,37] Conversely, the absence of anticentromere antibodies is associated with decreased likelihood of ILD.[30,38] In patients with RA, anti-citrullinated cyclic peptide (CCP) antibodies and high-titer rheumatoid factor predict ILD, with some studies demonstrating a correlation between anti-CCP titers and HRCT severity.[39–42] In patients with IIM, anti-tRNA synthetase antibodies are commonly detected, most frequently anti-Jo-1, anti-PL-7, and PL-12 antibodies. These antisynthetase antibodies are the hallmark of antisynthetase syndrome, which carries high risk of developing ILD, with reports of ILD in more than 90% of antisynthe-tase antibody-positive patients.[43,44] Another antibody found in patients with IIM is the (anti-MDA5/CADM-140), which characterizes a subset with clinically amyopathic myositis and high risk of ILD.[45–50] Unfortunately, many of these antibodies tend to signal overall disease extent and risk of ILD, rather than the presence of ILD.

Beyond clinically approved autoantibodies, multiple investigations have focused on molecular markers of lung epithelial cell dysfunction, aberrant immunity (cytokines and chemokines), and abnormal lung remodeling (collagen peptides/extracellular matrix biomarkers) in patients with CTD-ILD. Among those with the best described test performance characteristics is Krebs von den Lungen 6 (KL-6), which is strongly expressed on regenerating type II pneumocytes and thought to be a marker of epithe-lial injury.[51] At various cutoff points, the sensitivity of KL-6 ranges from 73% to 87% and specificity ranges from 70% to 100% for discriminating CTD-ILD among patients with CTD.[52–60] The area under the curve (AUC), which describes global discrimination without a cutoff threshold, ranges from 0.86 to 0.90, depending on the cohort in which the test is applied. Another well-studied marker of lung epithelial damage and turnover is surfactant protein D (SP-D). As a biomarker of ILD in patients with CTD, sensitivity ranges from 68% to 89.4% and specificity ranges from 70% to 83% depending on the dichotomization threshold used, with an AUC of 0.72 to 0.983.[41,52,53,61] In studies comparing KL-6 and SP-D in the same cohort, the specificity of SP-D is generally lower than that of KL-6.[52,53,62]

Other well-studied blood-based biomarkers are described in **Table 1** and include SP-A[62,63]; club cell secreted protein 16[54]; pulmonary and activation-regulated chemo-kine (PARC)[41]; interleukin (IL)-6, 8, and 10[64]; tumor necrosis factor-α[64]; metalloprotei-nase (MMP)-7[41]; and Wnt Family member 5a (Wnt5a).[65] Although test performance characteristics are not reported for all biomarkers listed, studies have shown that circulating concentration of these biomarkers are higher in patients with CTD-ILD compared with those with CTD without ILD. Despite the advances made studying these blood-based biomarkers, none have been implemented clinically. Given the complexity of ILD pathogenesis, it is likely that biomarkers from multiple pathways are needed to achieve sufficient test performance to justify clinical implementation. Doyle and colleagues[41] demonstrated the promise of this approach in detecting RA-ILD. A model composed of clinical factors including demographics and autoanti-bodies, combined with a biomarker signature composed of MMP-7, PARC, and SP-D, outperformed the clinical signature alone or any of the stand-alone biomarkers.

The emergence of machine learning has further improved risk prediction and is likely to become an important tool in the diagnosis of CTD-ILD. Machine learning comprises mathematical algorithms that build, train, and self-evaluate iterative models to self-improve predictive power.[66] Kass and colleagues[67] demonstrated the promise of machine-learning in patients with RA, showing that biomarker signatures derived

Table 1
Novel blood-based diagnostic CTD-ILD biomarkers

Biomarker	Reference(s)	Diagnostic Test Performance (CTD-ILD from CTD Without ILD)
Lung epithelial cell dysfunction		
CA 125	RA[128]	RA[128]: cutoff 35 U/mL, sens 60.71%, spec 79.52%, AUC 0.78
CC16	SSc[54]	SSc[54]: cutoff 46.0 ng/mL, sens 51.8%, spec 88.8%, AUC 0.76
CCL18	SSc[129]	
E-Selectin	SSc[130,131] RA[132] IIM & SSc[133]	
ET-1	SSc[130]	
ICAM-1	SSc[134]	
KL-6	SSc[52–54,135,136] RA[55,56,137,57] IIM[62,58,138,139,60,140] SS[141] CTD[59]	SSc[52]: cutoff 602 U/mL, sens 73%, spec 70% SSc[53]: cutoff 500 U/mL, sens 78.8%, spec 90.0%, AUC 0.90 SSc[54]: cutoff 302 U/mL, sens 85.5%, spec 85.3%, AUC 0.89 RA[55]: cutoff 277.5 U/mL, sens 86.7%, spec 88%, AUC 0.88 RA[56]: cutoff 399 U/mL, sens 85.71%, spec 90.91%, AUC 0.92 RA[57]: AUC 0.81 IIM[58]: cutoff 437 U/mL, sens 87%, spec 96%, AUC 0.97 CTD[59]: cutoff 275.1 U/mL, sens 79.4%, spec 79.9%, AUC 0.86 IIM[60]: cutoff 549 U/mL, sens 83%, spec 100%
SP-A	SSc[63] IIM[62]	SSc[63]: Cutoff 43.8 ng/mL, sens 33%, spec 100% IIM[62]: Cutoff 39.5 ng/mL, PPV = 70%
SP-D	SSc[52–54] RA[41,137] IIM[62]	SSc[52]: cutoff 62.2 ng/mL, sens 68%, spec 70% SSc[53]: cutoff 90 ng/mL, sens 89.4%, spec 80.0%, AUC 0.983 Ssc[54]: cutoff 91.0 ng/mL, sens 71.4%, spec 77.2%, AUC 0.72 SSc: cutoff 110 ng/mL, sens 77%, spec 83% RA[41]: AUC 0.75 RA[41]: AUC 0.91
VEGF	SSc[130]	
Aberrant immunity		
CCL2	IIM[62,142] SSc[61]	
CX3CL1	SSc[143]	
CXCL10/IP-10	SSc[144,145] RA[146] IIM[147,142] CTD[148]	
CXCL11	CTD[148] IIM[142]	

(continued on next page)

Table 1 (*continued*)		
Biomarker	**Reference(s)**	**Diagnostic Test Performance (CTD-ILD from CTD Without ILD)**
CXCL12		
CXCL13	SS[149]	
CXCL16	SSc[150]	
CXCL4	SSc[151]	
CXCL9/MIG	SSc[67] CTD[148]	
IL-04	SSc[152]	
IL-06	SS[64] IIM[147]	SS[64]: cutoff 7.109 pg/mL, sens 90.88%, spec 62.75%, AUC 0.67
IL-08	SS[64,153] IIM[147]	SS[64]: cutoff 20.094 pg/mL, sens 90.9%, spec 62.8%, AUC 0.71
IL-10	SS[64]	SS[64]: cutoff 5.162 pg/mL, sens 87.54%, spec 78.63%, AUC 0.89
IL-15		
IL-23	SSc[154]	
IL-33	SSc[155]	
IL-35	SSc[156]	
PARC	SSc[135] RA[41]	RA[41]: AUC 0.80 RA[41]: AUC 0.70
TNF-α	SS[64] IIM[147]	SS[64]: cutoff 9.116 pg/mL, sens 80.6%, spec 73.2%, AUC 0.73
Wnt5a	RA[65]	RA[65]: cutoff 4.49, sens 55.6%, spec 4.9%, AUC 0.75
Abnormal lung remodeling		
MMP-7	SSc[157,158] RA[41,146,137] IIM[159]	RA[41]: AUC 0.86, RA[41]: AUC 0.83
MMP-12	SSc[160]	
TIMP-1	SSc[161]	
CCN2/CTGF	RA[162] SSc[163]	
GDF-15	SSc[164–166]	
YKL-40	SSc[167]	

Abbreviations: CC16, club cell secreted protein 16; CCL18, C-C motif chemokine ligand 18; IL, interleukin; MMP, metalloproteinase; PARC, pulmonary and activation-regulated chemokine; sens, sensitivity; spec, specificity; TNF, tumor necrosis factor; YKL-40, chitinase-3-like-1.

using this method could effectively discriminate ILD in these patients with higher sensitivity and specificity than stand-alone proteins. Although this approach can result in a highly in-sample predictive classifier, overfitting remains an issue and out-of-sample validation is required. Kass and colleagues[67] demonstrated this challenge, showing that the highly predictive diagnostic signatures developed in independent RA cohorts differed greatly, with little overlap in covariates. Qin and colleagues[57] pursued a similar approach in patients with RA, showing that 3 machine learning algorithms discriminated ILD with AUC of at least 0.95. These results have yet to be externally validated, however.

BLOOD-BASED PROGNOSTIC BIOMARKERS

As with diagnosis, the use of peripheral blood-based biomarkers holds promise as a prognostic tool in CTD-ILD. The outcomes of progression in CTD-ILD studies have generally been survival, lung function decline including forced vital capacity (FVC) and diffusing capacity of carbon monoxide (DLCO), or a composite end point of these measures (**Table 2**). With the recent publication of consensus definitions to define progressive pulmonary fibrosis,[68] substantial research is expected in the coming years to optimally define progression in this population.

Clinically approved autoantibodies have been studied in the prognosis of patients with CTD. In a large SSc outcome study, the presence of anti-Scl-70 antibody in patients predicted a faster rate of FVC decline.[31] Conversely, presence of anti-PM/Scl antibodies has been associated with less FVC decline and better survival compared with patients with anti-Scl-70.[69] In patients with anti-Jo or anti-MDA-5 antibody, the concurrent positivity with anti-SSA/Ro portends worse ILD and mortality compared with patients without dual antibodies.[70,71] Patients with IIM with anti-MDA-5 positivity have been well described to have rapidly progressive and fatal ILD among Japanese cohorts, with 33% to 66% experiencing 6-month and antibody positivity portending a 6-fold risk of death.[45-48] However, in predominantly Caucasian cohorts in the United States, patients with ILD with anti-MDA5 did not have the rapidly progressive ILD described in Japanese cohorts.[50]

Several studies of novel biomarkers have also evaluated prognosis in CTD-ILD. KL-6 again is among the best studied across common CTD-ILD subtypes.[59,72-74] Among 82 patients with SSc-ILD in the Genetics versus Environment Scleroderma Outcome Study (GENISOS), higher baseline KL-6 levels were predictive of faster progression, with patients averaging 7% more decline in annualized percent change of FVC when baseline KL-6 was greater than the cutoff value.[75] Chitinase-3-like-1 (YKL-40), C-C motif chemokine ligand 18 (CCL18), and IL-6, along with several other biomarkers previously linked to progression in idiopathic pulmonary fibrosis (IPF), have also been shown to predict worse outcome among patients with CTD-ILD (see **Table 2**). Like diagnostic biomarker studies, investigators have just begun to harness the power of composite biomarkers in risk prediction. In a multicenter retrospective cohort of Japanese patients with IIM-ILD, Gono and colleagues[76] showed that a prediction model based on anti-MDA-5 status, C-reactive protein level, and KL-6 level differentiated survival more effectively than anti-MDA-5 antibody testing alone. In the tocilizumab phase 3 trial, elevated acute phase reactants, as an entry criterion, were associated with marked decline in FVC during 1 year in the placebo group in those with ILD (257 mL in placebo group vs 6.5 mL in active group).[22]

Our group recently completed the first proteomic analysis of patients with non-IPF ILD, which included 245 patients with CTD-ILD across 3 centers.[77] Relative plasma concentration of 368 biomarkers was determined using a medium-throughput proteomic platform, 31 of which were found to be associated with near-term ILD progression, defined as death, lung transplant, or 10% or greater relative FVC decline within 1 year of blood draw. Of these 31 proteins identified in the derivation cohort, 17 maintained association in an independent validation cohort, with consistent outcome association in each of the ILD subgroups assessed. Using machine learning, we then derived a 12-analyte proteomic signature, which discriminated 1-year ILD progression with good sensitivity and negative predictive value across cohorts, suggesting this tool could effectively identify patients at low risk of ILD progression, justifying a conservative strategy in this population. Notably, those with a low-risk proteomic signature experienced an increase in FVC over 1 year, whereas those with a high-risk signature

Table 2 Novel blood-based prognostic CTD-ILD biomarkers	
Biomarker	Prognostic
	CTD-ILD subtype (reference): outcome of progression
Lung epithelial cell dysfunction	
CA 125	CTD[168]: composite FVC and survival
CC16	SSc[169]: composite FVC and survival
CCL18	SSc[170]: FVC, D$_{LCO}$, and survival SSc[136]: FVC and radiologic progression
ICAM-1	SSc[134]: FVC
IGFBP-2	SSc[171]: D$_{LCO}$
KL-6	SSc[75]: FVC SSc[172]: composite FVC, oxygen supplementation, survival IIM[72]: survival SS[73]: survival CTD[74]: survival CTD[59]: HRCT progression
SP-D	CTD[168]: composite (lung function and survival) SSc[173]: FVC
Aberrant immunity	
CCL2	Ssc[174]: FVC, survival IIM[142]: survival
CX3CL1	SSc[143]: composite survival, FVC, and HRCT
CXCL10/IP-10	IIM[142]: survival
CXCL11	IIM[142]: survival
CXCL12	CTD[168]: composite FVC and survival
CXCL13	CTD[168]: composite FVC and survival
CXCL4	SSc[175]: FVC SSc[151]: D$_{LCO}$
IL-06	SSc[176]: FVC, D$_{LCO}$, survival IIM[177]: survival CTD[178]: survival
IL-08	IIM[147]: survival
IL-10	Ssc[174]: FVC IIM[179]: survival
IL-15	IIM[179]: survival IIM[180]: exacerbation, survival
Neopterin	IIM[181]: survival
Abnormal lung remodeling	
MMP-7	SSc[158]: survival IIM[159]: survival
YKL-40	CTD[168]: composite FVC and survival IIM[182]: survival IIM[183]: survival

experienced an FVC loss of 227 mL, which mirrored that of placebo-treated patients from IPF clinical trials[78,79] (**Fig. 1**). Prospective validation of these findings could result in a clinically actionable biomarker to inform clinical decision making in patients with CTD-ILD and other fibrosing ILDs.

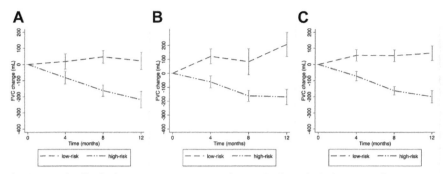

Fig. 1. Longitudinal plots comparing 1-year change in forced vital capacity between patients with high-risk and low-risk proteomic signature in the derivation (*A*), validation (*B*), and combined cohorts (*C*). (*Reprinted with permission from* Elsevier. The Lancet Respiratory Medicine, June 2022, 10 (6), 593-602.)

HIGH-RESOLUTION COMPUTED TOMOGRAPHY: CONNECTIVE TISSUE DISEASE-INTERSTITIAL LUNG DISEASE DIAGNOSIS AND PROGNOSIS

HRCT is a crucial component of the diagnostic evaluation of CTD-ILD, with thin slices and reconstruction algorithms tailored to the detection of patterns and distributions of interstitial, parenchymal, and airway abnormalities.[80,81] With the poor sensitivity of chest radiography [82,83] and PFT,[25,27] reliance on these measures to diagnose or rule out ILD in a patient with CTD is inadequate. An interdisciplinary expert consensus panel recently recommended that all patients with SSc be screened with HRCT at baseline, and the authors recommend a similar approach for all CTDs in which ILD commonly manifests. Major educational efforts have been undertaken to promote HRCT screening,[84,85] which will be critical to reduce the well-described diagnostic delays that occur in patients with ILD.[86,87]

With HRCT as our best tool for diagnosing ILD in patients with CTD, several groups have also investigated the role of HRCT as a predictor of CTD-ILD outcome. Extent of fibrotic disease on baseline HRCT, including the extent of reticulation, traction bronchiectasis, and honeycombing, is consistently associated with worse survival across CTD-ILD subtypes.[40,88–93] Walsh and colleagues[94] evaluated HRCTs and pulmonary function variables in 168 patients with CTD-ILD, and identified severity of traction bronchiectasis and extent of honeycombing as indices independently predictive of mortality. In patients with SSc-ILD, a higher extent of fibrosis on baseline HRCT was associated with subsequent lung function decline in the placebo group of the Scleroderma Lung Study.[95] A cutoff of 20% fibrotic extent has been proposed as an optimal predictor of mortality in patients with SSc-ILD, forming the basis of the Goh simple staging system for mortality risk.[96,97] It should be noted that by combining HRCT and PFTs in this staging system by using an FVC threshold when HRCT fibrotic extent was indeterminate, the risk prediction considerably improved beyond either HRCT or PFTs alone.

An additional question has been the role of the HRCT pattern of abnormality. There are many patterns described in CTD-ILD, with the 2 important patterns being that of nonspecific interstitial pneumonia (NSIP) and usual interstitial pneumonia (UIP).[98] The radiologic pattern of NSIP, characterized by bibasilar ground-glass opacities, is well recognized in patients with CTD-ILD, and is the most common pattern in patients with SSc-ILD and IIM-ILD.[99,100] In contrast, the radiologic pattern of UIP, with bibasilar reticulation and fibrotic architectural distortion, is most commonly observed among patients with RA-ILD.[40,101,102] The radiologic pattern of UIP is classically associated with IPF, the prototypic ILD characterized by poor prognosis, so naturally the question of whether UIP portends worse prognosis in the setting of non-IPF ILD arises. Several groups have found that a UIP pattern is associated with worse survival in patients with CTD-ILD.[40,88,94,103–106] In a cohort of patients with RA-ILD evaluated at National Jewish Health, Solomon and colleagues[107] also found that patients with UIP pattern had a shorter survival time than those with radiologic NSIP. However, in all multivariate Cox models that included key clinical variables or pulmonary physiology, baseline HRCT pattern was no longer a predictor of survival.[107] Rather, baseline FVC and evidence of FVC decline were independent predictors of worse survival. It remains unclear what additional information UIP pattern on HRCT provides, other than being a by-product of pulmonary fibrosis.

Although HRCT in cross-section may predict outcome, serial acquisition of HRCT may provide more clues about disease trajectory. Patients with SSc who had an increase in fibrotic extent on serial HRCT were more likely to experience further fibrotic progression and lung function decline[92]; this is congruent with our findings that worsening fibrosis extent on HRCT is a poor prognostic sign, with patients experiencing near-term FVC decline and a 2-fold increased risk of mortality after showing radiologic progression.[108,109] However, the radiation exposure of serial HRCT remains a consideration, especially among younger individuals with CTD-ILD, and in particular women due to radiation exposure to the breast tissue.

RADIOMICS AND QUANTITATIVE HIGH-RESOLUTION COMPUTED TOMOGRAPHY

The widespread use of visual HRCT assessment as biomarker in patients with CTD-ILD is currently limited due to low interobserver agreement.[110,111] Although semiquantitative scoring classifications have been proposed to judge the extent of fibrosis, discrepancy has been observed between radiologists' scoring, even after training.[97] Furthermore, the best studied candidate predictors of progression on HRCT—fibrotic extent and the UIP pattern—are both by-products of progressive pulmonary fibrosis. Tools that more effectively predict CTD-ILD progression before progression has occurred are more likely to be of clinical value.

One possible strategy to obviate interobserver variation is computer-based radiomic analysis. Radiomics is an emerging field that converts medical images into high-dimensional quantitative data and has high potential to serve as a novel avenue for ILD subphenotyping and outcome prediction. Quantification of HRCT features, density, and texture, along with algorithms developed by machine learning, has the potential to not only standardize the role of HRCT interpretation but also detect diagnostic and prognostic data not visually detectable by humans. Deep learning, which is a unique machine learning algorithm that incorporates multiple layers of learning architecture to create increasingly complex schema to improve autonomously, has emerged as a useful approach to modeling radiomic data.

In 2016, Anthimopoulos and colleagues[112] trained and tested a deep learning algorithm using HRCT examinations in 120 patients to detect ground-glass opacity, reticulation, consolidation, micronodules, and honeycombing, which had been manually labeled by 2 thoracic radiologists. This deep learning algorithm had an accuracy of 85% in classifying these imaging features. Using a similar approach, Kim and colleagues[113] employed a deep learning algorithm that achieved 95% accuracy for classifying these features of interest on HRCT images of patients with ILD. Advancing beyond individual HRCT features and toward HRCT pattern recognition, Walsh and colleagues[114] used a deep learning algorithm to detect classification of UIP based on the 2011 consensus guidelines. Their algorithm showed an accuracy of 76.4% for the classification of UIP in the derivation cohort, and an accuracy of 73.3% in an external validation cohort. Although promising, these investigations continue to rely on visual assessment as the gold standard, limiting their use to what can be detected by the human eye.

Evaluation of HRCT using density histogram analysis evaluates the lung according to simple density characteristics, deriving metrics of histogram skewness and kurtosis. Although Ash and colleagues[115] demonstrated a 3-fold increased risk of death or transplant in patients with IPF with higher mean lung density, the addition of quantitative HRCT density did not significantly augment prognostication beyond visual assessment of baseline lung fibrosis.[116] A more complex approach is texture-based analysis, which incorporates morphologic features. A quantitative lung fibrosis score can be generated using automated computer-aided diagnosis systems developed for assessing ILD using texture features. In patients with IPF, this texture-based score correlated with longitudinal FVC change, whereas HRCT density alone did not.[117] Kim and colleagues[118] applied this score to the HRCT examinations of 129 patients with SSc-ILD and showed good accuracy for detecting fibrosis when compared with visual assessment. Oh and colleagues[119] applied the quantitative lung fibrosis score to HRCT images of 144 patients with RA-ILD, and found that it predicted 5-year mortality. At a cutoff of 12% of total lung volume, higher quantitative lung fibrosis scores predicted survival similar to patients with IPF.[119] In addition, use of texture-based radiomic features in cluster analysis can predict different disease stages with moderate sensitivity and excellent specificity in patients with SSc-ILD.[120] In a recent study of 90 patients with SSc, texture-based radiomic features were extracted and cluster analysis performed to reveal 2 distinct patient clusters. Despite similar scores on the Goh simple staging system between clusters (based on visual assessment of HRCT and FVC), one texture-based radiomic cluster had significantly more impaired lung function. A radiomic risk score predicted faster disease progression and worse survival.[121]

For well over a decade, advances in CT scanner acquisition speed have led to the increase of volumetric HRCT scans, which can be acquired in a single breath-hold of 5 to 10 seconds, which bypasses the traditional issue of interspaced HRCT images with gaps of 1 cm or more between images, and allows for more precise evaluation of patterns such as honeycombing. Computer Aided Lung Informatics for Pathology Evaluation and Rating (CALIPER) is a tool that employs volumetric structural and textural analysis of the lung, trained to label and measure volumetric HRCT data as normal, ground glass, reticulation, low-attenuation, honeycombing, and vessel-related structures.[122] Jacob and colleagues[119] applied this tool in a study of 203 patients with CTD-ILD, with the CALIPER variable of vessel-related structure volume being the one most strongly associated with mortality (**Fig. 2**).[123] This same CALIPER variable has been shown to best predict mortality in patients with IPF.[122,124,125] Given that IPF mortality is worse than CTD-ILD mortality, Chung and colleagues[126] postulated that CALIPER may be able to differentiate CTD-ILD from IPF in the setting of a UIP pattern, finding that the vessel-related structure volume was greater in patients with IPF than patients with CTD-ILD, potentially showing its promise as a marker to differentiate CTD-ILD from IPF.[126]

CALIPER variables can be integrated into current classification schemes for prognosis in CTD-ILD. The CALIPER algorithm allows unbiased identification of CTD-ILD patient phenotypes using automated stratification. The substitution of this automated CALIPER model in place of pulmonary function variables in the ILD-GAP score, a validated staging score in ILD, resulted in a more sensitive predictor of 1- and 2-year

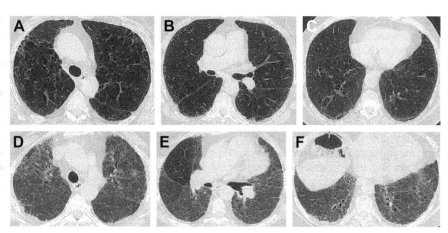

Fig. 2. Axial HRCT image color maps demonstrating CALIPER-derived vessel-related structures (VRS; red). VRS represent pulmonary arteries and veins (excluding hilar vessels) and connected tubular structures, the latter primarily reflecting adjoining regions of fibrosis. (A–C) Axial sections in a 71-year-old female 30-pack-year exsmoker with upper lobe emphysema and fibrosis visible in the lower lobes (VRS 2.1%); (D–F) axial sections in a 62-year-old female never smoker with upper lobe-predominant fibrosis (VRS 7.0%). Nonvascular region captures in the VRS signal are visible in the upper lobes (D) and adjacent to the right hemidiaphragm (F). (Reproduced with permission of the © ERS 2024: European Respiratory Journal 53 (1) 1800869; https://doi.org/10.1183/13993003.00869-2018 Published 3 January 2019.)

mortality.[123] In addition, Jacob and colleagues[127] conducted a study of 157 patients with RA-ILD to compare 3 prediction models based on HRCT: the Goh scleroderma simple staging system, the Fleischner Society IPF diagnostic guidelines, and CALIPER scores of vessel-related structures. Although all 3 models strongly predicted outcome, combining the CALIPER vessel-related structures threshold with the visual scoring from the Goh and Fleischner systems improved outcome modeling, predicting 4-year survival indistinguishable from a comparator group of patients with IPF.[127]

Although early, these studies are promising and suggest that radiomics has high potential to inform clinical decision making once widespread automation of one or more of these algorithms becomes possible. With machine learning, data extracted from quantitative HRCT carries the potential to develop new imaging biomarkers not discernible by humans and bypass the inherent problems of visual assessment. Radiomics is likely to provide complementary diagnostic and prognostic information with exciting potential for outcome prediction.

UNMET RESEARCH NEEDS AND STRATEGIES FOR BIOMARKER OPTIMIZATION

Although there has been impressive progress in biomarker discovery, unmet needs remain. At present, there are few biomarkers reliably predicting the presence of ILD in patients with CTD, and even fewer have been validated to predict CTD-ILD progression before it occurs. Although we reviewed emerging blood-based and HRCT biomarkers, none have been incorporated into clinical practice, reflecting modest test performance characteristics for most; this stems in large part from a paucity of validation testing for most biomarkers, because most candidate studies have been performed in retrospective single-center studies. Validation of these promising biomarkers in external cohorts will be key in biomarker investigation going forward. Equally important will be the assessment of test performance characteristics, which will allow clinicians to weigh the clinical utility of any biomarker advanced for clinical implementation. Furthermore, before clinical application, it will be essential that well-designed, prospective, multicenter studies be conducted.

As multicohort investigations become standard in biomarker investigation, it will be essential to ensure that the outcomes chosen in future studies are uniform and well-defined, particularly in studies of prognostic biomarkers. Understandably, survival should remain to be an important outcome. However, near-term progression should also be prioritized in future biomarker investigation. Near-term lung function decline has clinical implications, because patients may necessitate earlier intervention, as well as implications for drug development in clinical trials. At present, large sample sizes are required to ensure adequate power to detect differences in lung function decline, so the ability to predict near-term progression would allow clinical trial enrichment and more efficient recruitment.

Last, there is increased potential when modeling biomarkers in aggregate. The combination of multiple biomarkers across multiple modalities, perhaps combining clinical, blood-based, and radiomic biomarkers, holds high potential in CTD-ILD risk prediction. Machine learning can seamlessly tackle increasingly large datasets and the rapidly growing number of candidate biomarkers. After deriving and validating candidate signatures retrospectively, it will be necessary to quantify identified biomarkers and to prospectively validate specific thresholds that define individual risk most precisely.

SUMMARY

A number of biomarkers have been proved to be informative in patients with CTD-ILD, derived from blood-based and HRCT data. The development of large blood-based platforms, the refinement of radiomic algorithms, and the use of machine learning have shown early promise in the diagnosis and prognosis of CTD-ILD. A rapid expansion of investigation with aggregate biomarkers is expected in the coming years, making precision medicine closer to reality and improving outcomes in patients with CTD-ILD.

CLINICS CARE POINTS

- HRCT is the screening and diagnostic tool of choice for patients with CTDs. When screening for ILD, PFT and chest radiography are insufficient and an HRCT should be ordered.

- There are no single blood-based biomarkers validated for the diagnosis or prognosis of CTD-associated ILD. When caring for patients with CTD-ILD, making clinical decisions based on single laboratory tests should be avoided.

- The best prognostic radiographic markers are extent of fibrosis and evidence of progression on serial HRCT. When a patient has a large extent of fibrosis or shows worsening fibrosis on HRCT, the likelihood of future ILD progression is high.

FUNDING

NHLBI T32 HL007749 (Pugashetti).

REFERENCES

1. Juge PA, Lee JS, Ebstein E, et al. MUC5B Promoter Variant and Rheumatoid Arthritis with Interstitial Lung Disease. N Engl J Med 2018;379(23):2209–19.

2. Gabbay E, Tarala R, Will R, et al. Interstitial lung disease in recent onset rheumatoid arthritis. Am J Respir Crit Care Med 1997;156(2 Pt 1):528–35.
3. Walker UA, Tyndall A, Czirjak L, et al. Clinical risk assessment of organ manifestations in systemic sclerosis: a report from the EULAR Scleroderma Trials And Research group database. Ann Rheum Dis 2007;66(6):754–63.
4. Fathi M, Dastmalchi M, Rasmussen E, et al. Interstitial lung disease, a common manifestation of newly diagnosed polymyositis and dermatomyositis. Ann Rheum Dis 2004;63(3):297–301.
5. Reiseter S, Gunnarsson R, Mogens Aalokken T, et al. Progression and mortality of interstitial lung disease in mixed connective tissue disease: a long-term observational nationwide cohort study. Rheumatology (Oxford) 2018;57(2): 255–62.
6. Flament T, Bigot A, Chaigne B, et al. Pulmonary manifestations of Sjogren's syndrome. Eur Respir Rev 2016;25(140):110–23.
7. Castelino FV, Varga J. Interstitial lung disease in connective tissue diseases: evolving concepts of pathogenesis and management. Arthritis Res Ther 2010; 12(4):213.
8. Flaherty KR, Wells AU, Cottin V, et al. Nintedanib in Progressive Fibrosing Interstitial Lung Diseases. The New Engl J Med 2019. https://doi.org/10.1056/NEJMoa1908681.
9. Cottin V, Wollin L, Fischer A, et al. Fibrosing interstitial lung diseases: knowns and unknowns. Eur Respir Rev 2019;28(151). https://doi.org/10.1183/16000617.0100-2018.
10. Adegunsoye A, Oldham JM, Bellam SK, et al. Computed Tomography Honeycombing Identifies a Progressive Fibrotic Phenotype with Increased Mortality across Diverse Interstitial Lung Diseases. Ann Am Thorac Soc 2019;16(5): 580–8.
11. Tashkin DP, Elashoff R, Clements PJ, et al. Cyclophosphamide versus placebo in scleroderma lung disease. N Engl J Med 2006;354(25):2655–66.
12. Tashkin DP, Roth MD, Clements PJ, et al. Mycophenolate mofetil versus oral cyclophosphamide in scleroderma-related interstitial lung disease (SLS II): a randomised controlled, double-blind, parallel group trial. Lancet Respir Med 2016;4(9):708–19.
13. Fischer A, Brown KK, Du Bois RM, et al. Mycophenolate mofetil improves lung function in connective tissue disease-associated interstitial lung disease. J Rheumatol 2013;40(5):640–6.
14. Oldham JM, Lee C, Valenzi E, et al. Azathioprine response in patients with fibrotic connective tissue disease-associated interstitial lung disease. Respir Med 2016;121:117–22.
15. Huapaya JA, Silhan L, Pinal-Fernandez I, et al. Long-Term Treatment With Azathioprine and Mycophenolate Mofetil for Myositis-Related Interstitial Lung Disease. Chest 2019;156(5):896–906.
16. Sharma N, Putman MS, Vij R, et al. Myositis-associated Interstitial Lung Disease: Predictors of Failure of Conventional Treatment and Response to Tacrolimus in a US Cohort. J Rheumatol 2017;44(11):1612–8.
17. Witt LJ, Demchuk C, Curran JJ, et al. Benefit of adjunctive tacrolimus in connective tissue disease-interstitial lung disease. Pulm Pharmacol Ther 2016;36: 46–52.
18. Duarte AC, Cordeiro A, Fernandes BM, et al. Rituximab in connective tissue disease-associated interstitial lung disease. Clin Rheumatol 2019;38(7):2001–9.

19. Keir GJ, Maher TM, Hansell DM, et al. Severe interstitial lung disease in connective tissue disease: rituximab as rescue therapy. Eur Respir J 2012;40(3):641–8.

20. Koduri G, Norton S, Young A, et al. Interstitial lung disease has a poor prognosis in rheumatoid arthritis: results from an inception cohort. Rheumatology (Oxford) 2010;49(8):1483–9.

21. Steen VD, Medsger TA. Changes in causes of death in systemic sclerosis, 1972–2002. Ann Rheum Dis 2007;66(7):940–4.

22. Khanna D, Lin CJF, Furst DE, et al. Tocilizumab in systemic sclerosis: a randomised, double-blind, placebo-controlled, phase 3 trial. The Lancet Respir Med 2020;8(10):963–74.

23. Tashkin DP, Elashoff R, Clements PJ, et al. Cyclophosphamide versus placebo in scleroderma lung disease. The New Engl J Med 2006;354(25):2655–66.

24. Tashkin DP, Roth MD, Clements PJ, et al. Mycophenolate mofetil versus oral cyclophosphamide in scleroderma-related interstitial lung disease (SLS II): a randomised controlled, double-blind, parallel group trial. Lancet Respir Med 2016;4(9):708–19.

25. Pugashetti JV, Kitich A, Alqalyoobi S, et al. Derivation and Validation of a Diagnostic Prediction Tool for Interstitial Lung Disease. Chest 2020. https://doi.org/10.1016/j.chest.2020.02.044.

26. Bilgici A, Ulusoy H, Kuru O, et al. Pulmonary involvement in rheumatoid arthritis. Rheumatol Int 2005;25(6):429–35.

27. Suliman YA, Dobrota R, Huscher D, et al. Brief Report: Pulmonary Function Tests: High Rate of False-Negative Results in the Early Detection and Screening of Scleroderma-Related Interstitial Lung Disease. Arthritis Rheumatol 2015; 67(12):3256–61.

28. Wu AC, Kiley JP, Noel PJ, et al. Current Status and Future Opportunities in Lung Precision Medicine Research with a Focus on Biomarkers. An American Thoracic Society/National Heart, Lung, and Blood Institute Research Statement. Am J Respir Crit Care Med 2018;198(12):e116–36.

29. Reveille JD, Solomon DH. American College of Rheumatology Ad Hoc Committee of Immunologic Testing G. Evidence-based guidelines for the use of immunologic tests: anticentromere, Scl-70, and nucleolar antibodies. Arthritis Rheum 2003;49(3):399–412.

30. Nihtyanova SI, Schreiber BE, Ong VH, et al. Prediction of Pulmonary Complications and Long-Term Survival in Systemic Sclerosis. Arthritis Rheumatol 2014; 66(6):1625–35.

31. Jandali B, Salazar GA, Hudson M, et al. The Effect of Anti-Scl -70 Antibody Determination Method on Its Predictive Significance for Interstitial Lung Disease Progression in Systemic Sclerosis. ACR Open Rheumatol 2022;4(4):345–51.

32. Walker UA, Tyndall A, Czirjak L, et al. Clinical risk assessment of organ manifestations in systemic sclerosis: a report from the EULAR Scleroderma Trials And Research group database. Ann Rheum Dis 2007;66(6):754–63.

33. Liaskos C, Marou E, Simopoulou T, et al. Disease-related autoantibody profile in patients with systemic sclerosis. Autoimmunity 2017;50(7):414–21.

34. Mitri GM, Lucas M, Fertig N, et al. A comparison between anti-Th/To- and anti-centromere antibody-positive systemic sclerosis patients with limited cutaneous involvement. Arthritis Rheum 2003;48(1):203–9.

35. Lazzaroni M-G, Marasco E, Campochiaro C, et al. The clinical phenotype of systemic sclerosis patients with anti-PM/Scl antibodies: results from the EUSTAR cohort. Rheumatology 2021;60(11):5028–41.

36. Hudson M, Pope J, Mahler M, et al. Clinical significance of antibodies to Ro52/TRIM21 in systemic sclerosis. Arthritis Res Ther 2012;14(2):R50.
37. Mierau R, Moinzadeh P, Riemekasten G, et al. Frequency of disease-associated and other nuclear autoantibodies in patients of the German network for systemic scleroderma: correlation with characteristic clinical features. Arthritis Res Ther 2011;13(5):R172.
38. Wangkaew S, Euathrongchit J, Wattanawittawas P, et al. Incidence and predictors of interstitial lung disease (ILD) in Thai patients with early systemic sclerosis: Inception cohort study. Mod Rheumatol 2016;26(4):588–93.
39. Kamiya H, Panlaqui OM. Systematic review and meta-analysis of the risk of rheumatoid arthritis-associated interstitial lung disease related to anti-cyclic citrullinated peptide (CCP) antibody. BMJ Open 2021;11(3):e040465.
40. Kelly CA, Saravanan V, Nisar M, et al. Rheumatoid arthritis-related interstitial lung disease: associations, prognostic factors and physiological and radiological characteristics–a large multicentre UK study. Rheumatology (Oxford) 2014;53(9):1676–82.
41. Doyle TJ, Patel AS, Hatabu H, et al. Detection of Rheumatoid Arthritis–Interstitial Lung Disease Is Enhanced by Serum Biomarkers. Am J Respir Crit Care Med 2015;191(12):1403–12.
42. Giles JT, Danoff SK, Sokolove J, et al. Association of fine specificity and repertoire expansion of anticitrullinated peptide antibodies with rheumatoid arthritis associated interstitial lung disease. Ann Rheum Dis 2014;73(8):1487–94.
43. Richards TJ, Eggebeen A, Gibson K, et al. Characterization and peripheral blood biomarker assessment of anti-Jo-1 antibody-positive interstitial lung disease. Arthritis Rheum 2009;60(7):2183–92.
44. Marie I, Josse S, Decaux O, et al. Comparison of long-term outcome between anti-Jo1- and anti-PL7/PL12 positive patients with antisynthetase syndrome. Autoimmun Rev 2012;11(10):739–45.
45. Sato S, Hirakata M, Kuwana M, et al. Autoantibodies to a 140-kd polypeptide, CADM-140, in Japanese patients with clinically amyopathic dermatomyositis. Arthritis Rheum 2005;52(5):1571–6.
46. Tsuji H, Nakashima R, Hosono Y, et al. Multicenter Prospective Study of the Efficacy and Safety of Combined Immunosuppressive Therapy With High-Dose Glucocorticoid, Tacrolimus, and Cyclophosphamide in Interstitial Lung Diseases Accompanied by Anti–Melanoma Differentiation–Associated Gene 5–Pos. Arthritis Rheumatol 2020;72(3):488–98.
47. Hamaguchi Y, Kuwana M, Hoshino K, et al. Clinical Correlations With Dermatomyositis-Specific Autoantibodies in Adult Japanese Patients With Dermatomyositis. Arch Dermatol 2011;147(4):391.
48. Koga T, Fujikawa K, Horai Y, et al. The diagnostic utility of anti-melanoma differentiation-associated gene 5 antibody testing for predicting the prognosis of Japanese patients with DM. Rheumatology (Oxford) 2012;51(7):1278–84.
49. Fiorentino D, Chung L, Zwerner J, et al. The mucocutaneous and systemic phenotype of dermatomyositis patients with antibodies to MDA5 (CADM-140): A retrospective study. J Am Acad Dermatol 2011;65(1):25–34.
50. Hall JC, Casciola-Rosen L, Samedy L-A, et al. Anti-Melanoma Differentiation-Associated Protein 5-Associated Dermatomyositis: Expanding the Clinical Spectrum. Arthritis Care Res 2013;65(8):1307–15.
51. Ishikawa N, Hattori N, Yokoyama A, et al. Utility of KL-6/MUC1 in the clinical management of interstitial lung diseases. Respir Investig 2012;50(1):3–13.

52. Asano Y, Ihn H, Yamane K, et al. Clinical significance of surfactant protein D as a serum marker for evaluating pulmonary fibrosis in patients with systemic sclerosis. Arthritis Rheum 2001;44(6):1363–9.
53. Hant FN, Ludwicka-Bradley A, Wang H-J, et al. Surfactant Protein D and KL-6 as Serum Biomarkers of Interstitial Lung Disease in Patients with Scleroderma. The J Rheumatol 2009;36(4):773–80.
54. Hasegawa M, Fujimoto M, Hamaguchi Y, et al. Use of Serum Clara Cell 16-kDa (CC16) Levels as a Potential Indicator of Active Pulmonary Fibrosis in Systemic Sclerosis. The J Rheumatol 2011;38(5):877–84.
55. Fotoh DS, Helal A, Rizk MS, et al. Serum Krebs von den Lungen-6 and lung ultrasound B lines as potential diagnostic and prognostic factors for rheumatoid arthritis–associated interstitial lung disease. Clin Rheumatol 2021;40(7):2689–97.
56. Zheng M, Lou A, Zhang H, et al. Serum KL-6, CA19-9, CA125 and CEA are Diagnostic Biomarkers for Rheumatoid Arthritis-Associated Interstitial Lung Disease in the Chinese Population. Rheumatol Ther 2021;8(1):517–27.
57. Qin Y, Wang Y, Meng F, et al. Identification of biomarkers by machine learning classifiers to assist diagnose rheumatoid arthritis-associated interstitial lung disease. Arthritis Res Ther 2022;24(1). https://doi.org/10.1186/s13075-022-02800-2.
58. Takanashi S, Nishina N, Nakazawa M, et al. Usefulness of serum Krebs von den Lungen-6 for the management of myositis-associated interstitial lung disease. Rheumatology 2019;58(6):1034–9.
59. Lee JS, Lee EY, Ha Y-J, et al. Serum KL-6 levels reflect the severity of interstitial lung disease associated with connective tissue disease. Arthritis Res Ther 2019;21(1). https://doi.org/10.1186/s13075-019-1835-9.
60. Fathi M, Barbasso Helmers S, Lundberg IE. KL-6: a serological biomarker for interstitial lung disease in patients with polymyositis and dermatomyositis. J Intern Med 2012;271(6):589–97.
61. Hasegawa M, Fujimoto M, Matsushita T, et al. Serum chemokine and cytokine levels as indicators of disease activity in patients with systemic sclerosis. Clin Rheumatol 2011;30(2):231–7.
62. Chen F, Lu X, Shu X, et al. Predictive value of serum markers for the development of interstitial lung disease in patients with polymyositis and dermatomyositis: a comparative and prospective study. Intern Med J 2015;45(6):641–7.
63. Takahashi H, Kuroki Y, Tanaka H, et al. Serum levels of surfactant proteins A and D are useful biomarkers for interstitial lung disease in patients with progressive systemic sclerosis. Am J Respir Crit Care Med 2000;162(1):258–63.
64. Yang H. Cytokine expression in patients with interstitial lung disease in primary Sjogren's syndrome and its clinical significance. Am J Transl Res 2021;13(7):8391–6.
65. Yu M, Guo Y, Zhang P, et al. Increased circulating Wnt5a protein in patients with rheumatoid arthritis-associated interstitial pneumonia (RA-ILD). Immunobiology 2019;224(4):551–9.
66. Maher TM, Nambiar AM, Wells AU. The role of precision medicine in interstitial lung disease. Eur Respir J 2022;60(3):2102146.
67. Kass DJ, Nouraie M, Glassberg MK, et al. Comparative Profiling of Serum Protein Biomarkers in Rheumatoid Arthritis-Associated Interstitial Lung Disease and Idiopathic Pulmonary Fibrosis. Arthritis Rheumatol 2020;72(3):409–19.
68. Raghu G, Remy-Jardin M, Richeldi L, et al. Idiopathic Pulmonary Fibrosis (an Update) and Progressive Pulmonary Fibrosis in Adults: An Official ATS/ERS/

JRS/ALAT Clinical Practice Guideline. Am J Respir Crit Care Med 2022;205(9): e18–47.

69. Guillen-Del Castillo A, Pilar Simeon-Aznar C, Fonollosa-Pla V, et al. Good outcome of interstitial lung disease in patients with scleroderma associated to anti-PM/Scl antibody. Semin Arthritis Rheum 2014;44(3):331–7.

70. Xu A, Ye Y, Fu Q, et al. Prognostic values of anti-Ro52 antibodies in anti-MDA5-positive clinically amyopathic dermatomyositis associated with interstitial lung disease. Rheumatology (Oxford) 2021;60(7):3343–51.

71. Bauhammer J, Blank N, Max R, et al. Rituximab in the Treatment of Jo1 Antibody-associated Antisynthetase Syndrome: Anti-Ro52 Positivity as a Marker for Severity and Treatment Response. J Rheumatol 2016;43(8):1566–74.

72. Arai S, Kurasawa K, Maezawa R, et al. Marked increase in serum KL-6 and surfactant protein D levels during the first 4 weeks after treatment predicts poor prognosis in patients with active interstitial pneumonia associated with polymyositis/dermatomyositis. Mod Rheumatol 2013;23(5):872–83.

73. Kamiya Y, Fujisawa T, Kono M, et al. Prognostic factors for primary Sjögren's syndrome-associated interstitial lung diseases. Respir Med 2019;159:105811.

74. Satoh H, Kurishima K, Ishikawa H, et al. Increased levels of KL-6 and subsequent mortality in patients with interstitial lung diseases. J Intern Med 2006; 260(5):429–34.

75. Salazar GA, Kuwana M, Wu M, et al. KL-6 But Not CCL-18 Is a Predictor of Early Progression in Systemic Sclerosis-related Interstitial Lung Disease. The J Rheumatol 2018;45(8):1153–8.

76. Gono T, Masui K, Nishina N, et al. Risk Prediction Modeling Based on a Combination of Initial Serum Biomarker Levels in Polymyositis/Dermatomyositis–Associated Interstitial Lung Disease. Arthritis Rheumatol 2021;73(4):677–86.

77. Bowman WS, Newton CA, Linderholm AL, et al. Proteomic biomarkers of progressive fibrosing interstitial lung disease: a multicentre cohort analysis. Lancet Respir Med 2022. https://doi.org/10.1016/S2213-2600(21)00503-8.

78. Noble PW, Albera C, Bradford WZ, et al. Pirfenidone in patients with idiopathic pulmonary fibrosis (CAPACITY): two randomised trials. Comparative Study Multicenter Study Randomized Controlled Trial Research Support. Non-U.S Gov't *Lancet* 2011;377(9779):1760–9.

79. Richeldi L, Du Bois RM, Raghu G, et al. Efficacy and Safety of Nintedanib in Idiopathic Pulmonary Fibrosis. New Engl J Med 2014;370(22):2071–82.

80. Mayo JR. CT evaluation of diffuse infiltrative lung disease: dose considerations and optimal technique. J Thorac Imaging 2009;24(4):252–9.

81. Kazerooni EA. High-resolution CT of the lungs. AJR Am J Roentgenol 2001; 177(3):501–19.

82. Ghodrati S, Pugashetti JV, Kadoch MA, et al. Diagnostic Accuracy of Chest Radiography for Detecting Fibrotic Interstitial Lung Disease. Ann Am Thorac Soc 2022. https://doi.org/10.1513/AnnalsATS.202112-1377RL.

83. Schurawitzki H, Stiglbauer R, Graninger W, et al. Interstitial lung disease in progressive systemic sclerosis: high-resolution CT versus radiography. Radiology 1990;176(3):755–9. https://doi.org/10.1148/radiology.176.3.2389033.

84. Hoffmann-Vold A-M, Maher TM, Philpot EE, et al. The identification and management of interstitial lung disease in systemic sclerosis: evidence-based European consensus statements. Lancet Rheumatol 2020;2(2):e71–83. https://doi.org/10.1016/s2665-9913(19)30144-4.

85. Bruni C, Chung L, Hoffmann-Vold AM, et al. High-resolution computed tomography of the chest for the screening, re-screening and follow-up of systemic

sclerosis-associated interstitial lung disease: a EUSTAR-SCTC survey. Clin Exp Rheumatol 2022. https://doi.org/10.55563/clinexprheumatol/7ry6zz.

86. Pritchard D, Adegunsoye A, Lafond E, et al. Diagnostic test interpretation and referral delay in patients with interstitial lung disease. Respir Res 2019;20(1): 253. https://doi.org/10.1186/s12931-019-1228-2.

87. Cano-Jiménez E, Vázquez Rodríguez T, Martín-Robles I, et al. Diagnostic delay of associated interstitial lung disease increases mortality in rheumatoid arthritis. Scientific Rep 2021;11(1). https://doi.org/10.1038/s41598-021-88734-2.

88. Kim EJ, Elicker BM, Maldonado F, et al. Usual interstitial pneumonia in rheumatoid arthritis-associated interstitial lung disease. Eur Respir J 2010;35(6): 1322–8.

89. Nurmi HM, Kettunen H-P, Suoranta S-K, et al. Several high-resolution computed tomography findings associate with survival and clinical features in rheumatoid arthritis-associated interstitial lung disease. Respir Med 2018;134:24–30.

90. Yamakawa H, Sato S, Tsumiyama E, et al. Predictive factors of mortality in rheumatoid arthritis-associated interstitial lung disease analysed by modified HRCT classification of idiopathic pulmonary fibrosis according to the 2018 ATS/ERS/JRS/ALAT criteria. J Thorac Dis 2019;11(12):5247–57.

91. Winstone TA, Assayag D, Wilcox PG, et al. Predictors of mortality and progression in scleroderma-associated interstitial lung disease: a systematic review. Chest 2014;146(2):422–36.

92. Hoffmann-Vold A-M, Aaløkken TM, Lund MB, et al. Predictive Value of Serial High-Resolution Computed Tomography Analyses and Concurrent Lung Function Tests in Systemic Sclerosis. Arthritis Rheumatol 2015;67(8):2205–12.

93. Kocheril SV, Appleton BE, Somers EC, et al. Comparison of disease progression and mortality of connective tissue disease-related interstitial lung disease and idiopathic interstitial pneumonia. Arthritis Rheum 2005;53(4):549–57.

94. Walsh SLF, Sverzellati N, Devaraj A, et al. Connective tissue disease related fibrotic lung disease: high resolution computed tomographic and pulmonary function indices as prognostic determinants. Thorax 2014;69(3):216–22.

95. Khanna D, Tseng C-H, Farmani N, et al. Clinical course of lung physiology in patients with scleroderma and interstitial lung disease: Analysis of the Scleroderma Lung Study Placebo Group. Arthritis Rheum 2011;63(10):3078–85.

96. Moore OA, Goh N, Corte T, et al. Extent of disease on high-resolution computed tomography lung is a predictor of decline and mortality in systemic sclerosis-related interstitial lung disease. Rheumatology 2013;52(1):155–60.

97. Goh NS, Desai SR, Veeraraghavan S, et al. Interstitial lung disease in systemic sclerosis: a simple staging system. Am J Respir Crit Care Med 2008;177(11): 1248–54.

98. Raghu G, Remy-Jardin M, Myers JL, et al. Diagnosis of Idiopathic Pulmonary Fibrosis. An Official ATS/ERS/JRS/ALAT Clinical Practice Guideline. Am J Respir Crit Care Med 2018;198(5):e44–68.

99. Desai SR, Veeraraghavan S, Hansell DM, et al. CT features of lung disease in patients with systemic sclerosis: comparison with idiopathic pulmonary fibrosis and nonspecific interstitial pneumonia. Radiology 2004;232(2):560–7.

100. Travis WD, Costabel U, Hansell DM, et al. An official American Thoracic Society/European Respiratory Society statement: Update of the international multidisciplinary classification of the idiopathic interstitial pneumonias. Am J Respir Crit Care Med 2013;188(6):733–48.

101. Bendstrup E, Moller J, Kronborg-White S, et al. Interstitial Lung Disease in Rheumatoid Arthritis Remains a Challenge for Clinicians. J Clin Med 2019;8(12). https://doi.org/10.3390/jcm8122038.

102. Tanaka N, Kim JS, Newell JD, et al. Rheumatoid arthritis-related lung diseases: CT findings. Radiology 2004;232(1):81–91.

103. Assayag D, Lubin M, Lee JS, et al. Predictors of mortality in rheumatoid arthritis-related interstitial lung disease. Respirology 2014;19(4):493–500.

104. Liu H, Xie S, Liang T, et al. Prognostic factors of interstitial lung disease progression at sequential HRCT in anti-synthetase syndrome. Eur Radiol 2019;29(10): 5349–57.

105. Maillet T, Goletto T, Beltramo G, et al. Usual interstitial pneumonia in ANCA-associated vasculitis: A poor prognostic factor. J Autoimmun 2020;106: 102338. https://doi.org/10.1016/j.jaut.2019.102338.

106. Kim HC, Lee JS, Lee EY, et al. Risk prediction model in rheumatoid arthritis-associated interstitial lung disease. Respirology 2020;25(12):1257–64.

107. Solomon JJ, Chung JH, Cosgrove GP, et al. Predictors of mortality in rheumatoid arthritis-associated interstitial lung disease. Eur Respir J 2016;47(2):588–96.

108. Pugashetti JV, Adegunsoye A, Wu Z, et al. Validation of Proposed Criteria for Progressive Pulmonary Fibrosis. Am J Respir Crit Care Med 2023;207(1):69–76.

109. Oldham JM, Lee CT, Wu Z, et al. Lung function trajectory in progressive fibrosing interstitial lung disease. Eur Respir J 2021. https://doi.org/10.1183/13993003. 01396-2021.

110. Watadani T, Sakai F, Johkoh T, et al. Interobserver variability in the CT assessment of honeycombing in the lungs. Radiology 2013;266(3):936–44.

111. Nathan SD, Pastre J, Ksovreli I, et al. HRCT evaluation of patients with interstitial lung disease: comparison of the 2018 and 2011 diagnostic guidelines. Ther Adv Respir Dis 2020;14. 175346662096849.

112. Anthimopoulos M, Christodoulidis S, Ebner L, et al. Lung Pattern Classification for Interstitial Lung Diseases Using a Deep Convolutional Neural Network. IEEE Trans Med Imaging 2016;35(5):1207–16.

113. Kim GB, Jung K-H, Lee Y, et al. Comparison of Shallow and Deep Learning Methods on Classifying the Regional Pattern of Diffuse Lung Disease. J Digital Imaging 2018;31(4):415–24.

114. Walsh SLF, Calandriello L, Silva M, et al. Deep learning for classifying fibrotic lung disease on high-resolution computed tomography: a case-cohort study. Lancet Respir Med 2018;6(11):837–45.

115. Ash SY, Harmouche R, Vallejo DLL, et al. Densitometric and local histogram based analysis of computed tomography images in patients with idiopathic pulmonary fibrosis. Respir Res 2017;18(1). https://doi.org/10.1186/s12931-017-0527-8.

116. Best AC, Meng J, Lynch AM, et al. Idiopathic pulmonary fibrosis: physiologic tests, quantitative CT indexes, and CT visual scores as predictors of mortality. Radiology 2008;246(3):935–40.

117. Kim HJ, Brown MS, Chong D, et al. Comparison of the quantitative CT imaging biomarkers of idiopathic pulmonary fibrosis at baseline and early change with an interval of 7 months. Acad Radiol 2015;22(1):70–80.

118. Kim HG, Tashkin DP, Clements PJ, et al. A computer-aided diagnosis system for quantitative scoring of extent of lung fibrosis in scleroderma patients. Clin Exp Rheumatol 2010;28(5 Suppl 62):S26–35.

119. Oh JH, Kim GHJ, Cross G, et al. Automated quantification system predicts survival in rheumatoid arthritis-associated interstitial lung disease. Rheumatology (Oxford) 2022. https://doi.org/10.1093/rheumatology/keac184.

120. Martini K, Baessler B, Bogowicz M, et al. Applicability of radiomics in interstitia lung disease associated with systemic sclerosis: proof of concept. Eur Radio 2021;31(4):1987–98.

121. Schniering J, Maciukiewicz M, Gabrys HS, et al. Computed tomography-based radiomics decodes prognostic and molecular differences in interstitial lung disease related to systemic sclerosis. Eur Respir J 2022;59(5):2004503.

122. Jacob J, Bartholmai BJ, Rajagopalan S, et al. Automated Quantitative Computed Tomography Versus Visual Computed Tomography Scoring in Idiopathic Pulmonary Fibrosis: Validation Against Pulmonary Function. J Thorac Imaging 2016;31(5):304–11.

123. Jacob J, Bartholmai BJ, Rajagopalan S, et al. Evaluation of computer-based computer tomography stratification against outcome models in connective tissue disease-related interstitial lung disease: a patient outcome study. BMC Med 2016-12-01 2016;14(1). https://doi.org/10.1186/s12916-016-0739-7.

124. Jacob J, Bartholmai BJ, Rajagopalan S, et al. Mortality prediction in idiopathic pulmonary fibrosis: evaluation of computer-based CT analysis with conventional severity measures. Eur Respir J 2017;49(1):1601011.

125. Jacob J, Bartholmai BJ, Rajagopalan S, et al. Predicting Outcomes in Idiopathic Pulmonary Fibrosis Using Automated Computed Tomographic Analysis. Am J Respir Crit Care Med 2018;198(6):767–76.

126. Chung JH, Adegunsoye A, Cannon B, et al. Differentiation of Idiopathic Pulmonary Fibrosis from Connective Tissue Disease-Related Interstitial Lung Disease Using Quantitative Imaging. J Clin Med 2021;10(12):2663.

127. Jacob J, Hirani N, Van Moorsel CHM, et al. Predicting outcomes in rheumatoid arthritis related interstitial lung disease. Eur Respir J 2019;53(1):1800869.

128. Wang T, Zheng XJ, Ji YL, et al. Tumour markers in rheumatoid arthritis-associated interstitial lung disease. Clin Exp Rheumatol 2016;34(4):587–91.

129. Prasse A, Pechkovsky DV, Toews GB, et al. CCL18 as an indicator of pulmonary fibrotic activity in idiopathic interstitial pneumonias and systemic sclerosis. Arthritis Rheum 2007;56(5):1685–93.

130. Kuryliszyn-Moskal A, Klimiuk PA, Sierakowski S. Soluble adhesion molecules (sVCAM-1, sE-selectin), vascular endothelial growth factor (VEGF) and endothelin-1 in patients with systemic sclerosis: relationship to organ systemic involvement. Clin Rheumatol 2005;24(2):111–6.

131. Ihn H, Sato S, Fujimoto M, et al. Increased serum levels of soluble vascular cell adhesion molecule-1 and E-selectin in patients with systemic sclerosis. Br J Rheumatol 1998;37(11):1188–92.

132. Ates A, Kinikli G, Turgay M, et al. Serum-Soluble Selectin Levels in Patients with Rheumatoid Arthritis and Systemic Sclerosis. Scand J Immunol 2004;59(3):315–20.

133. Kumanovics G, Minier T, Radics J, et al. Comprehensive investigation of novel serum markers of pulmonary fibrosis associated with systemic sclerosis and dermato/polymyositis. Clin Exp Rheumatol 2008;26(3):414–20.

134. Hasegawa M, Asano Y, Endo H, et al. Serum Adhesion Molecule Levels as Prognostic Markers in Patients with Early Systemic Sclerosis: A Multicentre, Prospective, Observational Study. PLoS ONE 2014;9(2):e88150.

135. Kodera M, Hasegawa M, Komura K, et al. Serum pulmonary and activation-regulated chemokine/CCL18 levels in patients with systemic sclerosis: A sensitive indicator of active pulmonary fibrosis. Arthritis Rheum 2005;52(9):2889–96.
136. Elhai M, Hoffmann-Vold AM, Avouac J, et al. Performance of Candidate Serum Biomarkers for Systemic Sclerosis–Associated Interstitial Lung Disease. Arthritis Rheumatol 2019;71(6):972–82.
137. Moon J, Lee JS, Yoon YI, et al. Association of Serum Biomarkers With Pulmonary Involvement of Rheumatoid Arthritis Interstitial Lung Disease: From KORAIL Cohort Baseline Data. J Rheum Dis 2021;28(4):234–41.
138. Bandoh S. Sequential changes of KL-6 in sera of patients with interstitial pneumonia associated with polymyositis/dermatomyositis. Ann Rheum Dis 2000;59(4):257–62.
139. Kubo M, Ihn H, Yamane K, et al. Serum KL-6 in adult patients with polymyositis and dermatomyositis. Rheumatology 2000;39(6):632–6.
140. Wang Y, Chen S, Lin J, et al. Lung ultrasound B-lines and serum KL-6 correlate with the severity of idiopathic inflammatory myositis-associated interstitial lung disease. Rheumatology 2020;59(8):2024–9.
141. Chiu Y-H, Chu C-C, Lu C-C, et al. KL-6 as a Biomarker of Interstitial Lung Disease Development in Patients with Sjögren Syndrome: A Retrospective Case-Control Study. J Inflamm Res 2022;15:2255–62.
142. Oda K, Kotani T, Takeuchi T, et al. Chemokine profiles of interstitial pneumonia in patients with dermatomyositis: a case control study. Scientific Rep 2017;7(1). https://doi.org/10.1038/s41598-017-01685-5.
143. Hoffmann-Vold A-M, Weigt SS, Palchevskiy V, et al. Augmented concentrations of CX3CL1 are associated with interstitial lung disease in systemic sclerosis. PLOS ONE 2018;13(11):e0206545.
144. Tiev KP, Chatenoud L, Kettaneh A, et al. [Increase of CXCL10 serum level in systemic sclerosis interstitial pneumonia]. Rev Med Interne 2009;30(11):942–6. Augmentation de CXCL10 dans le serum au cours de la pneumopathie interstitielle de la sclerodermie systemique.
145. Antonelli A, Ferri C, Fallahi P, et al. CXCL10 (alpha) and CCL2 (beta) chemokines in systemic sclerosis–a longitudinal study. Rheumatology (Oxford) 2008;47(1):45–9.
146. Chen J, Doyle TJ, Liu Y, et al. Biomarkers of Rheumatoid Arthritis-Associated Interstitial Lung Disease. Arthritis Rheumatol 2015;67(1):28–38.
147. Gono T, Kaneko H, Kawaguchi Y, et al. Cytokine profiles in polymyositis and dermatomyositis complicated by rapidly progressive or chronic interstitial lung disease. Rheumatology (Oxford) 2014;53(12):2196–203.
148. Kameda M, Otsuka M, Chiba H, et al. CXCL9, CXCL10, and CXCL11; biomarkers of pulmonary inflammation associated with autoimmunity in patients with collagen vascular diseases–associated interstitial lung disease and interstitial pneumonia with autoimmune features. PLOS ONE 2020;15(11):e0241719.
149. Nishikawa A, Suzuki K, Kassai Y, et al. Identification of definitive serum biomarkers associated with disease activity in primary Sjögren's syndrome. Arthritis Res Ther 2016;18(1). https://doi.org/10.1186/s13075-016-1006-1.
150. Cossu M, Andracco R, Santaniello A, et al. Serum levels of vascular dysfunction markers reflect disease severity and stage in systemic sclerosis patients. Rheumatology (Oxford) 2016;55(6):1112–6.
151. Van Bon L, Affandi AJ, Broen J, et al. Proteome-wide Analysis and CXCL4 as a Biomarker in Systemic Sclerosis. New Engl J Med 2014;370(5):433–43.

152. Khadilkar PV, Khopkar US, Nadkar MY, et al. Fibrotic Cytokine Interplay in Evaluation of Disease Activity in Treatment Naive Systemic Sclerosis Patients from Western India. J Assoc Physicians India 2019;67(8):26–30.
153. Abdel-Magied RA, Kamel SR, Said AF, et al. Serum interleukin-6 in systemic sclerosis and its correlation with disease parameters and cardiopulmonary involvement. Sarcoidosis Vasc Diffuse Lung Dis 2016;33(4):321–30.
154. Olewicz-Gawlik A, Danczak-Pazdrowska A, Kuznar-Kaminska B, et al. Interleukin-17 and interleukin-23: importance in the pathogenesis of lung impairment in patients with systemic sclerosis. Int J Rheum Dis 2014;17(6):664–70.
155. Yanaba K, Yoshizaki A, Asano Y, et al. Serum IL-33 levels are raised in patients with systemic sclerosis: association with extent of skin sclerosis and severity of pulmonary fibrosis. Clin Rheumatol 2011;30(6):825–30.
156. Tang J, Lei L, Pan J, et al. Higher levels of serum interleukin-35 are associated with the severity of pulmonary fibrosis and Th2 responses in patients with systemic sclerosis. Rheumatol Int 2018;38(8):1511–9.
157. Moinzadeh P, Krieg T, Hellmich M, et al. Elevated MMP-7 levels in patients with systemic sclerosis: correlation with pulmonary involvement. Exp Dermatol 2011; 20(9):770–3.
158. Matson SM, Lee SJ, Peterson RA, et al. The prognostic role of matrix metalloproteinase-7 in scleroderma-associated interstitial lung disease. Eur Respir J 2021;58(6):2101560.
159. Nakatsuka Y, Handa T, Nakashima R, et al. Serum matrix metalloproteinase levels in polymyositis/dermatomyositis patients with interstitial lung disease. Rheumatology 2019;58(8):1465–73.
160. Manetti M, Guiducci S, Romano E, et al. Increased serum levels and tissue expression of matrix metalloproteinase-12 in patients with systemic sclerosis: correlation with severity of skin and pulmonary fibrosis and vascular damage. Ann Rheum Dis 2012;71(6):1064–72.
161. Kikuchi K, Kubo M, Sato S, et al. Serum tissue inhibitor of metalloproteinases in patients with systemic sclerosis. J Am Acad Dermatol 1995;33(6):973–8.
162. Ren J, Sun L, Sun X, et al. Diagnostic value of serum connective tissue growth factor in rheumatoid arthritis. Clin Rheumatol 2021;40(6):2203–9.
163. Sato S, Nagaoka T, Hasegawa M, et al. Serum levels of connective tissue growth factor are elevated in patients with systemic sclerosis: association with extent of skin sclerosis and severity of pulmonary fibrosis. J Rheumatol 2000;27(1): 149–54.
164. Lambrecht S, Smith V, De Wilde K, et al. Growth differentiation factor 15, a marker of lung involvement in systemic sclerosis, is involved in fibrosis development but is not indispensable for fibrosis development. Arthritis Rheumatol 2014;66(2):418–27.
165. Gamal SM, Elgengehy FT, Kamal A, et al. Growth Differentiation Factor-15 (GDF-15) Level and Relation to Clinical Manifestations in Egyptian Systemic Sclerosis patients: Preliminary Data. Immunol Invest 2017;46(7):703–13.
166. Yanaba K, Asano Y, Tada Y, et al. Clinical significance of serum growth differentiation factor-15 levels in systemic sclerosis: association with disease severity. Mod Rheumatol 2012;22(5):668–75.
167. Nordenbæk C, Johansen JS, Halberg P, et al. High serum levels of YKL-40 in patients with systemic sclerosis are associated with pulmonary involvement. Scand J Rheumatol 2005;34(4):293–7.

168. Alqalyoobi S, Adegunsoye A, Linderholm A, et al. Circulating Plasma Biomarkers of Progressive Interstitial Lung Disease. Am J Respir Crit Care Med 2020;201(2):250–3.
169. Rivière S, Hua-Huy T, Tiev KP, et al. High Baseline Serum Clara Cell 16 kDa Predicts Subsequent Lung Disease Worsening in Systemic Sclerosis. The J Rheumatol 2018;45(2):242–7.
170. Volkmann ER, Tashkin DP, Kuwana M, et al. Progression of Interstitial Lung Disease in Systemic Sclerosis: The Importance of Pneumoproteins Krebs von den Lungen 6 and CCL18. Arthritis Rheumatol 2019;71(12):2059–67.
171. Guiot J, Njock M-S, André B, et al. Serum IGFBP-2 in systemic sclerosis as a prognostic factor of lung dysfunction. Scientific Rep 2021;11(1). https://doi.org/10.1038/s41598-021-90333-0.
172. Kuwana M, Shirai Y, Takeuchi T. Elevated Serum Krebs von den Lungen-6 in Early Disease Predicts Subsequent Deterioration of Pulmonary Function in Patients with Systemic Sclerosis and Interstitial Lung Disease. The J Rheumatol 2016;43(10):1825–31.
173. Kennedy B, Branagan P, Moloney F, et al. Biomarkers to identify ILD and predict lung function decline in scleroderma lung disease or idiopathic pulmonary fibrosis. Sarcoidosis Vasc Diffuse Lung Dis 2015;32(3):228–36.
174. Wu M, Baron M, Pedroza C, et al. CCL2 in the Circulation Predicts Long-Term Progression of Interstitial Lung Disease in Patients With Early Systemic Sclerosis: Data From Two Independent Cohorts. Arthritis Rheumatol 2017;69(9):1871–8.
175. Volkmann ER, Tashkin DP, Roth MD, et al. Changes in plasma CXCL4 levels are associated with improvements in lung function in patients receiving immunosuppressive therapy for systemic sclerosis-related interstitial lung disease. Arthritis Res Ther 2016;18(1). https://doi.org/10.1186/s13075-016-1203-y.
176. De Lauretis A, Sestini P, Pantelidis P, et al. Serum interleukin 6 is predictive of early functional decline and mortality in interstitial lung disease associated with systemic sclerosis. J Rheumatol 2013;40(4):435–46.
177. Nara M, Komatsuda A, Omokawa A, et al. Serum interleukin 6 levels as a useful prognostic predictor of clinically amyopathic dermatomyositis with rapidly progressive interstitial lung disease. Mod Rheumatol 2014;24(4):633–6.
178. Lee JH, Jang JH, Park JH, et al. The role of interleukin-6 as a prognostic biomarker for predicting acute exacerbation in interstitial lung diseases. PLOS ONE 2021;16(7):e0255365.
179. Takada T, Ohashi K, Hayashi M, et al. Role of IL-15 in interstitial lung diseases in amyopathic dermatomyositis with anti-MDA-5 antibody. Respir Med 2018;141:7–13.
180. Shimizu T, Koga T, Furukawa K, et al. IL-15 is a biomarker involved in the development of rapidly progressive interstitial lung disease complicated with polymyositis/dermatomyositis. J Intern Med 2021;289(2):206–20.
181. Peng Q-L, Zhang Y-M, Liang L, et al. A high level of serum neopterin is associated with rapidly progressive interstitial lung disease and reduced survival in dermatomyositis. Clin Exp Immunol 2020;199(3):314–25.
182. Hozumi H, Fujisawa T, Enomoto N, et al. Clinical Utility of YKL-40 in Polymyositis/dermatomyositis-associated Interstitial Lung Disease. The J Rheumatol 2017;44(9):1394–401.
183. Jiang L, Wang Y, Peng Q, et al. Serum YKL-40 level is associated with severity of interstitial lung disease and poor prognosis in dermatomyositis with anti-MDA5 antibody. Clin Rheumatol 2019;38(6):1655–63.

Imaging of Rheumatic Diseases Affecting the Lower Limb

Aurea Valeria Rosa Mohana-Borges, MD[a],
Christine B. Chung, MD[a,b,*]

KEYWORDS

- Imaging • MR imaging • Ultrasound • CT • Conventional radiography
- Osteoarthritis • Rheumatoid arthritis • Gout

KEY POINTS

- MR imaging and ultrasonography can identify early findings of joint inflammation and structural damage associated with arthritis and are of paramount importance in the management of inflammatory rheumatic diseases.
- MR imaging is the best imaging modality for assessment of whole organ abnormalities associated with osteoarthritis.
- Ultrasonography and dual-energy computed tomography are biomarkers for evaluation of gouty arthritis.

INTRODUCTION
Discussion of Problem/Clinical Presentation

The successful use of disease-modifying antirheumatic drugs, which interrupt the inflammatory cascade, provided strong motivation for identification of biomarkers of inflammation, subclinical disease, and earliest objective findings of active disease. In this context, imaging methods capable of detecting inflammation, such as MR imaging and ultrasound (US), are of paramount importance in rheumatic disease management, not only for diagnostic purposes but also for monitoring disease activity and treatment response. The purpose of this review is to provide an overview of imaging of some of the most prevalent inflammatory rheumatic diseases affecting the lower limb (osteoarthritis [OA], rheumatoid arthritis [RA], and gout) and up-to-date recommendations regarding imaging diagnostic workup.

This article previously appeared in *Radiologic Clinics* volume 61 issue 2 March 2023.
[a] Department of Radiology, University of California San Diego, 9427 Health Sciences Drive, La Jolla, CA 92093, USA; [b] Department of Radiology, VA San Diego, 3350 La Jolla Village Drive, La Jolla, CA 92161, USA
* Corresponding author. Department of Radiology, University of California San Diego, 9427 Health Sciences Drive, La Jolla, CA 92093
E-mail address: cbchung@health.ucsd.edu

OSTEOARTHRITIS
Background

OA is the most prevalent form of arthritis, with a chronic and progressive course. In the 2019 Global Health Data Exchange, OA had an estimated global prevalence of more than 527.8 million cases surpassing common conditions of the modern world, such as depression, anxiety, and interpersonal violence. A large proportion of the OA burden is caused by involvement of joints of the lower limbs, such as knee and hip, which account for approximately 60.6% and 5.5%, respectively, of years lived with disability attributed to the disease.[1] OA can lead to undesirable long-term opioid addiction as a "side effect" of chronic pain therapy and to joint replacement at end stage of the disease.[2] As we might expect, joint replacement surgeries have become one of the most common orthopedic procedures worldwide, especially total knee arthroplasty.[3]

OA was traditionally considered a degenerative articular disease, caused by "wear and tear." However, new molecular biology techniques in association with findings of advanced imaging methods progressively changed the way the scientific community has come to view the disease. It is now considered a much more complex condition affecting the whole joint, with both biomechanical and inflammatory drivers.[4] Several risk factors are implicated to trigger a low-grade inflammation in the joint inducing structural damage. They include, but are not limited to, age, female gender, prior joint injury, obesity, genetic predisposition, and mechanical factors, such as malalignment and abnormal joint shape.[5]

Imaging Findings

Findings of inflammation and structural damage can be identified by several imaging methods (**Fig. 1**). Joints often compromised in the lower limb are knee, hip, and first metatarsophalangeal joint. Osteoarthritic changes elsewhere in the foot, such as the subtalar joint, are usually caused by altered mechanics from congenital or acquired abnormalities (eg, pes planus, coalition, trauma) or are secondary to another underlying arthropathy (eg, psoriasis, reactive arthritis).[6]

Radiography

Radiography in OA can directly identify structural damage by the presence of osteophytes (bone outgrowths), subchondral bone sclerosis, and bone cysts. Joint space narrowing is another important radiographic finding but should be considered the indirect and nonspecific sequelae of cartilage loss, meniscal volume reduction, and/or meniscus extrusion. In OA, joint space narrowing is usually asymmetric as opposed to the symmetric joint reduction observed in RA. In the knee, asymmetric distribution more often predominates in the medial compartment. In the hip, superior joint space narrowing predominates (**Fig. 2**). On weight-bearing knee radiographs, a finding of joint space greater than 5 mm is considered normal and less than 3 mm, an absolute indication of joint space narrowing.

Subchondral sclerosis occurs as cartilage loss increases and appears as an area of increased density on the radiograph. In the advanced stage of the disease, subchondral remodeling with collapse of the joint may occur; however, ankylosis is usually not present in patients with primary OA.[6] Subchondral cysts usually have a sclerotic border and may or may not communicate with the joint space and can occur before cartilage loss.[6] However, the last two findings are best visualized by MR imaging.

In 1952, Kellgren and Lawrence (KL) introduced a 5-grade radiographic classification system for OA[7] (**Figs. 3** and **4**). In KL classification, the most important radiographic finding for diagnosis is the definite presence of osteophyte, and to estimate

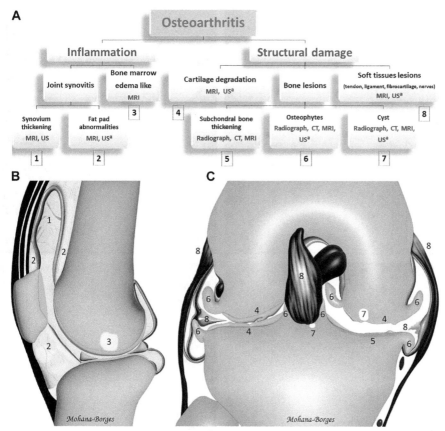

Fig. 1. (*A*) Flowchart of alterations observed in OA with best imaging methods for diagnosis. Accompanying diagrams in (*B*) lateral and (*C*) anterior views. Note. There are limitations in the use of US in the evaluation of deep-seated structures. However, US can be reliably used to evaluate superficial joint pathologies such as marginal erosions and marginal synovial cysts.

the severity of the disease, the narrowing of the joint space. KL grading system continues to be used today for diagnosis and disease progression. Additional OA classification systems and atlas were proposed by Ahlbäck,[8] Osteoarthritis Research Society International,[9] and Altman and colleagues.[10]

Advantages of radiography are low-cost, wide availability, and short imaging time. Disadvantages are the use of ionizing radiation and detection of more advanced disease as it is unable to directly visualize synovium and cartilage as well as insensitive to detect soft tissues abnormalities.[11] Radiographs are also subjected to a lack of reproducibility of joint space measurements in longitudinal assessment.[11]

MR Imaging

MR imaging can directly identify joint inflammation and structural damage, being suitable for diagnosis of both early and advanced OA. Detection of early OA by MR imaging is a window of opportunity to prevent further articular damage and avoid pain sensitization. In addition to the conventional morphologic joint evaluation,[12] MR imaging can also be applied in semiquantitative (SQ) scoring systems of the whole joint,[13–15] quantitative analysis of the biochemical composition of the joint tissues

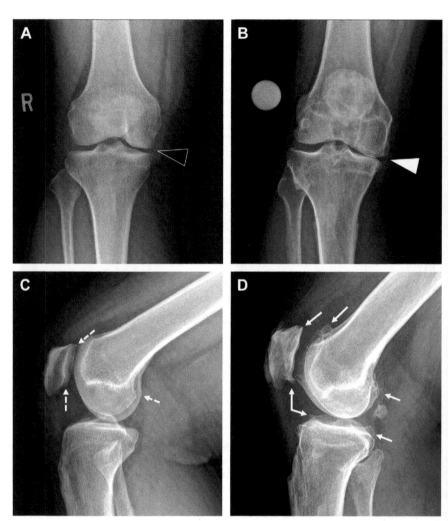

Fig. 2. Radiographic findings of knee OA. (*A, B*) Anteroposterior view. (*C, D*) Lateral view. (*A*) and (*C*) demonstrate a mild OA, with possible reduction of the medial joint space (*open arrowhead*) and tiny osteophytes (*dotted arrows*). (*B*) and (*D*) demonstrate a moderate to severe OA with reduction of the medial joint space (*arrowhead*) and moderate to large-sized osteophytes (*arrows* in *D*). Marginal subchondral bone sclerosis is observed in the medial tibial plateau with slight bone deformity associated. Also note irregularity in contour of the femoral trochlea in lateral view (*D*). This case demonstrates findings of bicompartmental OA, involving the medial femorotibial and patellofemoral compartments.

(compositional MR imaging),[16] and quantitative volumetric analyses of cartilage and other tissues (quantitative MR imaging)[17,18] (**Box 1, Table 1**). Disadvantages of MR imaging are the higher cost and longer time for imaging in comparison with radiographs, US, and computed tomography (CT).

Morphologic MR Imaging

Synovitis is characterized by synovial thickening and enhancement in post-contrast imaging and may be accompanied by variable amounts of joint fluid (effusion).[19,20]

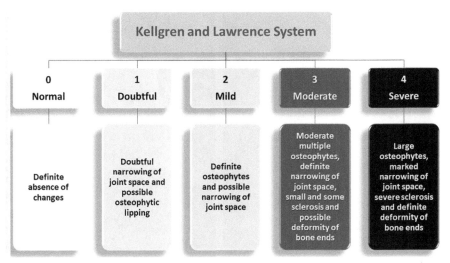

Fig. 3. Radiographic classification of OA by Kellgren and Lawrence. OA is diagnosed in grades ≥2.

On conventional MR imaging, synovitis and synovial fluid can be difficult to distinguish as the synovium typically appears hyperintense on T2-weighted sequences and hypo- to isointense to skeletal muscle and cartilage on T1-weighted sequences.[20] More recently, promising novel non-contrast enhanced assessment of synovitis was proposed with sequences such as fluid attenuated inversion recovery (FLAIR) with fat-saturated, quantitative double-echo in steady state (qDESS), and dual inversion recovery (DIR).[20]

In the knee, synovitis may be associated with areas of edema and contour irregularities in fat pads, such as prefemoral, suprapatellar, and Hoffa's fat pad. However, edema in fat pads seems to be a nonspecific measure of synovitis when contrast enhancement is used as the reference.[19]

Bone marrow lesions (BMLs), also called bone marrow edema (BME), are ill-defined areas of altered signal intensity best seen as hyperintensities on fluid-sensitive sequences.[21] Some authors avoid the term BME because the altered signal in OA is due to a combination of several non-characteristic histologic abnormalities that include bone marrow necrosis, bone marrow fibrosis, and trabeculae abnormalities.[22] In OA, BMLs are frequently detected in conjunction with areas of cartilage damage (**Fig. 5**). The identification of BMLs is relevant because they are associated with pain and greater OA severity. Furthermore, their presence may predict OA progression.[23]

Regarding structural damage, the T1-weighted sequence is the best sequence for evaluation of osteophytes (bone outgrowths) and subchondral bone remodeling. However, cartilage is best evaluated on fluid-sensitive sequences, especially intermediate-weighted fast spin-echo sequences.[24,25] Cartilage lesions usually have higher signal intensity in comparison to normal cartilage signal, which is caused by damage to collagenous ultrastructure and increased free water. This mechanism is elegantly exploited in compositional MR imaging.

Semiquantitative MR Imaging

Several SQ MR imaging grading systems have been developed for evaluation of OA in the knee (Whole Organ Magnetic Resonance Score [WORMS], KOSS, BLOKS, MOAKS, ROAMES), hip (HOAMS, SHOMRI), and hand (OHOA, HOAMRIS)[26,27]

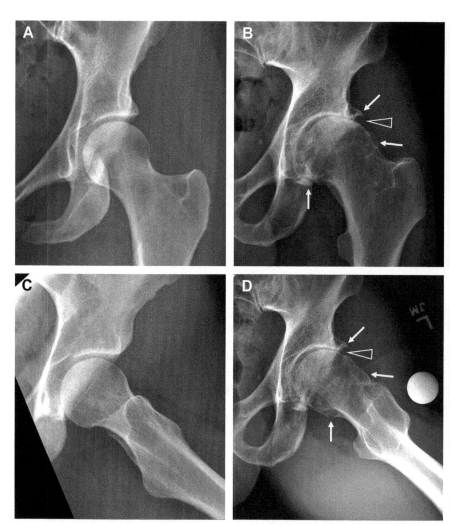

Fig. 4. Radiographic findings of hip OA. (*A, B*) Anteroposterior (AP) view. (*C, D*) Lateral view. (*A*) and (*C*) demonstrate normal hip joint (KG 0) with preservation of joint space and absence of osteophytes. (*B*) and (*D*) show marked osteoarthritic (KG 4) changes with large marginal osteophytes (*arrows*), marked narrowing of the superior joint space (*open arrowhead*), severe sclerosis in the lateral aspect of the femoral head and acetabulum, and femoral head deformity.

(**Fig. 6**). The first comprehensive MR imaging-based SQ scoring system was published in 2004 and received the name WORMS.[13] WORMS is a complex and detailed system with features evaluated in 15 different regions subdivided by anatomic landmarks.[26] WORMS protocol is time-consuming and developed in a research environment. The last published MR imaging grading system, ROAMES, on the other hand, was proposed to be a simplified version of previous systems, with less features to be evaluated and less subdivisions of anatomic regions for analysis. In ROAMES, investigators introduced five different imaging phenotypes (inflammatory, subchondral bone, meniscus/cartilage, atrophic, and hypertrophic), aimed to explore potential targets for clinical trials of disease-modifying OA drug.[28]

Box 1
MR imaging sequences for evaluation of cartilage lesions

Cartilage Lesion
  Morphologic
    Fluid-sensitive sequences (fat-saturated PD-weighted and T2-weighted and short tau
    inversion recovery [STIR]) 2D and 3D:
      Detects cartilage loss and abnormal signal intensity
  Compositional
    T2 and T2*-mapping:
      Detects increased water content associated with early cartilage (collagen matrix)
      degradation
    T1-rho:
      Measures GAG/proteoglycan content
    dEMERIC(delayed gadolinium-enhanced MR imaging of cartilage):
      Measures GAG/proteoglycan content
    Diffusion-weighted and diffusion tensor imaging
      Detects increased free water content associated with cartilage degradation
    Sodium imaging:
      Measures GAG/proteoglycan content
    gagCEST (Chemical exchange saturation transfer of glycosaminoglycans):
      Measures GAG/proteoglycan content
    UTE (quantitative ultrashort echo time) T2*, ZTE, MT:
      Measures GAG/proteoglycan content
  Quantitative volumetric
    3D-sequences, such as 3D-SPGR (spoiled gradient recalled echo) and 3D-DESS (dual-echo
    steady state), with segmentation software assistance

Abbreviations: GAG, glycosaminoglycan; MT, magnetization transfer; PD, proton density; ZTE,
zero echo time.

Table 1
MR imaging sequences for evaluation of (A) synovitis and (B) bone

Synovitis	Bone Lesion
Morphologic	Morphologic
Fluid-sensitive sequences (fat-saturated PD-weighted and T2-weighted and STIR):	T1-weighted:
	Detects bone erosion, attrition, and fracture
Detects articular fluid produced by synovium	Fluid-sensitive sequences (PD-weighted and T2-weighted and STIR):
T1-contrasted enhanced:	Detects bone marrow edema-like cysts
Detects enhancement in areas of synovitis	T1-contrasted enhanced:
Compositional	Detects enhancement in areas of osteitis/ bone marrow edema like
Diffusion tensor imaging:	Compositional
Restricted motion of water in joints as a result of inflammatory cell aggregation	UTE (quantitative ultrashort echo time) T2*, ZTE, MT:
Functional	Detects alterations in composition of osteochondral junction and bone
Dynamic contrast-enhanced MR imaging:	
Characterize the uptake and washout of gadolinium-based contrast agents in synovium, providing biomarkers of tissue perfusion, capillary permeability, and blood and interstitial volume	

Abbreviations: GAG, glycosaminoglycan; MT, magnetization transfer; PD, proton density; ZTE, zero
echo time.

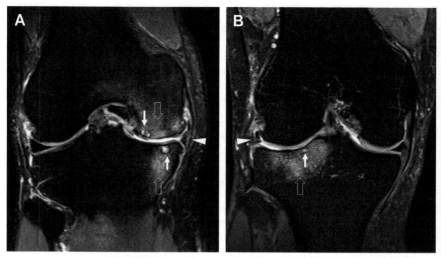

Fig. 5. MR imaging findings of OA in the knee. (*A*) Medial compartment OA and (*B*) lateral compartment OA. Note bone marrow lesions (*open arrows*) with associated subchondral bone cysts (*arrows*). In (*A*) cartilage lesions are more pronounced in the femoral condyle and in (*B*) in the tibial plateau. Note associated meniscal lesions (*arrowhead*) in both cases.

Compositional MR Imaging

Compositional MR imaging aims to identify early damage and breakdown of cartilage exploring changes that occur in cartilage macromolecules. In OA, proteoglycan and collagen content are reduced. This disrupts the collagen network and results in matrix degradation and increased water content.[29] Compositional MR imaging sequences can be divided into collagen-sensitive, for example, T2 and T2* mapping, and proteoglycan-sensitive, for example, T1-rho and dGEMRIC (delayed gadolinium-enhanced MR imaging of cartilage)[30] (**Fig. 7**). In T2–T2* mapping and T1-rho, increased values are associated with decreased collagen and proteoglycan content in hyaline cartilage and meniscus.[31]

Ultrasonography

Like MR imaging, US can identify synovitis and much of the structural damage associated with OA. It is cheaper and faster than MR imaging and without nonionizing radiation. However, there are limitations associated with the acoustic window and wave penetration, with only partial visualization of deeper joint tissues. In knee OA, US adds

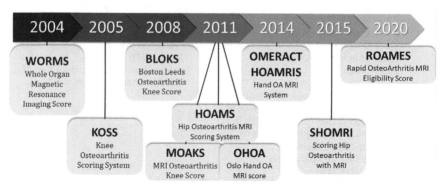

Fig. 6. Timeline of MR imaging semiquantitative grading systems for OA.

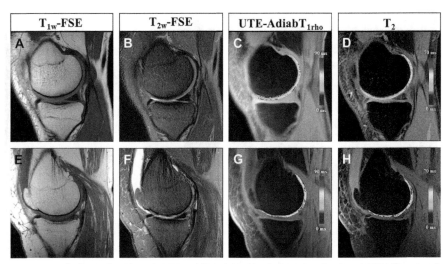

Fig. 7. Morphologic (*A, B*) and compositional (*C, D*) MR imaging in OA. Sagittal images in the medial femorotibial compartment demonstrate cartilage findings in (*A–D*) a 23-year-old male and (*E–H*) 74-year-old female with diagnosis of OA. In both cases, compositional MR imaging can identify changes in the cartilage (*C, D, G, H*) characterized by areas of increased T1-rho and T2 values (*yellow and red*), more pronounced in established OA (*G, H*). Morphologic sequences in (*A*) and (*B*) were insensitive to cartilage abnormalities. (*Courtesy* of Y Ma, PhD, San Diego, California.)

diagnostic information over radiographs primarily by its ability to directly visualize cartilage and meniscus as well as to sensitively depict effusion and synovitis.[27] The Outcome Measures in Rheumatology Clinical Trials (OMERACT) of US created a grading system for cartilage loss (**Table 2**) and osteophytes (varying from 0 normal to 3 severe) to assess OA in finger, which can also be applied to other joints.

Computed Tomography

Like radiographs, conventional CT can identify structural damage (**Fig. 8**). Identification of soft tissue abnormalities with CT is better than with radiograph, but less sensitive than with MR imaging. However, techniques such as CT arthrography and PET/CT add value in the investigation of the soft tissues and synovitis. A recent novel use of CT arthrography is the ability to measure sulfated glycosaminoglycans (GAGs) in a similar

Table 2 Outcome measures in rheumatology clinical ultrasound semiquantitative scoring system for cartilage abnormalities in osteoarthritis		
Grade	**Classification**	**Finding**
Grade 0	Normal joint	Normal cartilage (anechoic structure, normal margins of cartilage)
Grade 1	Small cartilage loss	Loss of anechoic structure and/or focal thinning of cartilage layer OR irregularities and/or loss of sharpness of at least one cartilage margin
Grade 2	Moderate cartilage loss	Loss anechoic structure and/or focal thinning of cartilage layer AND irregularities and/or loss of sharpness of at least one cartilage margin
Grade 3	Severe cartilage loss	Focal absence or complete loss of the cartilage layer

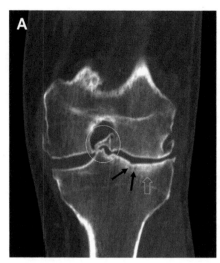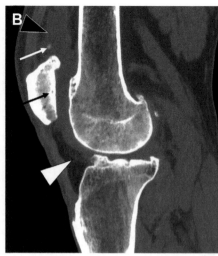

Fig. 8. Conventional CT in OA. CT directly identifies structural damage related to bone and indirectly damage to cartilage and meniscus by means of evaluation of joint space narrowing. Note (*A*) bridging hypertrophic osteophytes in the region of the intercondylar (*circle*) notch resulting in mass effect on and impingement of the cruciate ligaments. Joint space narrowing in the lateral femorotibial compartment is associated with subchondral sclerosis (*open large arrow*) and cysts (*black arrows*). Subchondral cysts are manifested as well-marginated lucent foci, in this case of small size (*black arrows* in *A* and *B*). (*B*) Joint effusion (black *arrowhead*) and soft tissue abnormalities, such as infiltration of Hoffa's fat pad (*white arrowhead*) are usually better identified by CT than radiography but not as well visualized as by MR imaging. However, small intra-articular bodies (*white arrow*) are better visualized by CT than MR imaging.

way of compositional MR imaging, such as dGEMRIC. Contrast agent uptake and GAG content correlate negatively for anionic agents, that is, the higher the uptake the lower the GAG content, and positively for cationic agents, that is, the higher uptake, the higher the GAG content.[32]

RHEUMATOID ARTHRITIS
Background

RA is the typical synovium-based inflammatory arthritis. RA is a systemic chronic autoimmune disease with production of autoantibodies, such as rheumatoid factor and anti-citrullinated protein antibody. The current understanding of the pathophysiology of RA has progressed and proposes a genetic predisposition resulting in autoreactive T cells and B cells, and a triggering event providing antigen-presenting cells to activate the autoreactive lymphocytes.[33]

Unlike OA, which typically affects one specific joint or fewer joints at presentation, RA is classically described as a symmetric small joint polyarthritis with additional involvement of large joints.[34] Joints commonly involved in the feet are metatarsal phalangeal joints (MTPs) and proximal interphalangeal joints. Jacoby and colleagues reported involvement of the knees, ankle, and MTP in 56%, 53%, and 48% of cases, respectively.[35] Positive RF is one of the best predictors of small joint erosions.

Imaging Findings

Imaging methods for RA diagnosis and follow-up that identify early synovial inflammation, such as US and MR imaging, are superior to the ones that only diagnosis later structural damage, such as conventional radiography and CT (**Fig. 9**).

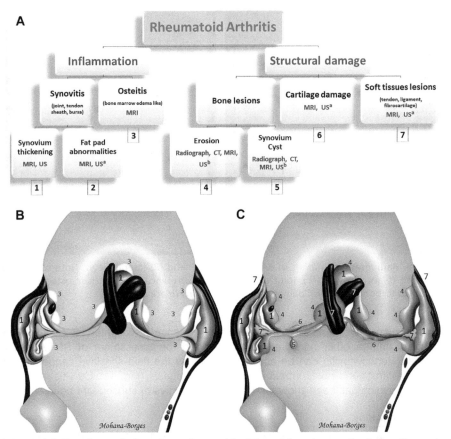

Fig. 9. (*A*) Flowchart of alterations observed in RA and imaging methods for diagnosis. Note. There are limitations in the use of US in the evaluation of deep-seated structures. However, US can be reliably used to evaluate superficial joint pathologies such as marginal erosions and marginal synovial cysts. Accompanying diagrams with findings of (*B*) inflammation and (*C*) inflammation and structural damage. Fat pad abnormalities (2) not shown.

Radiography

Radiographic analysis should start with the location and distribution of radiologic findings, considering that in the feet, RA affects more proximal joints compared with OA and psoriatic arthritis, which predominate in the distal joints. Early radiographic findings identified in RA are soft tissue swelling and osteoporosis. Findings of established disease and advanced damage are erosions, cysts, joint space narrowing, and deformity (**Fig. 10**). Detection of bone erosions at the time of RA diagnosis is related to a poor long-term functional and radiographic outcome, and the presence of erosions in early undifferentiated arthritis is a risk factor for developing persistent arthritis.[36]

MR Imaging

RA MR imaging scoring system proposed by the working group of OMERACT was initially developed and validated from 1998 to 2002 and updated in 2016.[37] Their recommendations for basic MR imaging sequences are T1-weighted images before and after IV gadolinium-contrast injection for detection of erosions and synovitis, with

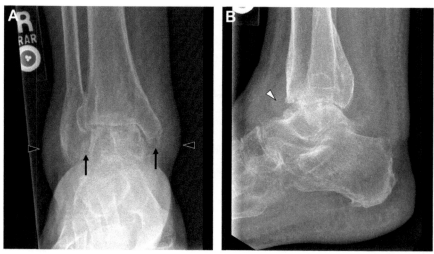

Fig. 10. Radiographic findings in RA. Ankle (*A*) AP and (*B*) lateral views. Note soft tissue swelling (*black arrowheads*), joint effusion (*white arrowhead*) and diffuse osteopenia, in addition to bone structural damage, such as erosions (*black arrows*).

visualization in two planes. The fluid-sensitive sequence T2-weighted fat-sat and STIR images, on the other hand, are recommended for assessment of BME/osteitis, whereas tenosynovitis can be assessed either by the fluid-sensitive sequences or by precontrast and postcontrast T1-weighted images[37] (**Fig. 11**). Osteitis identified by MR imaging has been shown to be highly predictive of subsequent bone erosion.

Ultrasonography

In 2017, the European League Against Rheumatisms (EULAR) in collaboration with OMERACT US task force published a consensus-based definition for synovitis in RA.[38] The consensus stated that synovial hypertrophy is necessary for synovitis even in the absence of Doppler signal. Greater than 90% of participants agreed not to consider effusion alone (ie, without concomitant synovial hypertrophy) as a sign of synovitis and not to define and score joint effusion and synovial hypertrophy together as components of a common process.[38]

Doppler US is used to evaluate soft tissue hyperemia and distinguish active from inactive inflammatory tissue. Ongoing angiogenesis in areas of synovial hypertrophy is responsible for the intra-articular Doppler signal. The continued presence of intensely perfused areas of synovial hypertrophy inside the joint is a reliable indicator of insufficient response to therapy and is predictive of the development of erosions.[39]

Computed Tomography

CT can detect bone erosions more accurately than other techniques, such as MR imaging, US, and radiography but is limited in the detection of synovitis and soft tissue abnormalities.[40] Another disadvantage of CT in routine clinical practice is the radiation exposure. One alternative to conventional CT in the evaluation of peripheral joints is the novel and sensitive technique high-resolution peripheral quantitative CT that is reported to have a very low radiation dose with maintenance of the high accuracy of conventional CT for erosion detection.[40]

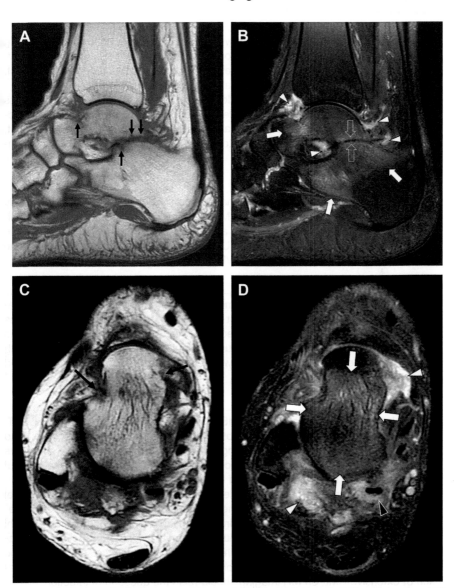

Fig. 11. MR imaging findings in RA. Ankle MR imaging with (*A* and *C*) T1-weighted and (*B*) and (*D*) fluid-sensitive sequences. The inclusion of T1-weighted sequence in the basic protocol for RA aim to improve the detection of erosions (*black arrows*) while the inclusion of fluid sensitive images, the detection of effusion (*white arrowhead*), bone marrow edema (*large white arrow*), and tenosynovitis (*black arrowhead*). Note in (*B*) the well depiction of joint space narrowing (*open large arrows*).

GOUT
Background

Gout is the second most prevalent form of arthritis, only behind OA, and is characterized by chronic deposition of monosodium urate (MSU) crystals, which form in the presence of increased urate concentrations. The clinical features of gout occur as a result of the inflammatory response to monosodium urate crystals.[41]

Gout is more common in men than in women with male to female sex ratio varying from 2:1 to 8:1 depending on the population-based studies.[41] The incidence and prevalence of gout also increase with age. Several risk factors are associated with gout, such as genetic, drugs, dietary, and metabolic syndrome.[41]

Acute gouty arthritis is typically of sudden onset, involving one or few joints (less frequently polyarticular), with a preference for inferior limbs (in 85% of cases), particularly for the first metatarsophalangeal space.[42] The predilection for the first MTP joint, a condition known as podagra, is related to local anatomic characteristic of lower temperature and repetitive physical trauma.

Imaging

Imaging in gout is traditionally focused on the detection of tophus, a chronic, foreign-body granulomatous inflammatory response to MSU crystals deposits,[41] and USG and dual-energy CT (DECT) have a high sensitivity and specificity for tophus detection and are the preferred method for diagnosis. Both US and DECT have been incorporated in the American College of Rheumatology (ACR)/EULAR 2015 gout classification criteria.[43]

Radiography

In acute gouty arthritis, radiographs are most of the time normal or display a nonspecific joint effusion and/or periarticular soft tissue edema. Some radiographic features seen in chronic gouty arthritis are intermediate to high-density tophi in subcutaneous or intraosseous location, well-defined, "punched-out" periarticular bone erosions with overhanging edges adjacent to tophus, with relative preservation of joint space and osseous mineralization.

MR Imaging

MR imaging cannot specifically identify MSU crystals, as in the case of US and DECT, but it provides important information about the presence of synovitis, erosions, and BME.[44] Another advantage of MR imaging is its ability to visualize deeper structures as well as intraosseous deposits, not accessible to US.[44] Some disadvantages of the method are the high cost and time of imaging.

MR imaging features of gout are variable. Tophi may have intermediate or low signal intensity on T1-weighted and heterogeneous signal intensity on fluid-sensitive sequences, depending on the degree of hydration and its calcium concentration.[45] Tophi show intense gadolinium enhancement due to hypervascular soft tissue and granulation tissue that surround tophi. A clue to the diagnosis of gout in the setting of generic inflammatory changes is that BME is uncommon and if present is often mild, the presence of extensive BME on MR imaging should raise the question of infection.[45]

Ultrasonography

Characteristic ultrasonographic findings in gout can be divided into general findings and gout-specific findings. The general ultrasonographic findings include synovitis and tenosynovitis along with subcutaneous edema which are common in patients with ongoing joint attacks. The gout-specific findings include visualization of the crystal deposits in both joints and tendons and definitions were provided by OMERACT US working group.[46] They include double contour, aggregated, tophus, and erosion (**Figs. 12–14**).

Computed Tomography and Dual-Energy Computed Tomography

In the early stages of gout, standard CT has little utility because it is not suitable for imaging the soft tissue inflammation that characterizes early gout. Later in the

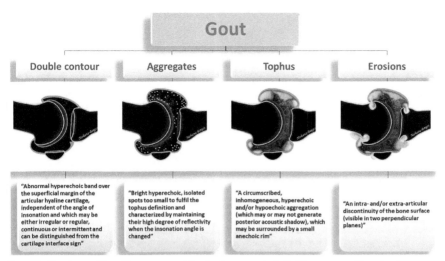

Fig. 12. Gout-specific ultrasonographic findings and definitions according to OMERACT USWG.

progression of the disease, bone erosions and tophi can be visualized and quantified.[47] Tophi have a characteristic density of around 160 Hounsfield units and volume and density measurements can be performed using CT.

DECT has revolutionized gout imaging. The technology can separate urate and calcium in a highly sensitive way because the tissues have different absorption spectra on 80-keV and 140/150-keV voltage.[48] Thus, DECT has become the recommended

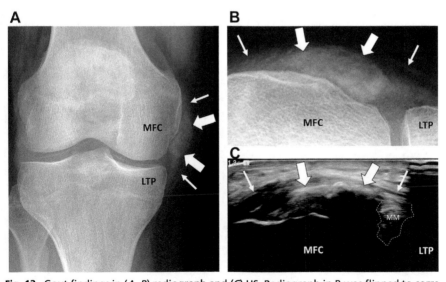

Fig. 13. Gout findings in (A, B) radiograph and (C) US. Radiograph in B was flipped to correspond to US image. Note the tophus (*large arrows*) compressing the joint capsule (*small arrows*). The tophus has a slightly higher density than surrounding soft tissues in radiograph (A and B). (C) The tophi in US have a globular inhomogeneous hyperechoic appearance associated with acoustic shadowing. LTP, lateral tibial plateau; MCF, medial femoral condyle; MM, medial meniscus. (*Courtesy of* Karen Chen, MD, San Diego, California.)

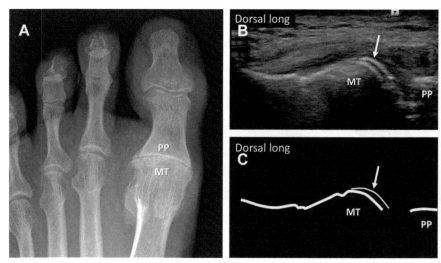

Fig. 14. (*A*) Radiography of the foot in AP with detail of the first ray in a person with gouty arthritis. Note joint space narrowing in the metatarsophalangeal joint and soft tissue swelling in the distal interphalangeal joint. (*B*) US of the metatarsophalangeal joint of the hallux demonstrates the double contour (*arrow*) at the level of the metatarsal head. (*C*) Corresponding diagram. (*Courtesy of* Karen Chen, MD, San Diego, California.)

modality to diagnose urate distribution around the joint in 3D and even automatically calculate the volume of urate along with any change of urate load after treatment (**Fig. 15**). In addition, with a bone algorithm, conventional CT images can be used to detect potential erosive changes with better sensitivity and in more detail than either radiograph or MR imaging.[48,49] DECT has reduced the need for aspiration of joint fluid

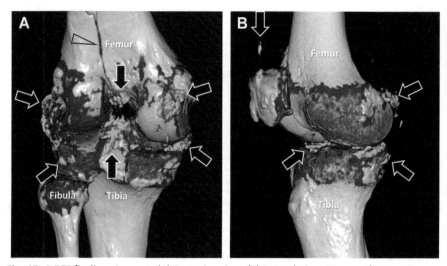

Fig. 15. DECT findings in gout. (*A*) Posterior view. (*B*) Lateral view. Monosodium urate crystal deposits are demonstrated in green (*arrows*). Note incidental fracture in the femur (*arrowhead*). (*Courtesy of* Karen Chen, MD, San Diego, California.)

and phase-contrast microscopic analysis to make the diagnosis and for these reasons has become part of the classification system for gout evaluation recommended by both ACR and EULAR.[48]

SUMMARY

The imaging diagnostic workup in arthritis is based on the identification of inflammation and structural damage. In practice, radiographs still a frequent method of investigation not because the ability for detection of abnormalities but availability and cost. MR imaging and US can detect synovium hypertrophy, increased vascularity, bone and cartilage damage, and intra-articular and extra-articular soft tissue abnormalities. However, US have some limitations in visualization of deeper joint tissues caused by bone interference in the acoustic window and the tradeoff of penetration and resolution. US and DECT are recommended as the first line of investigation of tophus because of high sensitivity and specificity in comparison with other imaging methods.

CLINICS CARE POINTS

- Clinicians should be aware of the limitations of radiographs in assessing inflammation in rheumatological diseases and the implications in patient treatment.
- BMLs and synovitis mediate pain in OA, and the best imaging method for the simultaneous evaluation of these findings is MR imaging.
- US and MR imaging can detect early findings of inflammation in RA, which is relevant for the clinical management of patients.
- US and DECT are recommended as the first line of investigation of the gouty tophus.

DISCLOSURE

The authors having nothing to disclosure.

REFERENCES

1. Long H, Liu Q, Yin H, et al. Prevalence trends of site-specific osteoarthritis from 1990 to 2019: findings from the Global Burden of Disease Study 2019. Arthritis Rheumatol 2022. https://doi.org/10.1002/art.42089.
2. Safiri S, Kolahi AA, Smith E, et al. Global, regional and national burden of osteoarthritis 1990-2017: A systematic analysis of the global burden of disease study 2017. Ann Rheum Dis 2020. https://doi.org/10.1136/annrheumdis-2019-216515.
3. Cisternas AF, Ramachandran R, Yaksh TL, et al. Unintended consequences of COVID-19 safety measures on patients with chronic knee pain forced to defer joint replacement surgery. Pain Rep 2020;5(6). https://doi.org/10.1097/PR9.0000000000000855.
4. Mobasheri A, Batt M. An update on the pathophysiology of osteoarthritis. Ann Phys Rehabil Med 2016;59(5-6):333-9.
5. Loeser RF, Goldring SR, Scanzello CR, et al. Osteoarthritis: A disease of the joint as an organ. Arthritis Rheum 2012;64(6):1697-707.
6. Swagerty DL, Hellinger D. Radiographic assessment of osteoarthritis. Am Fam Physician 2001;64(2):279-86. http://www.ncbi.nlm.nih.gov/pubmed/11476273.
7. KELLGREN JH, LAWRENCE JS. Rheumatism in miners. II. X-ray study. Br J Ind Med 1952;9(3):197-207.

8. Ahlbäck S. Osteoarthrosis of the knee. a radiographic investigation. Acta Radiol Diagn (Stockh) 1968;277:7–72. Available at: http://www.ncbi.nlm.nih.gov/pubmed/5706059.

9. Altman RD, Hochberg M, Murphy WA, et al. Atlas of individual radiographic features in osteoarthritis. Osteoarthritis Cartilage 1995;3:3–70.

10. Altman R, Asch E, Bloch D, et al. Development of criteria for the classification and reporting of osteoarthritis: Classification of osteoarthritis of the knee. Arthritis Rheum 1986;29(8):1039–49.

11. Guermazi A, Roemer FW, Burstein D, et al. Why radiography should no longer be considered a surrogate outcome measure for longitudinal assessment of cartilage in knee osteoarthritis. Arthritis Res Ther 2011;13(6). https://doi.org/10.1186/ar3488.

12. Bae W, Du J, Bydder G, et al. Conventional and ultrashort MRI of articular cartilage, meniscus and intervertebral disc. Top Magn Reson Imaging 2010;21(5): 275–89. Conventional.

13. Peterfy CG, Guermazi A, Zaim S, et al. Whole-organ magnetic resonance imaging score (WORMS) of the knee in osteoarthritis. Osteoarthr Cartil 2004;12(3): 177–90.

14. Kornaat PR, Ceulemans RYT, Kroon HM, et al. MRI assessment of knee osteoarthritis: knee osteoarthritis scoring system (KOSS) - inter-observer and intra-observer reproducibility of a compartment-based scoring system. Skeletal Radiol 2005;34(2):95–102.

15. Hunter DJ, Lo GH, Gale D, et al. The reliability of a new scoring system for knee osteoarthritis MRI and the validity of bone marrow lesion assessment: BLOKS (Boston-Leeds Osteoarthritis Knee Score). Ann Rheum Dis 2008;67(2):206–11.

16. Ariyachaipanich A, Bae WC, Statum S, et al. Update on MRI pulse sequences for the knee: imaging of cartilage, meniscus, tendon, and hardware. Semin Musculoskelet Radiol 2017;21(2):45–62.

17. Wang Y-XJ. Non-invasive MRI assessment of the articular cartilage in clinical studies and experimental settings. World J Radiol 2010;2(1):44.

18. Eckstein F, Wirth W. Quantitative cartilage imaging in knee osteoarthritis. Arthritis 2011;2011:1–19.

19. Guermazi A, Roemer FW, Hayashi D, et al. Assessment of synovitis with contrast-enhanced MRI using a whole-joint semiquantitative scoring system in people with, or at high risk of, knee osteoarthritis: the MOST study. Ann Rheum Dis 2011;70(5):805–11.

20. Thoenen J, MacKay JW, Sandford HJC, et al. Imaging of synovial inflammation in osteoarthritis, from the AJR special series on inflammation. Am J Roentgenol 2022;218(3):405–17.

21. Roemer FW, Frobell R, Hunter DJ, et al. MRI-detected subchondral bone marrow signal alterations of the knee joint: terminology, imaging appearance, relevance and radiological differential diagnosis. Osteoarthr Cartil 2009;17(9):1115–31.

22. Zanetti M, Bruder E, Romero J, et al. Bone marrow edema pattern in osteoarthritic knees: Correlation between MR imaging and histologic findings. Radiology 2000; 215(3):835–40.

23. Link T, Li X. Bone marrow changes in osteoarthritis. Semin Musculoskelet Radiol 2011;15(03):238–46.

24. Disler DG, Recht MP, McCauley TR. MR imaging of articular cartilage. Skeletal Radiol 2000;29(7):367–77.

25. Link TM, Stahl R, Woertler K. Cartilage imaging: motivation, techniques, current and future significance. Eur Radiol 2007;17(5):1135–46.

26. Jarraya M, Hayashi D, Roemer FW, et al. MR imaging-based semi-quantitative methods for knee osteoarthritis. Magn Reson Med Sci 2016;15(2):153–64.
27. Roemer FW, Demehri S, Omoumi P, et al. State of the art imaging of osteoarthritis. Radiology 2020;47(3):2009.
28. Roemer FW, Collins J, Kwoh CK, et al. MRI-based screening for structural definition of eligibility in clinical DMOAD trials: Rapid OsteoArthritis MRI Eligibility Score (ROAMES). Osteoarthr Cartil 2020;28(1):71–81.
29. Braun HJ, Gold GE. Advanced MRI of articular cartilage. Imaging Med 2011;3(5): 541–55.
30. Chang EY, Ma Y, Du J. MR parametric mapping as a biomarker of early joint degeneration. Sports Health 2016;8(5):405–11.
31. Takao S, Nguyen TB, Yu HJ, et al. T1rho and T2 relaxation times of the normal adult knee meniscus at 3T: analysis of zonal differences. BMC Musculoskelet Disord 2017;18(1):1–9.
32. Freedman JD, Ellis DJ, Lusic H, et al. dGEMRIC and CECT comparison of cationic and anionic contrast agents in cadaveric human metacarpal cartilage. J Orthop Res 2020;38(4):719–25.
33. Lin Y-J, Anzaghe M, Schülke S. Update on the pathomechanism, diagnosis, and treatment options for rheumatoid arthritis. Cells 2020;9(4):880.
34. Llopis E, Kroon HM, Acosta J, et al. Conventional radiology in rheumatoid arthritis. Radiol Clin North Am 2017;55(5):917–41.
35. Jacoby RK, Jayson MIV, Cosh JA. Onset, early stages, and prognosis of rheumatoid arthritis: a clinical study of 100 patients with ii-year follow-up. Br Med J 1973; 2(5858):96–100.
36. Døhn UM, Ejbjerg BJ, Court-Payen M, et al. Are bone erosions detected by magnetic resonance imaging and ultrasonography true erosions? A comparison with computed tomography in rheumatoid arthritis metacarpophalangeal joints. Arthritis Res Ther 2006;8(4):1–9.
37. Østergaard M, Peterfy CG, Bird P, et al. The OMERACT rheumatoid arthritis magnetic resonance imaging (MRI) scoring system: Updated recommendations by the OMERACT MRI in arthritis working group. J Rheumatol 2017;44(11):1706–12.
38. D'Agostino MA, Terslev L, Aegerter P, et al. Scoring ultrasound synovitis in rheumatoid arthritis: a EULAR-OMERACT ultrasound taskforce - Part 1: Definition and development of a standardised, consensus-based scoring system. RMD Open 2017;3(1):1–9.
39. Šenolt L, Grassi W, Szodoray P. Laboratory biomarkers or imaging in the diagnostics of rheumatoid arthritis? BMC Med 2014;12(1):1–6.
40. Barile A, Arrigoni F, Bruno F, et al. Computed Tomography and MR Imaging in Rheumatoid Arthritis. Radiol Clin North Am 2017;55(5):997–1007.
41. Dalbeth N, Gosling AL, Gaffo A, et al. Gout Lancet 2021;397(10287):1843–55.
42. Jacques T, Michelin P, Badr S, et al. Conventional radiology in crystal arthritis: gout, calcium pyrophosphate deposition, and basic calcium phosphate crystals. Radiol Clin North Am 2017;55(5):967–84.
43. Neogi T, Jansen TLTA, Dalbeth N, et al. 2015 Gout classification criteria: an American college of rheumatology/European league against Rheumatism collaborative initiative. Ann Rheum Dis 2015;74(10):1789–98.
44. Araujo EG, Manger B, Perez-Ruiz F, et al. Imaging of gout: new tools and biomarkers? Best Pract Res Clin Rheumatol 2016;30(4):638–52.
45. Chowalloor PV, Siew TK, Keen HI. Imaging in gout: A review of the recent developments. Ther Adv Musculoskelet Dis 2014;6(4):131–43.

46. Gutierrez M, Schmidt WA, Thiele RG, et al. International consensus for ultrasound lesions in gout: Results of delphi process and web-reliability exercise. Rheumatol (United Kingdom) 2015;54(10):1797–805.
47. Buckens CF, Terra MP, Maas M. Computed Tomography and MR Imaging in Crystalline-Induced Arthropathies. Radiol Clin North Am 2017;55(5):1023–34.
48. Boesen M, Roemer FW, Østergaard M, et al. Imaging of common rheumatic joint diseases affecting the upper limbs. Radiol Clin North Am 2019;57(5):1001–34.
49. McQueen FM, Doyle A, Dalbeth N. Imaging in gout - what can we learn from MRI, CT, DECT and US? Arthritis Res Ther 2011;13(6):246.

Prospects of Disease-Modifying Osteoarthritis Drugs

Win Min Oo, MD, PhD[a,b,]*

KEYWORDS

- Osteoarthritis • DMOADs • Disease-modifying drugs
- Intra-articular therapy: endotype

KEY POINTS

- Despite the massive disease burden of osteoarthritis (OA), there is an immense unmet need owing to the absence of approved disease-modifying osteoarthritis drugs and only modest efficacy of current therapies.
- By virtue of lessons learned from failed clinical trials and insights gained through molecular and imaging research, some promising agents are progressing to late-stage clinical trials.
- International consensus on phenotype classification, appropriate selection criteria, and trial design for each specific targeted therapy, the innovation of drug delivery system, target validation, and linkage with the disease in preclinical research should be the focus.

INTRODUCTION

Osteoarthritis (OA) is the most prevalent arthritis with an estimated global prevalence in 2020 of 22.9% (95% confidence interval [CI], 19.8%-26.1%) in persons over 40 years of age (correspondingly 654.1 million individuals globally).[1] The disease burden impacts on OA patients are substantial in terms of pain, functional limitations, and quality of life, resulting in the 15th highest cause of years lived with disability worldwide. In addition, direct and indirect costs of OA range from 1% to 2.5% of the gross national product across most countries.[2]

This article previously appeared in *Clinics in Geriatric Medicine* volume 38 issue 2 May 2022.
Funding: No funding is acquired for this work.
Conflicts of Interest: Dr WMO has no conflict of interest.
[a] Department of Physical Medicine and Rehabilitation, Mandalay General Hospital, University of Medicine, Mandalay, Mandalay, Myanmar; [b] Rheumatology Department, Royal North Shore Hospital, Institute of Bone and Joint Research, Kolling Institute, The University of Sydney, Sydney, Australia
* Department of Physical Medicine and Rehabilitation, Mandalay General Hospital, University of Medicine, Mandalay, Mandalay, Myanmar.
E-mail addresses: wioo3335@uni.sydney.edu.au; drwinminoopmr@gmail.com

Despite the massive disease burden in OA populations, there are currently no disease-modifying osteoarthritis drugs (DMOADs) approved by regulatory bodies.[3] The current pharmacologic or nonpharmacologic management has revealed only modest efficacy at best,[4] and there are often safety concerns for the long-term use of commonly used analgesics in elderly patients who usually have comorbid diseases.[3] More than half of the patients with moderate and severe OA reported unsatisfactory pain relief,[5] suggesting an immense unmet need in the current therapies. Therefore, finding innovative, effective DMOAD therapies for OA patients is exquisitely urgent, given the global increase of the elderly population and prevalence of obesity.[6]

A DMOAD can be defined as a pharmaceutical agent that will delay or reverse the progression of the structural damage of the joint, thereby leading to clinical translation of improvement in symptoms, manifested either by pain reduction or by benefits in physical function.[7] So far, there is no effective DMOAD approved by the regulatory bodies.

This narrative review focuses on the DMOAD candidates currently undergoing or having completed the active phase 2 and 3 clinical trials within the last 5 years (Fig. 1) related to 3 main molecular endotypes: (1) inflammation-driven endotype, (2) bone-driven endotype, (3) cartilage-driven endotype. Although the assignment of a specific drug on account of its predominant activity was made only to 1 specific endotype, some drugs may have broader endotype effects, and where present, these are duly described. The electronic and manual searches were conducted on the https://clinicaltrials.gov/ site for detecting the phase 2/3 clinical trials, which are either active or have been completed within the last 5 years (Table 1). Moreover, the PubMed and Embase via Ovid trials from the inception to August 31, 2021 were used for electronic database searches for publications of these phase 2/3 clinical trials with the following MESH or keywords: osteoarthritis OR osteoarthrosis AND disease-modifying osteoarthritis drugs/OR DMOAD/OR structure modification. Then, the current challenges and potential research opportunities are discussed by using the PICO (population, intervention, control, and outcomes) approach commonly applied to formulate a research question in evidence-based medicine (Fig. 2).

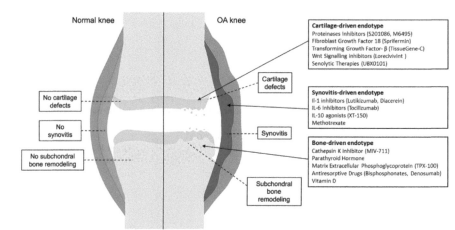

Fig. 1. Active drugs related to the 3 main OA endotypes (phase 2 and 3 RCT). Drug Design, Development and Therapy 2021:15 2921-2945 - Originally published by and used with permission from Dove Medical Press Ltd.

Table 1
Summary of disease-modifying osteoarthritis drugsclinical trials that are active or finished within 5 y in osteoarthritis (phase 2 and 3)

Targeted Endotype	Drug Class	Name of Investigational Drug	Route	OA Site	Active Trial IDs/Estimated Completion Date	Completed Trial IDs/Completed Date
Inflammation	Anti-IL-1	Lutikizumab (ABT-981)	SC	Hand		NCT02087904 (Dec 2016) NCT02384538 (July 2016) NCT02688400 (Dec 2019) NCT02477059 (Feb 2019)
	Anti-IL-6	Diacerein	Oral	Knee		
		Tocilizumab	IV	Hand		
	DNA plasmid with IL10 transgene	XT-150	IA	Knee	NCT04124042 (Feb 2022)	
	DMARD	Methotrexate	Oral	Knee	NCT03815448 (Dec 2022)	ISRCTN77854383 (2018)
Subchondral bone	Cathepsin K inhibitors	MIV-711	Oral	Knee		NCT02705625 (May 2017) NCT03037489 (Nov 2017)
	Parathyroid hormone	Teriparatide	SC	Knee	NCT03072147 (Oct 2022)	
	Matrix extracellular phosphoglycoprotein	TPX-100	IA	Knee		NCT01925261 (Sept 2016) NCT02837900 (Aug 2017)
	Anti-resorptives	Zoledronic acid	IV	Hip	NCT04303026 (Mar 2022)	
		Denosumab	SC	Hand	NCT02771860 (May 2021)	
		Vitamin D	Oral	Knee	NCT04739592 (Jul 2024)	
Cartilage	ADAMTS-5 inhibitors	GLPG1972/s201086	Oral	Knee		NCT03595618 (Jul 2020) NCT01919164 (May 2019)
	Fibroblast growth factor	Sprifermin (AS902330)	IA	Knee	NCT03291470 (Sept 2021) NCT03203330 (Oct 2024)	
	Gene therapy	TissueGene-C	IA	Knee	NCT03928184 (Aug 2021) NCT03727022 (Sept 2021) NCT04385303 (Sept 2021) NCT03706521 (Dec 2021) NCT04520607 (Sept 2022)	
	Wnt/β-catenin signaling pathway inhibitors	Lorecivivint SM04690	IA	Knee		NCT02536833 (April 2017) NCT03122860 (April 2018)
	Senolytic agents	UBX0101	IA	Knee		NCT04129944 (Aug 2020) NCT04349956 (Nov 2020)

Abbreviations: IV, intravenous; SC, subcutaneous.

OSTEOARTHRITIS SUBTYPES: PHENOTYPES AND ENDOTYPES

Because of marked heterogeneity in clinical and structural manifestations and the complexity of the pathobiological mechanism of the OA disease process, targeting a particular subtype of the OA population would be meaningful for a target therapy in drug development.[8] Broadly, OA disease can be divided into either a phenotype based on observable traits (ie, similar clinically observable characteristics, such as etiologic factors, risk factors), or an endotype that possesses a distinct pathophysiologic mechanism via cellular, molecular, and biomechanical signaling pathways.[9] As a note, a given clinical OA phenotype may reveal overlapping molecular endotypes at some stages of the disease process.[7] From the perspective of drug development, there seems to be a consensus on the presence of 3 endotypes, namely synovitis-driven endotype, bone-driven endotype, and cartilage-driven endotype.

SYNOVITIS-DRIVEN ENDOTYPE

The synovium in OA patients undergoes infiltration of mononuclear cells,[10] synovial hypertrophy, and generation of inflammatory cytokines, such as tumor necrosis factor-alpha (TNF-α), interleukin-1β (IL-1β), and IL-6,[11] leading to the synovitis evidenced by the histologic studies[12] and imaging modalities.[13] As synovitis may be associated with pain and radiographic progression,[14] investigating the anti-inflammatory agents is a promising approach for a subset of the OA population with predominant inflammation (**Tables 2 and 3**).

INTERLEUKIN-1 INHIBITORS

IL-1 can induce the production of proteinases[15] in chondrocytes and synoviocytes, leading to cartilage destruction, and it also inhibits the generation of proteoglycan and collagen type II.[16] Therefore, inhibition of the IL-1 pathway can be considered a promising target.[17] Phase 2/3 clinical trials for 2 investigational drugs that can inhibit IL-1 pathway have finished recently.

Lutikizumab (ABT-981)

Lutikizumab is a novel human dual-variable domain immunoglobulin, which demonstrated simultaneous blockage of both IL-1a and IL-1b in a mouse OA model.[18] In a

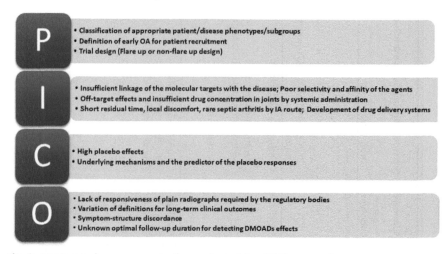

Fig. 2. Barriers to be overcome in the context of the PICO approach.

Table 2
Published results of phase 2/3 clinical trials related to the symptomatic efficacy of pharmaceutical agents in synovitis-driven endotype

Authors/Ref.	ClinialTrials.gov Identifier	OA Site	Dosage, Route of Interventions	N	Follow-Up Duration	Efficacy in Symptomatic Modification		Phase of Development
						Pain (0–50) (WOMAC if not Denoted Otherwise)	Function (0–170) (WOMAC if not Denoted Otherwise)	
Lutikizumab (ABT-981)								
Fleischmann et al,[19] 2019	NCT02087904	Knee	Placebo / Lutikizumab 25 mg SC q2w / Lutikizumab 100 mg SC q2w / Lutikizumab 200 mg SC q2w	85 / 89 / 87 / 89	16 wk	−8.1 (−10.44, −5.79) / −10.3 (−12.58, −8.08) / −11.7 (−14.17, −9.26)* / −11.9 (−14.11, −9.66)*	−29.1 (−36.46, −21.82) / −31.4 (−38.53, −24.34) / −36.3 (−43.99, −28.53) / −32.6 (−39.61, −25.52)	Phase 2
Kloppenburg et al,[20] 2019	NCT02384538	Hand	Placebo / Lutikizumab 200 mg SC q2w	67 / 64	16 wk	−10.7 (−15.4 to −6.0) / −9.2 (−13.8 to −4.6) AUSCAN pain range 0–50	−17.2 (−24.9 to −9.4) / −14.6 (−22.1 to −7.1) AUSCAN function ranges 0—90	Phase 2
Diacerein								
Pelletier et al,[22] 2020	NCT02688400	Knee	Diacerein 50 mg OD for 1 mo and then BD / Celecoxib 200 mg OD	140 / 148	6 mo	−11.1 (0.9) / −11.8 (0.9)	−27.2 (39.0) / −29.3 (39.8)	Phase 2
Tocilizumab								
Richette et al,[28] 2021	NCT02477059	Hand	Placebo / Tocilizumab 8 mg/kg IV at weeks 0 and 4	41 / 42	6 wk	−9.9 (SD 20.1) / −7.9 (SD 19.4) VAS pain range 0–100	0.2 ± 0.6 / −0.04 ± 0.6 FIHOA (0—30)	Phase 3

(continued on next page)

Table 2
(continued)

Authors/Ref.	ClinialTrials. gov Identifier	OA Site	Dosage, Route of Interventions	N	Follow-Up Duration	Efficacy in Symptomatic Modification		Phase of Development
						Pain (0–50) (WOMAC if not Denoted Otherwise)	Function (0–170) (WOMAC if not Denoted Otherwise)	
Methotrexate								
Kingsbury et al,[33] 2019	ISRCTN77854383	Knee	Placebo 10 mg to 25 mg over 8 wk and then maintenance at 25 mg	68 66	6 mo	−0.83 (−1.55, −0.10) (mean difference, NRS pain)	−5.01 (−8.74, −1.29)	Phase 3

Abbreviations: AUSCAN, the Australian Canadian Osteoarthritis Hand Index; BD, ; FIHOA, Functional Index for Hand Osteoarthritis; NRS, numerical rating scale; OD, ; SD, standard deviation.

Table 3
Published results of phase 2/3 clinical trials related to the structural efficacy of pharmaceutical agents in synovitis-driven endotype

Authors/Ref.	ClinialTrials.gov Identifier	OA Site	Dosage, Route of Interventions	N	Follow-Up Duration (wk)	Efficacy in Structural Modification		Phase of Development
						Plain Radiographs	MRI	
Lutikizumab (ABT-981)								
Fleischmann et al,[19] 2019	NCT02087904	Knee	Placebo Lutikizumab 25 mg SC every 2 wk Lutikizumab 100 mg SC every 2 wk Lutikizumab 200 mg SC every 2 wk	85 89 87 89	26 wk for MRI synovitis 52 wk for radiographs	No significant difference in medal or lateral JSN except for Lutikizumab 25 mg	No significant difference in synovial thickness, synovial fluid volume, and WORMS semiquantitative synovitis/effusion volume	Phase 2
Kloppenburg et al,[20] 2019	NCT02384538	Hand	Placebo Lutikizumab 200 mg SC q2w	67 64	26 wk	No significant changes in JSN	No significant changes in HOAMRIS MRI scores	Phase 2
Methotrexate								
Kingsbury et al,[33] 2019	ISRCTN77854383	Knee	Placebo 10 mg to 25 mg over 8 wk and then maintenance at 25 mg	68 66	6 mo	NA	14.89 (−18.19, 47.96) (mean difference, mm³)	Phase 3

Abbreviations: HOAMRIS, Hand Osteoarthritis Magnetic Resonance Imaging Scoring System; NA, nonavailable; WORMS, .

phase 2 study in 347 patients with knee OA with MRI- or ultrasound-detected synovi-tis, Lutikizumab showed limited reduction in the Western Ontario and McMaster Universities Osteoarthritis Index (WOMAC) pain score at week 16 and no significant improvement in structural endpoints, such as MRI synovitis, at 26 weeks and joint space narrowing (JSN) on radiographs at week 52.[19] A preplanned subgroup analysis showed that Lutikizumab 100 mg had statistically significant improvement in pain among patients with K/L grade 3 knee OA, suggesting that more advanced disease may be more responsive from IL-1 blockage. Lutikizumab had more adverse events: injection site reactions (25.2% vs 15.3%) and neutropenia (27.5% vs 2.4%), compared with the placebo. In another phase 2 study evaluating its efficacy in erosive hand OA with ≥3 tender and/or swollen hand joints (n = 132), Lutikizumab demonstrated no symptomatic or structural benefits assessed with multiple imaging scoring systems,[20] in agreement with the previous study in knee OA.

Diacerein

Diacerein acts by suppressing the IL-1b system and related downstream pathways. In mice, diacerein (5.0–25.0 mg/kg) also inhibits IL-1β in a dose-dependent manner and reduces TNF-α–induced nociception.[21] Recently, in an international, multi-center, double-blind randomized clinical trial (RCT) (NCT02688400), the efficacy and safety of administering diacerein 50 mg once per day for 1 month and twice daily thereafter (n = 140), or celecoxib 200 mg once per day for 6 months (n = 148), were compared in moderate and severe knee OA. A similar treatment effect on WOMAC pain and function was detected, starting at 2 months' follow-up and maintained for the entire duration of the study. However, the study did not include the outcomes measures for structural modification. In the diacerein group, gastrointestinal side effects (diarrhea) were more common (10.2% vs 3.7%), and 1 patient had symptoms suggestive of possible hepatitis.[22] The EMA's Pharmacovigilance Risk Assessment Committee recommended restrictions of its use to limit risks of severe diarrhea and hepatotoxicity in 2014.[23] In a recent meta-analysis investigating the adverse effects of OA medications, compared with placebo, diacerein was significantly related to gastrointestinal disorders (odds ratio [OR], 2.53; 95% CI, 1.43–4.46) and renal disorders (OR, 3.16; 95% CI, 1.93–5.15) even when concomitant OA medications were not allowed.[24]

ANTI-INTERLEUKIN-6 INHIBITORS

IL-6 played a direct role in regulating chondrocyte function and cartilage metabolism and seems to have a differential effect on OA pathophysiology depending on the signal via the classic (protective) or transsignaling (inflammatory and catabolic) pathway.[25] In the destabilization of the medial meniscus (DMM) mouse model, neutralizing antibody of the IL-6 receptor reduced osteophyte formation, cartilage lesions, and synovitis.[26]

Tocilizumab

Tocilizumab, an IL-6 antagonist, leads to cartilage preservation in a mouse model of ischemic osteonecrosis.[27] However, in a recent phase 3 clinical trial (n = 83), which evaluated the efficacy of tocilizumab in refractory hand OA with at least 3 painful joints, there was no significant benefits in pain and function.[28] This might suggest that removing IL-6 signaling alone in the short term is not sufficient for pain reduction in human OA. As a note, tocilizumab causes inhibition of all IL-6 signaling pathways, including classic and trans-signaling.[25]

INTERLEUKIN-10 AGONISTS

IL-10 is a potent anti-inflammatory cytokine, which can suppress the generation of key proinflammatory cytokines, such as TNF-α, IL-1β, and IL-6, as well as reduce matrix metallopeptidases (MMPs) expression.[29]

XT-150

IL-10 protein possesses a short half-life in vivo and poor permeation into articular capsule upon systemic administration. Therefore, XT-150 was developed using plasmid DNA-based therapy for the generation of a long-acting human IL-10 variant.[30] XT150 administered into canine OA joints showed an increase in intra-articular (IA) IL-10 levels, showed improved pain, and is well tolerated.[31] Currently, a phase 2 clinical trial is ongoing for knee OA (NCT04124042).

METHOTREXATE

Methotrexate (MTX) is a traditional disease-modifying antirheumatic drug used in a variety of inflammatory rheumatic and autoimmune disorders.[32] In the phase 3 PROMOTE trial published as a 2019 OARSI conference abstract (n = 134), oral MTX showed significant improvement in knee pain and function at 6-month follow-up but not at 9 and 12 months with no change in synovial volume on contrast-enhanced MRI at 6 months.[33] Currently, a phase 3 study is active for symptomatic knee OA patients with effusion-synovitis grade of ≥2 (NCT03815448).

BONE-DRIVEN ENDOTYPE

Microstructural changes in subchondral bone are attributed to an uncoupled remodeling process owing to the spontaneous activation (in early-stage OA) or inactivation (in late-stage OA) of osteoclastic bone resorption activity.[34] An acidic microenvironment created by bone-resorbing osteoclasts via secreting H+ produced bone pain in animal models of bone metastasis.[35] During aberrant subchondral bone remodeling, Netrin-1 produced by osteoclasts can induce sensory innervation and genesis of OA pain by acting through its receptor DCC (deleted in colorectal cancer).[36] The agents acting through subchondral bone remodeling have reached late clinical trials (**Tables 4 and 5**).

CATHEPSIN K INHIBITOR

Cathepsin K is a lysosomal cysteine protease present in activated osteoclasts for degrading collagen and other matrix proteins during bone resorption.[37] Moreover, it is also involved in cartilage matrix degradation, and OA as a milder cartilage degradation occurred in cathepsin K–deficient mice after anterior cruciate ligament transection (ACLT) when compared with wild-type controls.[38]

MIV-711 is a potent selective cathepsin K inhibitor that revealed reduced subchondral bone loss and cartilage damage in ACLT-induced rabbit OA and partial-medial meniscectomy-induced dog OA.[39] In a 26-week phase 2 human trial in knee OA (n = 244), significant reductions in bone and cartilage OA progression were detected with no improvement in pain. The active treatment groups had 5 cardiovascular events, and skin disorders were more common in the active groups (100 mg/d: 7.3%; 200 mg/d: 12.2%; placebo: 2.5%).[40]

PARATHYROID HORMONE

Recombinant human parathyroid hormone, teriparatide, possesses a bone anabolic effect in the subchondral plate via acting on the osteoblasts. It increased proteoglycan

Table 4
Published results of phase 2/3 clinical trials related to the symptomatic efficacy of pharmaceutical agents in bone-driven endotype

Authors/Ref.	ClinialTrials.gov Identifier	OA Site	Dosage, Route of Interventions	N	Follow-up Duration (wk)	Efficacy in Symptomatic Modification		Phase of Development
						Pain (0–50) (WOMAC if not Denoted Otherwise)	Function (0–170) (WOMAC if not Denoted Otherwise)	
Cathepsin K inhibitors								
Conaghan et al,[40] 2020	NCT02705625 NCT03037489	Knee	Placebo MIV-711, 100 mg/d MIV-711, 200 mg/d	80 82 82	26 wk	−1.4 (−1.9 to −0.8) −1.7 (−2.3 to −1.2) −1.5 (−2.0 to −0.9) NRS (0–10)	NA	Phase 2
Matrix extracellular phosphoglycoprotein								
McGuire et al,[45] 2018	—	Knee	Placebo TPX-100 IA 200 mg 4 weekly injections	93 93	12 mo	— Significant WOMAC scores (no numerical data)	— Significant WOMAC scores (no numerical data)	Phase 2
Antiresorptives								
Frediani et al,[56] 2020	—	Knee	Clodronate IM 200 mg/d for 15 d and then q1w for next 2.5 mo Clodronate IM 200 mg/d for 15 d and then q1w for next 11.5 mo	37 37	12 mo	50.3 ± 31.9 (SD) 15.6 ± 9.8 (SD)* (VAS = 0–100)	24.0 ± 11.9 13.5 ± 5.7*	NA
Cai et al,[58] 2020	ACTRN12613000039785	Knee	Placebo saline IV zoledronic acid IV 5 mg baseline and 12 mo	110 113	24 mo	−16.8 (−22.0 to −11.6) −11.5 (−16.9 to −6.2) (VAS)	NA	Phase 3

MacFarlane et al,[60] 2020	NCT01351805	Knee	Placebo Cholecalciferol oral 2000 IU/d	630 591	4 y	34.6 ± 0.9 (SE) 32.7 ± 0.9	34.6 (0.9) (SE) 34.1 (1.0)	NA
Tu et al,[62] 2021	NCT01176344	Knee	Placebo Cholecalciferol oral 50,000 IU (1.25 mg) per month	204 209	2 y	Change from baseline 1.30 (0.51, 2.09) −0.03 (−0.80, 0.74)* (MFPDI range 0–34)	NA	Phase 3

Abbreviations: IM, intramuscular; IU, international units; MFPDI, Manchester Foot Pain and Disability Index scores; NRS, numerical rating scale; SE, .

Table 5
Published results of phase 2/3 clinical trials related to the structural efficacy of pharmaceutical agents in bone-driven endotype

Authors/ Ref.	ClinialTrials.gov Identifier	OA Site	Dosage, Route of Interventions	N	Follow-Up Duration (wk)	Plain Radiographs	MRI	Phase of Development
Cathepsin K inhibitors								
Conaghan et al,[40] 2020	NCT02705625 NCT03037489	Knee	Placebo MIV-711, 100 mg/d MIV-711, 200 mg/d	80 82 82	26 wk	NA	23.3 (15.7–30.9) 7.9 (0.5–15.3)** 8.6 (1.1–16.1)** (bone area, mm²) −0.066 (−0.119 to −0.013) 0.011 (−0.042–0.063)* −0.022 (−0.074–0.031) (cartilage thickness, mm)	Phase 2
Matrix extracellular phosphoglycoprotein								
McGuire et al,[45] 2018	—	Knee	Placebo TPX-100 IA 200 mg 4 weekly injections	93 93	12 mo	NA	No significance in cartilage thickness/volume on quantitative MRI (no numerical data)	Phase 2
McGuire et al,[46] 2020	—	Knee	Placebo TPX-100 IA 200 mg 4 weekly injections	78 78		NA	Significant decrease in pathologic bone shape change in the femur (no numerical data) >	Phase 2
Antiresorptives								
Frediani et al,[56] 2020	—	Knee	Clodronate IM 200 mg/d for 15 d and then q1w for next 2.5 mo Clodronate IM 200 mg/d for 15 d and then q1w for next 11.5 mo	37 37	12 mo	NA	5.9 ± 4.9 1.1 ± 0.8* (BML)	NA

Cai et al,[58] 2020	ACTRN12613000039785	Knee	Placebo saline IV zoledronic acid IV 5 mg baseline and 12 mo	110 113	24 mo	NA	NA	-919 (-1004 to -835) -878 (-963 to -793) (cartilage volume mm^3) -6 (-75–63) -33 (-104–39) (BML mm^2)	Phase 3
Perry et al,[61] 2021	—	Knee	Placebo Cholecalciferol oral 800 IU/d	26 24	24 mo	NA	NA	Change from baseline 61.5 (-1085.6–1208.6) 155.4 (-1097.3–1408.0) (synovial volume mm^3) -193.4 (-2845.7–2459.0) -506.9 (-3395.6–2381.9) (subchondral BML volume mm^3)	NA

Abbreviation: IV, intravenous.

content and inhibited cartilage degeneration in a mouse model of injury-induced knee OA.[41] It can reduce pain by ameliorating temporomandibular joint OA changes in aging mice,[42] decreasing chondrocyte apoptosis via autophagy-related proteins,[43] prostaglandin E2 production, and sensory innervation of subchondral bone in DMM mice.[44] A phase 2 clinical trial in knee OA is currently ongoing (NCT03072147).

MATRIX EXTRACELLULAR PHOSPHOGLYCOPROTEIN

TPX-100 is a matrix extracellular phosphoglycoprotein derivative having a novel 23-amino-acid peptide.[45] IA injections of TPX-100 stimulate articular cartilage proliferation in goats and reduced joint damage in rats. In a phase 2 study involving 93 patients with bilateral patellofemoral OA, 4 weekly injections of 200 mg TPX-100 demonstrated a significant difference in pain when ascending and descending stairs at 12 months but no structural benefits on quantitative MRI,[45] perhaps because of the small sample size. Another 2020 OARSI conference abstract described a reduction in pathologic bone shape change in the femur and stabilization in tibiofemoral cartilage.[46]

ANTIRESORPTIVE DRUGS: BISPHOSPHONATES AND DENOSUMAB

Research has established an association of OA developments and symptoms with bone marrow lesions (BML) on MRI,[47,48] an altered signal pattern related to increased vascularization, bone marrow necrosis, fibrosis, and less mineralized bone.[49] Histochemical analysis of BMLs revealed an abundance of matrix metalloproteinases, TNF-α, and substance P, which might induce pain receptor stimulation.[50] Therefore, antiresorptive agents seem to be a promising therapy because of their implications in pathogenesis and clinical manifestations in OA.

However, in both preclinical and clinical studies, inconsistent results are reported, which is reflected by significant heterogeneity across the studies in the systematic reviews.[51,52] In the latest reviews, bisphosphonates showed neither symptomatic relief nor improved radiographic progression in knee OA.[53,54] However, there may be some benefits in certain subgroups with early OA and high bone-turnover rates.[51,53] An individual patient data meta-analysis examining the effects of bisphosphonates in certain knee OA subgroups is still ongoing.[55]

In a small sample (n = 74), administration of intramuscular clodronate 200 mg daily for 15 days (higher dose than used in osteoporosis) and then once weekly for the next 11.5 months improved BML and pain in knee OA[56] compared with a shorter maintenance regimen (2.5 months).[56] In a propensity-matched retrospective cohort analysis of the Osteoarthritis Initiative in female participants (n = 346), bisphosphonate exposure showed a significant protective effect (51% relative reduction) against 2-year radiographic progression in nonoverweight patients (body mass index <25 kg/m^2) with early radiographic OA.[57]

Recently, in the 2-year Zoledronic Acid for Osteoarthritis Knee Pain (ZAP2) study conducted in 223 knee OA patients with significant knee pain and MRI-detected BMLs, twice yearly administration of 5 mg zoledronic acid (the most potent of all bisphosphonates) did not significantly improve knee pain, cartilage volume loss, or BML size. Although the clinical trial was designed and sufficiently powered for detecting disease-modifying effects on BMLs in the bone-driven subgroup, the more sensitive MRI-detected cartilage volume was measured as the primary outcome, and the follow-up is quite long (2 years).[58] On the exploratory subgroup analysis of the ZAP2 study, there was a greater symptomatic but not structure-modifying benefit in patients without radiographic JSN (n = 44) than those with JSN grade 1 to 2 (−13.5 vs 9.9 on a visual analogue scale [VAS] score).[58] The zoledronic acid group had more knee replacements (9%) compared with the placebo group (2%) over 2 years. Currently, there are 2 clinical trials examining the effects of zoledronic acid in hip OA (NCT04303026) and of denosumab in hand OA (NCT02771860).

VITAMIN D

Vitamin D stimulates proteoglycan synthesis in mature chondrocytes and reduces the production of inflammatory cytokine by activating AMPK/mTOR signaling.[59] In a VITAL (Vitamin D and Omega-3) Trial, which included a subset of patients with chronic knee pain (1,39), vitamin D supplementation neither reduces knee pain nor improves function at 4-year follow-up.[60] Vitamin D supplementation in patients with symptomatic knee OA showed no significant difference in MRI-detected synovial tissue volume and subchondral BML volume at 2-year follow-up (n = 50).[61] A recent post hoc study in patients with knee OA showed that foot pain scores remained unchanged in the vitamin D group (−0.03 [−0.80, 0.74]) (n = 209) over 2 years while worsening in the placebo group (1.30 [0.51, 2.09]) (n = 204).[62] A recent meta-analysis reported that it had symptomatic benefits but no structure-modifying effect in knee OA.[63] A small phase 4 clinical trial is ongoing (NCT04739592).

CARTILAGE-DRIVEN ENDOTYPE

Cartilage failure to maintain homeostasis between synthesis and degradation of extracellular matrix components is a major contributor to OA pathogenesis, leading to cartilage softening, fibrillation and fissuring of the superficial cartilage layers, and diminished cartilage thickness.[64] **Tables 6 and 7** show the DMOAD candidates for this endotype.

PROTEINASE INHIBITORS

Articular cartilage is formed by chondrocytes, which are embedded in an ECM that has an abundance of type II collagen fibrils and aggrecan. Collagenases, such as matrix metalloproteinases (MMPs), and aggrecanase, such as a disintegrin and metalloproteinases, with thrombospondin motifs (ADAMTSs) belong to the family of zinc endopeptidases and are responsible for degradation of triple-helical type II collagen fibrils (collagenolysis) and aggrecan, the major proteoglycan in articular cartilage.[65] As broad-spectrum MMP inhibitors with strong Zn^{2+} chelating properties, such as PG-116800, showed poor selectivity and caused adverse effects, such as musculoskeletal triad (arthralgia, myalgia, tendinitis), also known as the musculoskeletal syndrome (MSS), and gastrointestinal disorders perhaps owing to a nonselective inhibition of other metalloproteinases or a combined inhibition of a series of critical MMPs, further development has been terminated.[66]

Preclinical studies revealed overwhelming data on a potential role of MMP-13 in OA pathogenesis, and MMP 13 has been a potential target.[67] Because of the unusual presence of the large hydrophobic S1′ pocket of MMP-13, non-zinc-binding MMP-13 inhibitors with higher potency and superior selectivity profiles by occupying themselves deeper in the S1′ pocket have been developed to avoid MSS, but have not reached the phase 2 clinical trials owing to poor solubility, biodistribution, permeability, metabolic stability, or bioavailability.[68]

ADAMTS-5 has been a target for OA therapy, as it is the most potent aggrecanase in vitro (30-fold more potent than ADAMTS-4) and ADAMTS-5 ablation or inhibition prevents joint damage in mice and human chondrocytes.[69] S201086/GLPG1972 is orally administered and a potent active site inhibitor of ADAMTS5[69] with an 8-fold

Table 6
Published results of phase 2/3 clinical trials related to the symptomatic efficacy of pharmaceutical agents in cartilage-driven endotype

Authors/Ref.	ClinialTrials.gov Identifier	OA Site	Dosage, Route of Interventions	N	Follow-Up Duration (wk)	Efficacy in Symptomatic Modification		Phase of Development
						Pain (0–50) (WOMAC if not Denoted Otherwise)	Function (0–170) (WOMAC if not Denoted Otherwise)	
Proteinases inhibitors								
Galapagos and Servier,[71] 2020	NCT03595618	Knee	Placebo S201086/GLPG1972 low dose S201086/GLPG1972 medium dose S201086/GLPG1972 high dose (no numerical report)	932 (total)	52 wk	No significance (no numerical report)	No significance (no numerical report)	Phase 2
Fibroblast growth factor-18								
Lohmander et al,[80] 2014	NCT01033994	Knee	Placebo Sprifermin IA 10 μg 3 once weekly Sprifermin IA 30 μg 3 once weekly Sprifermin IA 100 μg 3 once weekly	42 21 42 63	12 mo	−5.56 (4.17) −4.10 (5.11) −3.54 (3.67) −2.87 (4.76)* (mean change from baseline, SD)	−17.02 (13.56) −15.76 (13.72) −12.12 (12.06) −11.28 (15.30)* (mean change from baseline, SD)	Phase 1b
Hochberg et al,[83] 2019	NCT01919164	Knee	Placebo Sprifermin IA 30 μg 3 once weekly q6 mo Sprifermin IA 30 μg 3 once weekly q12 mo Sprifermin IA 100 μg 3 once weekly q6 mo Sprifermin IA 100 μg 3 once weekly q12 mo	108 111 110 110 110	24 mo	NA 2.58 (−3.47, 8.64) 1.29 (−4.53, 7.10) −0.06 (−5.76, 5.65) 3.65 (−1.99, 9.28) (difference with placebo; total WOMAC score)	No numerical data for individual WOMAC scores	Phase 2

Study	NCT	Joint	Intervention	N	Duration			Phase
Eckstein et al,[86] 2021	NCT01919164	Knee	Placebo	108	60 mo	−22.38 (22.19)	−17.03 (24.15)	Phase 2
			Sprifermin IA 30 μg 3 once weekly q12 mo	110		−24.41 (22.48)	−18.74 (21.87)	
			Sprifermin IA 30 μg 3 once weekly q6 mo	111		−20.38 (22.49)	−18.55 (23.76)	
			Sprifermin IA 100 μg 3 once weekly q12 mo	110		−24.94 (19.95)	−18.82 (21.62)	
			Sprifermin IA 100 μg 3 once weekly q6 mo	110		−24.00 (22.38) (change from baseline at 5 y)	−18.56 (23.60)	
Gene therapy								
Lee et al,[94] 2020	NCT01221441	Knee	Placebo IA (2 mL normal saline 0.9%)	35	12 mo	Significant improvement in VAS pain	Significant improvement in IKDC scores	Phase 2
			TissueGene-C IA	67				
Kim et al,[95] 2018	—	Knee	Placebo IA (2 mL normal saline 0.9%)	81	12 mo	−10	NA	Phase 3
			TissueGene-C IA	78		−25*** (change from baseline, VAS pain score)		
Wnt/β-catenin signaling pathway inhibitors								
Yazici et al,[103] 2020	NCT02536833	Knee	Placebo	114	13 wk	−22.1 ± 2.1	NA	Phase 2
			Lorecivivint (SM04690) 0.03 mg	112		−23.3 ± 2.2		
			Lorecivivint (SM04690) 0.07 mg	117		−23.5 ± 2.1		
			Lorecivivint (SM04690) 0.23 mg	109		−23.5 ± 2.1 (mean ± SD change from baseline)		
Yazici et al,[104] 2021	NCT03122860	Knee	Dry needle	117	24 wk	NA	NA	Phase 2b
			Placebo	116		6.2 (1.0)	59.2 (9.8)	
			Lorecivivint (SM04690) 0.03 mg	116		6.2 (1.1)*	59.0 (10.9)	
			Lorecivivint (SM04690) 0.07 mg	115		6.1 (1.1)	58.1 (11.2)	
			Lorecivivint (SM04690) 0.15 mg	115		6.1 (1.0)	57.7 (11.1)	
			Lorecivivint (SM04690) 0.23 mg	116		6.1 (1.0)* (mean ± SD change from baseline, NRS pain)	57.3 (11.4)* (mean ± SD change from baseline)	

(continued on next page)

Table 6
(continued)

Authors/Ref.	ClinialTrials.gov Identifier	OA Site	Dosage, Route of Interventions	N	Follow-Up Duration (wk)	Efficacy in Symptomatic Modification		Phase of Development
						Pain (0–50) (WOMAC if not Denoted Otherwise)	Function (0–170) (WOMAC if not Denoted Otherwise)	
Senolytic agents								
UNITY Biotechnology,[110] 2021	NCT04129944	Knee	Placebo	46	12 wk	−1.017	NA	Phase 2
			UBX0101 IA 0.5 mg	45		−0.924		
			UBX0101 IA 2.0 mg mg	46		−1.052		
			UBX0101 IA 4.0 mg mg	46		−1.019 (mean change from baseline)		

Abbreviations: IKDC, international knee documentation committee scores; NRS, numerical rating scale.

Table 7
Published results of phase 2/3 clinical trials related to the structural efficacy of pharmaceutical agents in cartilage-driven endotype

Authors/Ref.	ClinialTrials.gov Identifier	OA Site	Dosage, Route of Interventions	N	Follow-up Duration (wk)	Efficacy in Structural Modification		Phase of Development
						Plain Radiographs	MRI	
Proteinases Inhibitors								
Galapagos and Servier,[71] 2020	NCT03595618	Knee	Placebo S201086/GLPG1972 low dose S201086/GLPG1972 medium dose S201086/GLPG1972 high dose (no numerical report)	932 (total)	52 wk	NA	−0.116 (0.27) −0.068 (0.20), −0.097 (0.27) 0.085 (0.22) change in cartilage thickness (in mm [SD])	Phase 2
Fibroblast growth factor-18								
Lohmander et al,[80] 2014	NCT01033994	Knee	Placebo Sprifermin IA10 µg 3 once weekly Sprifermin IA 30 µg 3 once weekly Sprifermin IA 100 µg 3 once weekly	42 21 42 63	12 mo	−0.02 (0.90) 0.05 (1.00) 0.03 (0.72) −0.04 (0.90) (mean change, MFTC JSW, mm) −0.18 (0.74) −0.02 (0.86) 1.0 (0.73) 0.34 (0.90)* (mean change, LFTC JSW, mm)	−0.11 (−0.20, −0.02) 0.02 (−0.18, 0.23) −0.11 (−0.18, −0.03) −0.03 (−0.11, 0.04) (mean change, cMFTC cartilage thickness, mm) −0.03 (−0.04, 0.01) 0.00 (−0.08, 0.08) −0.01 (−0.02, 0.01) 0.01 (0.00, 0.03)* (mean change, TFTC cartilage thickness, mm)	Phase 1b

(continued on next page)

Table 7
(continued)

Authors/Ref.	ClinialTrials.gov Identifier	OA Site	Dosage, Route of Interventions	N	Follow-up Duration (wk)	Efficacy in Structural Modification		Phase of Development
						Plain Radiographs	MRI	
			Proteinases Inhibitors					
Hochberg et al,[83] 2019	NCT01919164	Knee	Placebo	108	24 mo	NA	−0.02(−0.04, −0.01)	Phase 2
			Sprifermin IA 30 µg 3 once weekly q12 mo	110		0.08 mm (−0.08, 0.25)	0.00 (−0.02, 0.02)	
			Sprifermin IA 30 µg 3 once weekly q6 mo	111		0.04 mm (−0.13, 0.20)	−0.01(−0.03, 0.00)	
			Sprifermin IA 100 µg 3 once weekly q12 mo	110		0.26 mm (0.12, 0.40)**	0.03 (0.01, 0.04)	
			Sprifermin IA 100 µg 3 once weekly q6 mo	110		0.26 mm (0.12, 0.41)** (difference vs placebo, LFTC JSW, mm)	0.02 (0.00, 0.03)*** (mean change, TFTC cartilage thickness, mm)	
Eckstein et al,[86] 2021	NCT01919164	Knee	Placebo	108	60 mo	−0.38 (0.72); mean (SD)	—	Phase 2
			Sprifermin IA 30 µg 3 once weekly q12 mo	110		−0.47 (1.02)	—	
			Sprifermin IA 30 µg 3 once weekly q6 mo	111		−0.31 (0.75)	—*	
			Sprifermin IA 100 µg 3 once weekly q12 mo	110		−0.27 (0.75)	No numerical data reported for TFTC cartilage thickness	
			Sprifermin IA 100 µg 3 once weekly q6 mo	110		−0.16 (0.77)		
						Change from baseline at 5 y; MFTC JSW, mm		
						−0.13 (0.65)		
						−0.05 (0.60)		
						−0.03 (0.69)		
						0.03 (0.88)		
						0.02 (0.76)		
						Change from baseline at 5 y; LFTC JSW, mm		

Gene therapy

Study	NCT	Joint	Intervention (n)	Duration		Outcomes	Phase
Guermazi et al,[91] 2017	NCT01221441	Knee	Placebo IA (2 mL normal saline 0.9%) 29; TissueGene-C IA 57	12 mo	—	47.9% 34.6% Progression of cartilage morphology in any subregion 21.1% 9.6% Any worsening in Hoffa-synovitis/effusion-synovitis combined 60.6% 66.2% (any BML progression) 32.4% 31.6% any meniscal damage progression	Phase 2
Lee et al,[94] 2020	NCT01221441	Knee	Placebo IA (2 mL normal saline 0.9%) 35; TissueGene-C IA 67	12 mo	—	47.9% 34.6% Progression of cartilage morphology in any subregion 21.1% 9.6% Any worsening in Hoffa-synovitis/effusion-synovitis combined	Phase 2
Kim et al,[95] 2018	—	Knee	Placebo IA (2 mL normal saline 0.9%) 81; TissueGene-C IA 78	12 mo	Not significant (JSW)	No significant change in any of WORMS subscore	Phase 3

(continued on next page)

Table 7
(continued)

Authors/Ref.	ClinialTrials.gov Identifier	OA Site	Dosage, Route of Interventions	N	Follow-up Duration (wk)	Efficacy in Structural Modification		Phase of Development
						Plain Radiographs	MRI	
Proteinases Inhibitors								
Wnt/β-catenin signaling pathway inhibitors								
Yazici et al,[103] 2020	NCT02536833	Knee	Placebo IA	114	26 wk	−0.20 mm	NA	Phase 2
			Lorecivivint (SM04690) IA 0.03 mg	112		−0.07 mm		
			Lorecivivint (SM04690) IA 0.07 mg	117		−0.11 mm		
			Lorecivivint (SM04690) IA 0.23 mg	109		−0.02 mm* (mean ± SD change from baseline, medial JSW)		
Yazici et al,[104] 2021	NCT03122860	Knee	Dry needle IA	117	24 wk	NA	NA	Phase 2
			Placebo IA	116		3.44 (1.31)		
			Lorecivivint (SM04690) IA 0.03 mg	116		3.30 (1.26)		
			Lorecivivint (SM04690) IA 0.07 mg	115		3.16 (1.10)		
			Lorecivivint (SM04690) IA 0.15 mg	115		3.26 (1.24)		
			Lorecivivint (SM04690) IA 0.23 mg	116		3.27 (1.08) (mean ± SD change from baseline, medial JSW)		

Abbreviations: cMFTC, central medial femorotibial compartment; LFTC, lateral femorotibial compartment; TFTC, total femorotibial compartment.

selectivity over ADAMTS-4 in preclinical studies.[70] In a phase 2 study (Roccella study) including 932 knee OA patients, no significant difference was found between the active treatment arms (all 3 different dose levels) and placebo arm in both quantitative MRI cartilage thickness and clinical outcomes,[71] although the study was optimally designed by applying 2 radiologically based selection criteria for structural severity in the cartilage damage (ie, the combined Kellgren/Lawrence [KL] 2 or 3 and OARSI medial JSN 1 or 2 grading).[72] Phase 1 studies for an ADAMTS5 nanobody (M6495) were recently completed (NCT03583346, NCT03224702).

A major problem in the application of small molecules for directly targeting protease activity is the high degree of conservation in the sequence and structure of the active site, leading to unintended cross-inactivation of multiple metalloproteinases. This can result in possible short- and long-term side effects with systemic administration of the drug.[73] As an example, blocking the aggrecan degradation may be desired in the articular cartilage[74] but simultaneously may cause undesirable effects in tendons and the aorta, where aggrecan accumulation in tendons resulted in decreased mechanical properties,[75] and aggrecan and versican accumulation in thoracic aortic aneurysms can lead to aortic dissection and rupture.[76]

FIBROBLAST GROWTH FACTOR-18

Sprifermin is a recombinant human fibroblast growth factor-18 (FGF-18), which is a 19.83-kDa protein derived from the *Escherichia coli* expression system.[77] It induces the proliferation of chondrocytes and promotes hyaline extracellular matrix synthesis in preclinical models.[78] In 2007, a first-in-human trial (NCT00911469) for IA sprifermin administration was commenced in 73 end-stage knee OA patients who were scheduled for knee replacement within the next 6 months and showed positive effects on histologic cartilage parameters with no major safety issues over 24 weeks.[79] In the second proof-of-concept phase 1b trial (NCT01033994) conducted in 2008, a significant dose-dependent response in the sprifermin groups was detected in the secondary structural outcomes, such as radiographic JSW, and MRI-detected total and lateral tibiofemoral cartilage thickness over 12 months (n = 168).[80] The sprifermin also improved WOMAC pain score from baseline, but there was no significant difference, compared with the placebo group. The post hoc analyses of the same studies showed the structure-protective effects on cartilage damage and BMLs at 12-month follow-up.[81,82]

In the third phase 2 dose-ranging clinical trial (FGF18 Osteoarthritis Randomized Trial with Administration of Repeated Doses [FORWARD] study) (NCT01919164), there was a statistically significant dose-dependent improvement, but of uncertain clinical importance, in total tibiofemoral cartilage thickness in patients administered with a dose of 100 µg sprifermin every 6 and 12 months, but not with the dose of 30 µg at 2 years (n = 549). No symptomatic improvement is revealed in the active groups, compared with the placebo saline injection.[83] An exploratory analysis of the same study for 3-year follow-up (n = 442) revealed similar results. These findings were published in the *Journal of the American Medical Association* in 2019. In the post hoc analysis, a "subgroup at risk" with narrower medial or lateral minimum JSW and higher WOMAC pain than the overall study population at baseline (n = 161) showed a significant improvement in WOMAC pain on 3-year follow-up (−8.8 (−22.4, 4.9]) in the 100-µg Sprifermin group (n = 34) compared with the placebo (n = 33).[84] In another post hoc analysis using the cartilage thinning/thickening scores and ordered values on MRI over 24 months regardless of the location, 100-µg Sprifermin every 6 months causes cartilage thickening more than double and cartilage thinning almost reduced to that in healthy reference subjects from the Osteoarthritis Initiative data set (n = 82), supporting the structure-protective action of Sprifermin.[85]

Recently, a report on the 5-year efficacy and safety results from the FORWARD study (n = 494) revealed that sprifermin 100 µg every 6 months for 2 years maintained long-term structural protective effects on articular cartilage despite a treatment-free period of 3 years, with a good safety profile.[86] A recent meta-analysis published in 2021 included 8 reports from 3 original trials and confirmed the structure-protective effects of sprifermin and safety profile, although symptomatic modifications were inconclusive.[87] The reasons for its nonsignificant effect on symptom alleviations are largely unclear, which might be attributed to the heterogeneity of patient populations with a high proportion of low-pain and/or high-cartilage thickness at baseline and to the placebo effect of IA saline injections, which improved symptoms in the placebo group.[7,88] These structure-protective findings together with the symptomatic improvement in the subgroup at risk could pave the way for future phase 3 clinical trials in the specific target OA endotype.

TRANSFORMING GROWTH FACTOR-β

Transforming growth factor-β (TGF-β) contributes to early cartilage development and maintains cartilage homeostasis in later life by stimulating the extracellular matrix protein synthesis.[89] Moreover, osteocyte TGF-β signaling may be associated with regulating subchondral bone remodeling in advanced OA.[90] TissueGene-C (TG-C) is retrovirally transduced to promote TGF-β1 transcription (hChonJb#7 cells).[91] A recent study in a monosodium iodoacetate model of OA rats showed that TG-C produces an M2 macrophage-dominant proanabolic microenvironment, promoting cartilage regeneration.[92]

In a phase 2 trial (NCT01221441), the IA TG-C administration (n = 57) had a positive effect on the progression of the cartilage damage and inflammation markers but not on BML and meniscal damage on MRI compared with the placebo (n = 29) over 12 months.[91] In a 2017 poster abstract, a single IA administration of the TG-C caused symptomatic improvement, but its effects on the cartilage were inconclusive at 12-month follow-up (n = 156).[93] These findings were confirmed by another study in 102 OA patients.[94] In a phase 3 trial (NCT02072070), improvement in pain and function was reported in 163 OA patients but with no significant structural benefits.[95] Despite clinical holds in April 2019 over the concerns of chemistry, manufacturing, and control issues related to the potential mislabeling of ingredients, this was lifted in April 2020.[96] In analysis of observational long-term safety follow-up data, there was no evidence showing the association of TG-C administration with increased risk of cancer or other major safety concerns over an average of 10 years.[97] The results of 2 pivotal phase 3 trials (NCT03203330, NCT03291470) are still awaited.

WNT SIGNALING INHIBITORS

Increased Wnt signaling in the chondrocytes results in degeneration of cartilage, whereas stimulation of the Wnt pathway in subchondral bone promotes bone formation and sclerosis.[98,99] Moreover, increased Wnt signaling in the synovium causes increased generation of MMPs and thus OA disease progression.[100] Lorecivivint (SM04690) is a small-molecule CLK/DYRK1A Wnt signaling inhibitor and reduced the cartilage damage in animal studies.[101] In a 52-week, multicenter, phase 2 trial (NCT02536833), IA injection of 0.07 mg revealed significant symptomatic and radiographic improvement compared with IA placebo saline injection starting from week 13 through to the 52-week follow-up in 455 patients with unilateral symptomatic knee OA,[102] although the primary symptomatic endpoints were not met. This was also confirmed by another phase 2 clinical trial (NCT03122860) (n = 700), and the lowest optimal dose was determined as 0.07 mg.[103] The analysis of safety data after combining the 2 trials (848 = Lorecivivint-treated and 360 = control subjects) exhibited the favorable safety profile.[104] Two small phase 2 (NCT03727022, NCT03706521) and 3 phase 3 (NCT03928184, NCT04385303, NCT04520607) trials are active.

SENOLYTIC THERAPIES

Senescence, in which cells cease dividing, is newly implicated in the aging-related OA pathogenesis[105] via the production of proinflammatory cytokines, chemokines, and dysfunction of neighboring cells.[106,107] Therefore, senotherapeutics are being investigated as an emerging therapy for treating aging-related diseases, such as OA. UBX0101 is a potent senolytic, a p53/MDM2 interaction inhibitor, and showed increased chondrogenesis in preclinical studies.[108] Despite its promising findings in a phase 1 study (n = 48),[109] there was no significant change in pain and function in a 12-week phase 2 clinical study (NCT04129944) (n = 183).[110] Failure to meet the primary and secondary endpoints lead to termination of a long-term follow-up study of the previous trial (NCT04349956). Future development for improving the specificity of senolytics to certain types of senescent cells, alternative senolytics with higher potency, or a combination of senolytic agents should be considered.[111]

PERSPECTIVES

The costs of commercial research and development from discovery through to phase 3 trials for a commercially viable product are estimated to have increased 9-fold from 1979 (US$92 million) to 2010 (US$883.6 million).[112] In a recent study, an estimated cost to bring a new therapeutic agent to market is averaged at US$1335.9 million (in 2018 US dollars).[113] Despite active research and immense investment, DMOAD development has been entangled with several challenges.

Regulatory approval of any drug requires the demonstration, in a relevant and defined study population, of the efficacy of the drug under investigation (intervention) determined on a few selected endpoints in comparison with either a placebo or an active comparator. Therefore, careful considerations should be given to each of these factors to tackle the challenges in the drug development process. These are discussed as the 4 sections in terms of the formulation of a research question known as *PICO approach*: (1) population, (2) interventions, (3) comparison or placebo, and (4) outcomes.

Osteoarthritis Population or Phenotypes in Clinical Trials

OA can be defined as a complex heterogeneous disease involving different tissue targets with differing severities in a slowly progressive manner,[3] with the "one-size-fits-all" approach unlikely to work. Because of marked interpatient variability in clinical and structural presentations in the OA disease process,[114] investigation of a targeted therapy in an appropriate patient/disease phenotype according to the targeted pathogenetic pathways would be required for successful drug development. However, the classification of the OA phenotypes is not straightforward, as, during different phases of the OA disease, more than 1 pathogenetic mechanism may contribute to OA in the same patient at varying degrees and that 1 phenotype rarely exists in isolation.[115] Therefore, a new model of classifying OA subtypes that is internationally accepted should be formulated for selecting appropriate study subtypes in clinical trials. For example, for clinical trials to examine the efficacy of anti-inflammatory pharmaceutical agents, the study population with effusion and synovial hypertrophy would be optimal for meeting the trial endpoints.

Advanced OA with extensive structural changes may preclude successful halting or reversal of the disease process, suggesting that the treatment strategy should be initiated as soon as possible to prevent disease progression.[116] Currently, most DMOAD therapies are investigated in the knee OA with KL grade 2 or 3 on plain radiograph. However, such degree of radiographic evidence of OA is a relatively late phenomenon in the process of structural evolution, as alterations in the periarticular bone changes often precede the radiographic OA evidence by 5 to 10 years.[117] There is a lack of consensus definition for identifying either an "early OA" or the prestages of OA, whereby effective cure would be more feasible, although draft classification criteria of "early OA" in the primary setting were recently proposed based on the Knee Injury and Osteoarthritis Outcome Score, clinical signs for joint line tenderness or crepitus, and KL grade 0 or 1.[118]

As the symptomatic improvement translated through the structural protection is essential for defining a DMOADs, the use of the "flare design" (selecting only patients whose pain worsens after withdrawal of their usual pharmacologic treatment) versus "no flare design" may be considered for recruiting nonsteroidal anti-inflammatory drug responders with a more "inflammatory" phenotype in clinical trials, as this may influence the effect sizes of the active treatment.[119] However, a meta-analysis published in 2016 revealed no such difference in effect sizes between the 2 designs.[120]

Interventions

Most phase 2/3 drug development programs failed to show adequate efficacy because of no validated animal models, insufficient linkage of the molecular target with the disease, and use in indications based on insufficient biological rationale.[121] The poor translation of preclinical research into clinical use may result from the fact that animal models are usually young, male mice with injured joints, whereas the human disease occurs mostly in older women with no recent injury.[122] In addition, the crucial factor for targeted therapy to work as expected is the selectivity and affinity of the agents to their receptors as in differential effects of aggrecan degradation in articular cartilage versus tendon. The ideal drug should be fulfilled with the attributes of receptor or functional selectivity, specificity, and potency.[123]

OA is a slowly progressive disease usually found in the obese elderly with multiple comorbidities [4] and so the ideal therapeutic drug should be not only efficacious but also extremely safe in the long-term treatment in such a fragile population. Therefore, systemic drug treatment is not preferred because of off-target effects and systemic toxicity, as in the case of broad-spectrum MMP inhibitors.[124] Another obstacle toward the successful development of DMOADs is their insufficient concentration in OA joints upon systemic administration, leading to low therapeutic efficacy and potential systemic effects.[125]

Local therapy, such as IA administration, will directly target the recognized pathogenetic tissues within the joint and may require lower doses because of increased bioavailability. Still, the IA route has several issues, such as the pain and swelling during procedures, rare cases of septic arthritis, and short half-life of residual times of the agents in the joints owing to rapid clearance by the body. To prolong the residence time in the joint, a variety of drug delivery systems (DDS) have been developed. An ideal DDS should provide controlled and/or sustained drug release for facilitating long-term treatment with a reduced number of injections[126] and possess adequate disease modification, biocompatibility, and biodegradability.[127] New smart drug delivery strategies, using nanoparticles, microparticles, and hydrogels methods, may increase the opportunity for detecting the therapeutic potential of IA agents.[128]

Comparison or Placebo

Administration of placebo in the control group in the RCT is essential in demonstrating the efficacy of active treatment. However, all the placebos are not equal in pain improvement, with greater effect sizes in the IA placebo [0.29 (95% credible interval, 0.09–0.49)] and topical placebo (0.20 [credible interval, 0.02–0.38]) compared with oral placebo.[129] IA saline is a commonly used placebo for control groups in RCTs of injective procedures with remarkable pain relief that is potentially clinically meaningful to patients based on minimal clinically important difference values.[130] This was supported by the finding of a recent meta-analysis in the placebo effects of IA saline at 6-month follow-up, which revealed a significant pain reduction on 0 to 100 VAS (−13.4 [−21.7/−5.1]), improvement in WOMAC function sub-score (−10.1 [−12.2,-8.0]), and 56% in the pooled responder rate in terms of the OMERACT-OARSI criteria.[131] Therefore, the placebo effects of IA saline should be accounted for in planning the trial design when pain and function endpoints are used as the primary measures.[132]

In addition, as the IA saline injection is more than a "mere" placebo owing to dilution effects,[133] future robust studies investigating the underlying mechanisms and the predictors of the placebo responses as well as the comparative effects of sham injections versus saline injections are recommended.[7] In the context of the DMOAD definition, which requires structure-protective effects leading to the clinical translation of symptomatic improvement, the failure of active agents to meet the primary clinical endpoint compared with the placebo should be interpreted in light of large placebo responses. In addition, no active drug comparator can be used currently for noninferiority trial design, as there is a lack of DMOADs approved by the regulatory bodies.[134,135]

Outcome Measures

The issues for measuring the efficacy of DMOAD candidates in clinical trials include the lack of responsiveness of plain radiographs required by the regulatory bodies for DMOAD approval,[7] the absence of biomarkers for structure modifying endpoints,[136] and the variation of definitions for long-term clinical outcomes.[137] Another well-established hurdle is the symptom-structure discordance in OA disease process,[138] suggesting that a structure-protective agent may require long-term follow-up to detect the symptomatic benefits[7] but with no consensus on the threshold of optimal follow-up duration sufficient for detecting DMOAD effects. The recent progress in these areas include the Food and Drug Administration's formal recognition of OA as a serious disease,[139] the validation studies and extensive utilization of MRI in the clinical studies,[140,141] and the OA Biomarkers effort contributed by the FNIH Biomarkers Consortium, a major public-private biomedical research partnership.[136] Therefore, new insight into and discovery of biomarkers with optimal predictive validity and responsiveness will enable the development of recommendations for using specific biomarkers in clinical trials and establishment of efficacy of future DMOAD agents.

SUMMARY

OA contributes to an immense disease burden with an intense unmet need for effective and safe therapies. Lessons have been learned from the failure to find a meaningful disease-modifying agent despite massive efforts and investments in research and development pipelines, providing the progression in developing new strategies for overcoming the barriers. By virtue of lessons learned from past clinical trials and in-sights gained through preclinical research, several agents are revealing some prom-ising results in late-stage clinical trials. Further research should focus on the international consensuses on phenotype classification, appropriate selection criteria and trial design for each specific targeted therapy, the innovation of DDS for optimal drug residence in the joints, sufficient and appropriate procedures for target validation and linkage in preclinical research before progressing to clinical trials, and validation of imaging and biomarker outcomes.

ACKNOWLEDGMENTS

Dr WMO is supported by the Presidential Scholarship of Myanmar for his PhD course.

DISCLOSURE

Nothing to be disclosed.

REFERENCES

1. Cui A, Li H, Wang D, et al. Global, regional prevalence, incidence and risk fac-tors of knee osteoarthritis in population-based studies. EClinicalMedicine. 2020; 29-30:100587.
2. Leifer VP, Katz JN, Losina E. The burden of OA-health services and economics. Osteoarthritis and Cartilage 2021.
3. Oo WM, Yu SP, Daniel MS, et al. Disease-modifying drugs in osteoarthritis: cur-rent understanding and future therapeutics. Expert Opin emerging Drugs 2018; 23(4):331–47.
4. Hunter DJ, Bierma-Zeinstra S. Osteoarthritis. The Lancet 2019;393(10182): 1745–59.
5. Castro-Domínguez F, Vargas-Negrín F, Pérez C, et al. Unmet needs in the oste-oarthritis chronic moderate to severe pain management in Spain: a real word data study. Rheumatol Ther 2021;8(3):1113–27.
6. Malenfant JH, Batsis JA. Obesity in the geriatric population - a global health perspective. J Glob Health Rep 2019;3:e2019045.
7. Oo WM, Little C, Duong V, et al. The development of disease-modifying thera-pies for osteoarthritis (DMOADs): the evidence to date. Drug Des Devel Ther 2021;15:2921–45.
8. Felson DT. Identifying different osteoarthritis phenotypes through epidemiology. Osteoarthritis and cartilage. 2010;18(5):601–4.
9. Mobasheri A, van Spil WE, Budd E, et al. Molecular taxonomy of osteoarthritis for patient stratification, disease management and drug development: biochem-ical markers associated with emerging clinical phenotypes and molecular endo-types. Curr Opin Rheumatol 2019;31(1):80–9.
10. Prieto-Potin I, Largo R, Roman-Blas JA, et al. Characterization of multinucleated giant cells in synovium and subchondral bone in knee osteoarthritis and rheu-matoid arthritis. BMC Musculoskelet Disord 2015;16:226.
11. Wojdasiewicz P, Poniatowski Ł A, Szukiewicz D. The role of inflammatory and anti-inflammatory cytokines in the pathogenesis of osteoarthritis. Mediators In-flamm 2014;2014:561459.
12. de Lange-Brokaar BJ, Ioan-Facsinay A, van Osch GJ, et al. Synovial inflamma-tion, immune cells and their cytokines in osteoarthritis: a review. Osteoarthritis Cartilage. 2012;20(12):1484–99.

13. Oo WM, Linklater JM, Hunter DJ. Imaging in knee osteoarthritis. Curr Opin Rheumatol 2017;29(1):86–95.
14. Collins JE, Losina E, Nevitt MC, et al. Semiquantitative imaging biomarkers of knee osteoarthritis progression: data from the Foundation for the National Institutes of Health Osteoarthritis Biomarkers Consortium. Arthritis Rheumatol 2016; 68(10):2422–31.
15. Liacini A, Sylvester J, Li WQ, et al. Inhibition of interleukin-1-stimulated MAP kinases, activating protein-1 (AP-1) and nuclear factor kappa B (NF-κB) transcription factors down-regulates matrix metalloproteinase gene expression in articular chondrocytes. Matrix Biol 2002;21(3):251–62.
16. Hwang HS, Kim HA. Chondrocyte apoptosis in the pathogenesis of osteoarthritis. Int J Mol Sci 2015;16(11):26035–54.
17. Jenei-Lanzl Z, Meurer A, Zaucke F. Interleukin-1β signaling in osteoarthritis – chondrocytes in focus. Cell Signal 2019;53:212–23.
18. Kamath RV, Hart M, Conlon D, et al. 126 Simultaneous targeting OF IL-1A AND IL-1B by a dual-variable-domain immunoglobulin (DVD-IG(tm)) prevents cartilage degradation in preclinical models of osteoarthritis. Osteoarthritis and Cartilage. 2011;19:S64.
19. Fleischmann RM, Bliddal H, Blanco FJ, et al. A phase II trial of lutikizumab, an anti-interleukin-1α/β dual variable domain immunoglobulin, in knee osteoarthritis patients with synovitis. Arthritis Rheumatol 2019;71(7):1056–69.
20. Kloppenburg M, Peterfy C, Haugen IK, et al. Phase IIa, placebo-controlled, randomised study of lutikizumab, an anti-interleukin-1α and anti-interleukin-1β dual variable domain immunoglobulin, in patients with erosive hand osteoarthritis. 2019;78(3):413–420.
21. Gadotti VM, Martins DF, Pinto HF, et al. Diacerein decreases visceral pain through inhibition of glutamatergic neurotransmission and cytokine signaling in mice. Pharmacol Biochem Behav 2012;102(4):549–54.
22. Pelletier JP, Raynauld JP, Dorais M, et al. An international, multicentre, double-blind, randomized study (DISSCO): effect of diacerein vs celecoxib on symptoms in knee osteoarthritis. Rheumatology (Oxford). 2020;59(12):3858–68.
23. AgencyEM. PRAC re-examines diacerein and recommends that it remain available with restrictions. 2014.
24. Honvo G, Reginster J-Y, Rabenda V, et al. Safety of symptomatic slow-acting drugs for osteoarthritis: outcomes of a systematic review and meta-analysis. Drugs & Aging. 2019;36(1):65–99.
25. Wiegertjes R, van de Loo FAJ, Blaney Davidson EN. A roadmap to target interleukin-6 in osteoarthritis. Rheumatology (Oxford, England). 2020;59(10): 2681–94.
26. Latourte A, Cherifi C, Maillet J, et al. Systemic inhibition of IL-6/Stat3 signalling protects against experimental osteoarthritis. Ann Rheum Dis 2017;76(4):748–55.
27. Kamiya N, Kuroyanagi G, Aruwajoye O, et al. IL6 receptor blockade preserves articular cartilage and increases bone volume following ischemic osteonecrosis in immature mice. Osteoarthritis Cartilage. 2019;27(2):326–35.
28. Richette P, Latourte A, Sellam J, et al. Efficacy of tocilizumab in patients with hand osteoarthritis: double blind, randomised, placebo-controlled, multicentre trial. Ann Rheum Dis 2021;80(3):349–55.
29. Toyoda E, Maehara M, Watanabe M, et al. Candidates intra-articular adm ther therapies osteoarthritis. 2021;22(7):3594.
30. Broeren MGA, de Vries M, Bennink MB, et al. Suppression of the inflammatory response by disease-inducible interleukin-10 gene therapy in a three-

dimensional micromass model of the human synovial membrane. Arthritis Res Ther 2016;18:186.

31. Watkins LR, Chavez RA, Landry R, et al. Targeted interleukin-10 plasmid DNA therapy in the treatment of osteoarthritis: toxicology and pain efficacy assessments. Brain Behav Immun 2020;90:155–66.

32. Cronstein BN, Aune TM. Methotrexate and its mechanisms of action in inflammatory arthritis. Nat Rev Rheumatol 2020;16(3):145–54.

33. Kingsbury SR, Tharmanathan P, Keding A, et al. Significant pain reduction with oral methotrexate in knee osteoarthritis; results from the promote randomised controlled phase iii trial of treatment effectiveness. Osteoarthritis and Cartilage. 2019;27:S84–5.

34. Hu W, Chen Y, Dou C, et al. Microenvironment in subchondral bone: predominant regulator for the treatment of osteoarthritis. Ann Rheum Dis 2020;80(4): 413–22.

35. Nagae M, Hiraga T, Yoneda T. Acidic microenvironment created by osteoclasts causes bone pain associated with tumor colonization. J Bone Miner Metab 2007;25(2):99–104.

36. Zhu S, Zhu J, Zhen G, et al. Subchondral bone osteoclasts induce sensory innervation and osteoarthritis pain. The J Clin Invest 2019;129(3):1076–93.

37. Costa AG, Cusano NE, Silva BC, et al. Its skeletal actions and role as a therapeutic target in osteoporosis. Nat Rev Rheumatol 2011;7(8):447–56.

38. Hayami T, Zhuo Y, Wesolowski GA, et al. Inhibition of cathepsin K reduces cartilage degeneration in the anterior cruciate ligament transection rabbit and murine models of osteoarthritis. Bone. 2012;50(6):1250–9.

39. Lindström E, Rizoska B, Tunblad K, et al. The selective cathepsin K inhibitor MIV-711 attenuates joint pathology in experimental animal models of osteoarthritis. J translational Med 2018;16(1):56.

40. Conaghan PG, Bowes MA, Kingsbury SR, et al. Disease-modifying effects of a novel cathepsin K inhibitor in osteoarthritis: a randomized controlled trial. Ann Intern Med 2020;172(2):86–95.

41. Sampson ER, Hilton MJ, Tian Y, et al. Teriparatide as a chondroregenerative therapy for injury-induced osteoarthritis. Sci translational Med 2011;3(101). 101ra193-101ra193.

42. Cui C, Zheng L, Fan Y, et al. Parathyroid hormone ameliorates temporomandibular joint osteoarthritic-like changes related to age. Cell Prolif. 2020;53(4): e12755.

43. Chen C-H, Ho M-L, Chang L-H, et al. Parathyroid hormone-(1–34) ameliorated knee osteoarthritis in rats via autophagy. J Appl Physiol 2018;124(5):1177–85.

44. Sun Q, Zhen G, Li TP, et al. Parathyroid hormone attenuates osteoarthritis pain by remodeling subchondral bone in mice. eLife. 2021;10:e66532.

45. McGuire D, Lane N, Segal N, et al. TPX-100 leads to marked, sustained improvements in subjects with knee osteoarthritis: pre-clinical rationale and results of a controlled clinical trial. Osteoarthritis and Cartilage. 2018;26:S243.

46. McGuire D, Bowes M, Brett A, et al. Study TPX-100-5: significant reduction in femoral bone shape change 12 months after IA TPX-100 correlates with tibiofemoral cartilage stabilization. Osteoarthritis and Cartilage. 2020;28:S37–8.

47. Felson DT, Chaisson CE, Hill CL, et al. The association of bone marrow lesions with pain in knee osteoarthritis. Ann Intern Med 2001;134(7):541–9.

48. O'Neill TW, Felson DT. Mechanisms of osteoarthritis (OA) pain. Curr Osteoporos Rep 2018;16(5):611–6.

49. Zanetti M, Bruder E, Romero J, et al. Bone marrow edema pattern in osteoarthritic knees: correlation between MR imaging and histologic findings. Radiology 2000;215(3):835–40.

50. Singh V, Oliashirazi A, Tan T, et al. Clinical and pathophysiologic significance of MRI identified bone marrow lesions associated with knee osteoarthritis. Arch Bone Jt Surg 2019;7(3):211–9.

51. Fernández-Martín S, López-Peña M, Muñoz F, et al. Bisphosphonates as disease-modifying drugs in osteoarthritis preclinical studies: a systematic review from 2000 to 2020. Arthritis Res Ther 2021;23(1):60.

52. Moretti A, Paoletta M, Liguori S, et al. The rationale for the intra-articular administration of clodronate in osteoarthritis. Int J Mol Sci 2021;22(5):2693.

53. Vaysbrot EE, Osani MC, Musetti MC, et al. Are bisphosphonates efficacious in knee osteoarthritis? A meta-analysis of randomized controlled trials. Osteoarthritis Cartilage. 2018;26(2):154–64.

54. Eriksen EF, Shabestari M, Ghouri A, et al. Bisphosphonates as a treatment modality in osteoarthritis. Bone 2021;143:115352.

55. Deveza LA, Bierma-Zeinstra SMA, van Spil WE, et al. Efficacy of bisphosphonates in specific knee osteoarthritis subpopulations: protocol for an OA trial bank systematic review and individual patient data meta-analysis. BMJ open. 2018;8(12):e023889.

56. Frediani B, Toscano C, Falsetti P, et al. Intramuscular clodronate in long-term treatment of symptomatic knee osteoarthritis: a randomized controlled study. Drugs in R&D. 2020;20(1):39–45.

57. Hayes KN, Giannakeas V, Wong AKO. Bisphosphonate use is protective of radiographic knee osteoarthritis progression among those with low disease severity and being non-overweight: data from the Osteoarthritis Initiative. J Bone Mineral Res 2020;35(12):2318–26.

58. Cai G, Aitken D, Laslett LL, et al. Effect of intravenous zoledronic acid on tibiofemoral cartilage volume among patients with knee osteoarthritis with bone marrow lesions: a randomized clinical trial. JAMA. 2020;323(15):1456–66.

59. Kong C, Wang C, Shi Y, et al. Active vitamin D activates chondrocyte autophagy to reduce osteoarthritis via mediating the AMPK-mTOR signaling pathway. Biochem Cell Biol. 2020;98(3):434–42.

60. MacFarlane LA, Cook NR, Kim E, et al. The effects of vitamin D and marine omega-3 fatty acid supplementation on chronic knee pain in older US adults: results from a randomized trial. Arthritis Rheumatol 2020;72(11):1836–44.

61. Perry TA, Parkes MJ, Hodgson R, et al. Effect of vitamin D supplementation on synovial tissue volume and subchondral bone marrow lesion volume in symptomatic knee osteoarthritis. BMC Musculoskelet Disord 2019;20(1):76.

62. Tu L, Zheng S, Cicuttini F, et al. Effects of vitamin D supplementation on disabling foot pain in patients with symptomatic knee osteoarthritis. Arthritis Care Res 2021;73(6):781–7.

63. Zhao ZX, He Y, Peng LH, et al. Does vitamin D improve symptomatic and structural outcomes in knee osteoarthritis? A systematic review and meta-analysis. Aging Clin Exp Res 2021;33(9):2393–403.

64. Man GS, Mologhianu G. Osteoarthritis pathogenesis - a complex process that involves the entire joint. J Med Life 2014;7(1):37–41.

65. Yamamoto K, Wilkinson D, Bou-Gharios G. Targeting dysregulation of metalloproteinase activity in osteoarthritis. Calcif Tissue Int 2021;109(3):277–90.

66. Fields GB. The rebirth of matrix metalloproteinase inhibitors: moving beyond the dogma. Cells. 2019;8(9).

67. Wang M, Sampson ER, Jin H, et al. MMP13 is a critical target gene during the progression of osteoarthritis. Arthritis Res Ther 2013;15(1):R5.
68. Hu Q, Ecker M. Overview of MMP-13 as a promising target for the treatment of osteoarthritis. Int J Mol Sci 2021;22(4):1742.
69. Santamaria S. ADAMTS-5: a difficult teenager turning 20. Int J Exp Pathol 2020; 101(1–2):4–20.
70. Brebion F, Gosmini R, Deprez P, et al. Discovery of GLPG1972/S201086, a potent, selective, and orally bioavailable ADAMTS-5 inhibitor for the treatment of osteoarthritis. J Med Chem 2021;64(6):2937–52.
71. Galapagos and Servier report topline results for ROCCELLA phase 2 clinical trial with GLPG1972/S201086 in knee osteoarthritis patients. 2020.
72. vanderAar E, Deckx H, Van Der Stoep M, et al. Study design of a phase 2 clinical trial with a disease-modifying osteoarthritis drug candidate GLPG1972/ S201086: the Roccella trial. Osteoarthritis and Cartilage. 2020;28:S499–500.
73. Rose KWJ, Taye N, Karoulias SZ, et al. Regulation of ADAMTS proteases. Front Mol Biosciences. 2021;8(621).
74. Verma P, Dalal K. ADAMTS-4 and ADAMTS-5: key enzymes in osteoarthritis. J Cell Biochem. 2011;112(12):3507–14.
75. Wang VM, Bell RM, Thakore R, et al. Murine tendon function is adversely affected by aggrecan accumulation due to the knockout of ADAMTS5. J Orthopaedic Res 2012;30(4):620–6.
76. Cikach FS, Koch CD, Mead TJ, et al. Massive aggrecan and versican accumulation in thoracic aortic aneurysm and dissection. JCI Insight. 2018;3(5).
77. Song L, Huang Z, Chen Y, et al. High-efficiency production of bioactive recombinant human fibroblast growth factor 18 in Escherichia coli and its effects on hair follicle growth. Appl Microbiol Biotechnol 2014;98(2):695–704.
78. Hendesi H, Stewart S, Gibison ML, et al. Recombinant fibroblast growth factor-18 (sprifermin) enhances microfracture-induced cartilage healing. J orthopaedic Res : official Publ Orthopaedic Res Soc 2021.
79. Muurahainen N. Cartilage repair and the sprifermin story: mechanisms, preclinical and clinical study results, and lessons learned. Osteoarthritis and Cartilage. 2016;24:S4.
80. Lohmander LS, Hellot S, Dreher D, et al. Intraarticular sprifermin (recombinant human fibroblast growth factor 18) in knee osteoarthritis: a randomized, double-blind, placebo-controlled trial. Arthritis Rheumatol 2014;66(7):1820–31.
81. Roemer FW, Aydemir A, Lohmander S, et al. Structural effects of sprifermin in knee osteoarthritis: a post-hoc analysis on cartilage and non-cartilaginous tissue alterations in a randomized controlled trial. BMC Musculoskelet Disord 2016;17:267.
82. Eckstein F, Wirth W, Guermazi A, et al. Brief report: intraarticular sprifermin not only increases cartilage thickness, but also reduces cartilage loss: location-independent post hoc analysis using magnetic resonance imaging. Arthritis Rheumatol 2015;67(11):2916–22.
83. Hochberg MC, Guermazi A, Guehring H, et al. Effect of intra-articular sprifermin vs placebo on femorotibial joint cartilage thickness in patients with osteoarthritis: the FORWARD randomized clinical trial. JAMA. 2019;322(14):1360–70.
84. Hans Guehring JK, Moreau Flavie, Daelken Benjamin, et al, Hochberg cartilage thickness modification with sprifermin in knee osteoarthritis patients translates into symptomatic improvement over placebo in patients at risk of further structural and symptomatic progression: post-hoc analysis of a phase II trial. Arthritis Rheumatol 2019;71(suppl 10).

85. Eckstein F, Kraines JL, Aydemir A, et al. Intra-articular sprifermin reduces cartilage loss in addition to increasing cartilage gain independent of location in the femorotibial joint: post-hoc analysis of a randomised, placebo-controlled phase II clinical trial. Ann Rheum Dis 2020;79(4):525–8.

86. Eckstein F, Hochberg MC, Guehring H, et al. Long-term structural and symptomatic effects of intra-articular sprifermin in patients with knee osteoarthritis: 5-year results from the FORWARD study. Ann Rheum Dis 2021;80(8):1062–9.

87. Zeng N, Chen X-Y, Yan Z-P, et al. Efficacy and safety of sprifermin injection for knee osteoarthritis treatment: a meta-analysis. Arthritis Res Ther 2021; 23(1):107.

88. Li J, Wang X, Ruan G, et al. Sprifermin: a recombinant human fibroblast growth factor 18 for the treatment of knee osteoarthritis. Expert Opin Investig Drugs 2021;30(9):923–30.

89. Zhai G, Dore J, Rahman P. TGF-beta signal transduction pathways and osteoarthritis. Rheumatol Int 2015;35(8):1283–92.

90. Dai G, Xiao H, Liao J, et al. Osteocyte TGFβ1-Smad2/3 is positively associated with bone turnover parameters in subchondral bone of advanced osteoarthritis. Int J Mol Med 2020;46(1):167–78.

91. Guermazi A, Kalsi G, Niu J, et al. Structural effects of intra-articular TGF-beta1 in moderate to advanced knee osteoarthritis: MRI-based assessment in a randomized controlled trial. BMC Musculoskelet Disord 2017;18(1):461.

92. Lee H, Kim H, Seo J, et al. TissueGene-C promotes an anti-inflammatory microenvironment in a rat monoiodoacetate model of osteoarthritis via polarization of M2 macrophages leading to pain relief and structural improvement. Inflammopharmacology. 2020;28(5):1237–52.

93. Cho J, Kim T, Shin J, et al. A phase III clinical results of INVOSSA™ (TissueGene C): a clues for the potential disease modifying OA drug. Cytotherapy. 2017; 19(5):S148.

94. Lee B, Parvizi J, Bramlet D, et al. Results of a phase II study to determine the efficacy and safety of genetically engineered allogeneic human chondrocytes expressing TGF-β1. The J knee Surg 2020;33(2):167–72.

95. Kim MK, Ha CW, In Y, et al. A multicenter, double-blind, phase III clinical trial to evaluate the efficacy and safety of a cell and gene therapy in knee osteoarthritis patients. Hum Gene Ther Clin Dev 2018.

96. Kolon TissueGene cleared to resume US phase III trial for Invossa. The pharma letter 2020.

97. DHunter RM Wang, M Noh. Overall safety of TG-C: safety analysis of phase-1, phase-2 and long-term safety trials [Abstract]. Osteoarthritis and Cartilage 2020;28.

98. Lories RJ, Monteagudo S. Review article: is Wnt signaling an attractive target for the treatment of osteoarthritis? Rheumatol Ther 2020;7(2):259–70.

99. Kovács B, Vajda E, Nagy EE. Regulatory effects and interactions of the Wnt and OPG-RANKL-RANK signaling at the bone-cartilage interface in osteoarthritis. Int J Mol Sci 2019;20(18):4653.

100. Cherifi C, Monteagudo S, Lories RJ. Promising targets for therapy of osteoarthritis: a review on the Wnt and TGF-β signalling pathways. Ther Adv Musculoskelet Dis 2021;13. 1759720X211006959.

101. Deshmukh V, O'Green AL, Bossard C, et al. Modulation of the Wnt pathway through inhibition of CLK2 and DYRK1A by lorecivivint as a novel, potentially disease-modifying approach for knee osteoarthritis treatment. Osteoarthritis Cartilage. 2019;27(9):1347–60.

102. Yazici Y, McAlindon TE, Gibofsky A, et al. Lorecivivint, a novel intraarticular CDC-like kinase 2 and dual-specificity tyrosine phosphorylation-regulated kinase 1A inhibitor and Wnt pathway modulator for the treatment of knee osteoarthritis: a phase II randomized trial. Arthritis Rheumatol (Hoboken, NJ). 2020; 72(10):1694–706.
103. Yazici Y, McAlindon TE, Gibofsky A, et al. A Phase 2b randomized trial of lorecivivint, a novel intra-articular CLK2/DYRK1A inhibitor and Wnt pathway modulator for knee osteoarthritis. Osteoarthritis Cartilage. 2021;29(5):654–66.
104. Simsek I, Swearingen C, Kennedy S, et al. OP0188 Integrated safety summary of the novel, intra-articular agent lorecivivint (SM04690), a CLK/DYRK1A inhibitor that modulates the WNT pathway, in subjects with knee osteoarthritis. Ann Rheum Dis 2020;79(Suppl 1):117.
105. Loeser RF. Aging and osteoarthritis: the role of chondrocyte senescence and aging changes in the cartilage matrix. Osteoarthritis Cartilage. 2009;17(8): 971–9.
106. Coppé JP, Patil CK, Rodier F, et al. Senescence-associated secretory phenotypes reveal cell-nonautonomous functions of oncogenic RAS and the p53 tumor suppressor. PLoS Biol 2008;6(12):2853–68.
107. Ferreira-Gonzalez S, Lu WY, Raven A, et al. Paracrine cellular senescence exacerbates biliary injury and impairs regeneration. Nat Commun 2018;9(1):1020.
108. Jeon OH, Kim C, Laberge R-M, et al. Local clearance of senescent cells attenuates the development of post-traumatic osteoarthritis and creates a pro-regenerative environment. Nat Med 2017;23(6):775–81.
109. Hsu B, Lane NE, Li L, et al. Safety, tolerability, pharmacokinetics, and clinical outcomes following single- dose IA administration of UBX0101, a senolytic MDM2/p53 interaction inhibitor, in patients with knee OA [abstract]. Osteoarthritis and Cartilage. 2020;28.
110. UnityBiotechnology I. UNITY biotechnology announces 12-week data from UBX0101 phase 2 clinical study in patients with painful osteoarthritis of the knee. 2020.
111. Zhang X-X, He S-H, Liang X, et al. Aging, cell senescence, the pathogenesis and targeted therapies of osteoarthritis. Front Pharmacol 2021;12(2200).
112. Morgan S, Grootendorst P, Lexchin J, et al. The cost of drug development: a systematic review. Health Pol (Amsterdam, Netherlands). 2011;100(1):4–17.
113. Wouters OJ, McKee M, Luyten J. Estimated research and development investment needed to bring a new medicine to market, 2009-2018. JAMA. 2020; 323(9):844–53.
114. Bierma-Zeinstra SM, Verhagen AP. Osteoarthritis subpopulations and implications for clinical trial design. Arthritis Res Ther 2011;13(2):213.
115. Karsdal MA, Michaelis M, Ladel C, et al. Disease-modifying treatments for osteoarthritis (DMOADs) of the knee and hip: lessons learned from failures and opportunities for the future. Osteoarthritis Cartilage. 2016;24(12):2013–21.
116. Felson DT, Hodgson R. Identifying and treating preclinical and early osteoarthritis. Rheum Dis Clin North Am 2014;40(4):699–710.
117. Neogi T, Bowes MA, Niu J, et al. Magnetic resonance imaging-based three-dimensional bone shape of the knee predicts onset of knee osteoarthritis: data from the Osteoarthritis Initiative. Arthritis Rheum 2013;65(8):2048–58.
118. Luyten FP, Bierma-Zeinstra S, Dell'Accio F, et al. Toward classification criteria for early osteoarthritis of the knee. Semin Arthritis Rheum 2018;47(4):457–63.
119. Trijau S, Avouac J, Escalas C, et al. Influence of flare design on symptomatic efficacy of non-steroidal anti-inflammatory drugs in osteoarthritis: a meta-

analysis of randomized placebo-controlled trials. Osteoarthritis Cartilage. 2010; 18(8):1012–8.

120. Smith TO, Zou K, Abdullah N, et al. Does flare trial design affect the effect size of non-steroidal anti-inflammatory drugs in symptomatic osteoarthritis? A systematic review and meta-analysis. Ann Rheum Dis 2016;75(11):1971–8.

121. Hunter DJ, Little CB. The great debate: should osteoarthritis research focus on "mice" or "men"? Osteoarthritis Cartilage. 2016;24(1):4–8.

122. Oo WM, Hunter DJ. Disease modification in osteoarthritis: are we there yet? Clinical & Experimental Rheumatology 2019;37 Suppl 120(5):135–40.

123. Berg KA, Clarke WP. Making sense of pharmacology: inverse agonism and functional selectivity. Int J Neuropsychopharmacol 2018;21(10):962–77.

124. Krzeski P, Buckland-Wright C, Balint G, et al. Development of musculoskeletal toxicity without clear benefit after administration of PG-116800, a matrix metalloproteinase inhibitor, to patients with knee osteoarthritis: a randomized, 12-month, double-blind, placebo-controlled study. Arthritis Res Ther 2007;9(5): R109.

125. Oo WM, Liu X, Hunter DJ. Pharmacodynamics, efficacy, safety and administration of intra-articular therapies for knee osteoarthritis. Expert Opin Drug Metab Toxicol 2019;15(12):1021–32.

126. Maudens P, Jordan O, Allémann E. Recent advances in intra-articular drug delivery systems for osteoarthritis therapy. Drug Discov Today 2018;23(10): 1761–75.

127. Lima AC, Ferreira H, Reis RL, et al. Biodegradable polymers: an update on drug delivery in bone and cartilage diseases. Expert Opin Drug Deliv 2019;16(8): 795–813.

128. Gambaro FM, Ummarino A. Torres Andón F, Ronzoni F, Di Matteo B, Kon E. Drug delivery systems for the treatment of knee osteoarthritis: a systematic review of in vivo studies. Int J Mol Sci 2021;22(17).

129. Bannuru RR, McAlindon TE, Sullivan MC, et al. Effectiveness and implications of alternative placebo treatments: a systematic review and network meta-analysis of osteoarthritis trials. Ann Intern Med 2015;163(5):365–72.

130. Simsek I, Phalen T, Bedenbaugh A, et al. Adjusting for the intra-articular placebo effect in knee osteoarthritis therapies [Abstract]. 2018;77(Suppl 2):1135–1136.

131. Previtali D, Merli G. Di Laura Frattura G, Candrian C, Zaffagnini S, Filardo G. The long-lasting effects of "placebo injections" in knee osteoarthritis: a meta-analysis. Cartilage 2020. 1947603520906597.

132. Enck P, Bingel U, Schedlowski M, et al. The placebo response in medicine: minimize, maximize or personalize? Nat Rev Drug Discov 2013;12(3):191–204.

133. Altman RD, Devji T, Bhandari M, et al. Clinical benefit of intra-articular saline as a comparator in clinical trials of knee osteoarthritis treatments: a systematic review and meta-analysis of randomized trials. Semin Arthritis Rheum 2016;46(2): 151–9.

134. Fleming TR. Design and interpretation of equivalence trials. Am Heart J 2000; 139(4):S171–6.

135. Greene CJ, Morland LA, Durkalski VL, et al. Noninferiority and equivalence designs: issues and implications for mental health research. J Trauma Stress 2008; 21(5):433–9.

136. Hunter DJ, Nevitt M, Losina E, et al. Biomarkers for osteoarthritis: current position and steps towards further validation. Best Pract Res Clin Rheumatol 2014; 28(1):61–71.

137. Kraus VB, Blanco FJ, Englund M, et al. Call for standardized definitions of osteoarthritis and risk stratification for clinical trials and clinical use. Osteoarthritis and cartilage. 2015;23(8):1233–41.
138. Hannan MT, Felson DT, Pincus T. Analysis of the discordance between radiographic changes and knee pain in osteoarthritis of the knee. J Rheumatol 2000;27(6):1513–7.
139. OARSI TP-cCfOPo. OARSI white paper- OA as a serious disease. 2016.
140. Roemer FW, Collins J, Kwoh CK, et al. MRI-based screening for structural definition of eligibility in clinical DMOAD trials: rapid OsteoArthritis MRI Eligibility Score (ROAMES). Osteoarthritis and Cartilage. 2020;28(1):71–81.
141. Roemer FW, Kwoh CK, Hayashi D, et al. The role of radiography and MRI for eligibility assessment in DMOAD trials of knee OA. Nat Rev Rheumatol 2018; 14(6):372–80.

Beyond Coronary Artery Disease
Assessing the Microcirculation

Sonal Pruthi, MD[a], Emaad Siddiqui, MD[a],
Nathaniel R. Smilowitz, MD, MS[a,b,c,]*

KEYWORDS

- Coronary flow reserve • Coronary microvascular disease
- Coronary microvascular dysfunction • Coronary physiology
- Hyperemic microvascular resistance • Index of microcirculatory resistance
- Ischemia with nonobstructive coronary arteries • INOCA

KEY POINTS

- Coronary microvascular dysfunction (CMD) is an important cause of ischemia with nonobstructive coronary arteries (INOCA).
- The pathophysiology of CMD is not well established.
- Coronary flow reserve, the index of microcirculatory resistance, hyperemic microvascular resistance, and resistive reserve ratio are invasively measured indices to evaluate the microcirculation.
- CMD is associated with clinical outcomes in patients with INOCA and obstructive coronary artery disease.

BACKGROUND

Ischemic heart disease (IHD) affects more than 20 million adults in the United States and is a leading cause of death.[1] Stable IHD is associated with angina, decreased exercise tolerance, and adverse health-related quality of life. Although angina is classically attributed to atherosclerosis of the epicardial coronary arteries, recent evidence

This article previously appeared in *Clinics in Interventional Cardiology Clinics* volume 12 issue 1 January 2023.
[a] Division of Cardiology, Department of Medicine, NYU Langone Health, 550 First Avenue, New York, NY 10016, USA; [b] Cardiology Section, Department of Medicine, VA New York Harbor Healthcare System, 423 East 23rd Street, New York, NY 10010, USA; [c] The Leon H. Charney Division of Cardiology, NYU Langone Health, NYU School of Medicine, 423 East 23rd Street, 12-West, New York, NY 10010, USA
* Corresponding author. The Leon H. Charney Division of Cardiology, NYU Langone Health, NYU School of Medicine, 423 East 23rd Street, 12-West, New York, NY 10010.
E-mail address: nathaniel.smilowitz@nyulangone.org

Rheum Dis Clin N Am 50 (2024) 519–533
https://doi.org/10.1016/j.rdc.2024.03.004
0889-857X/24/Published by Elsevier Inc.

rheumatic.theclinics.com

suggests that nearly half of patients who undergo invasive coronary angiography for the evaluation of angina do not have obstructive coronary disease.[2,3] This perplexing clinical scenario, first described in 1967 and later termed *cardiac Syndrome X*, is now referred to as ischemia with nonobstructive coronary arteries (INOCA).[4] Underlying mechanisms of INOCA include microvascular angina with coronary microvascular dysfunction (CMD), epicardial coronary spasm, and noncardiac chest pain.[5,6] Recent American and European clinical practice guidelines recognize the impact of INOCA and recommend functional assessment of the coronary microcirculation to determine mechanisms of ischemia and guide pharmacologic therapy.[7–9] The objective of this review is to (1) outline the anatomy of the coronary circulation and the pathophysiology of CMD, (2) describe current approaches to assess the coronary microcirculation in the cardiac catheterization laboratory, and (3) examine the clinical implications of CMD in INOCA and other cardiovascular disorders.

Anatomy and Physiology of the Coronary Microcirculation

Anatomy

From the epicardial vessels to the myocardium, the coronary circulation can be divided into 3 distinct "compartments" (**Fig. 1**). Blood enters the coronary circulation via the major epicardial coronary arteries, vessels 500 μm to 5 mm in size that course predominantly along the surface of the myocardium and can be easily visualized by coronary angiography. Epicardial coronary arteries have been the focus of coronary interventions for more than half a century. Despite their important role as proximal conduit vessels, the epicardial coronaries only directly supply 5% to 10% of the myocardium. In normal physiologic conditions, epicardial coronary arteries offer little resistance to blood flow due to their relatively large diameters. Nitric oxide-mediated vasodilation of the epicardial coronaries accommodates increased blood flow in times of high metabolic demand. Atherosclerotic plaques in the epicardial coronaries can lead to dramatic increases in resistance to flow.[10] The epicardial coronary arteries branch and taper into a vast network of arterioles to supply the myocardium.

Extramyocardial prearteriolar vessels, which range in diameter from 100 to 500 μm, form the intermediate compartment of the coronary circulation. These prearteriolar vessels run in parallel, leading to physiologic drops in pressures.[11] Proximal prearterioles in this compartment are most sensitive to changes in intravascular flow, whereas distal vessels are sensitive to changes in pressure. Vasoconstriction and vasodilation of the prearterioles maintains constant arteriolar pressures.[12] This compartment may be responsible for CMD in patients with INOCA.

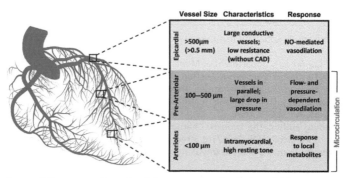

Fig. 1. Anatomy of the compartments of the coronary circulation. CAD, coronary artery disease; NO, nitric oxide.

The third and final compartment of the coronary circulation consists of innumerable intramural arterioles less than 100 μm in diameter. These vessels directly supply low-pressure myocardial capillary beds that serve as the site for nutrient and gas exchange. Arterioles in the coronary circulation have a high resting tone and dilate in response to local metabolites produced by the surrounding myocardium, including adenosine, nitric oxide, and prostaglandins.[11] Thus, arterioles are responsible for the metabolic regulation of myocardial blood flow.

In normal circumstances, the 3 compartments of the coronary circulation work in concert to regulate myocardial blood flow in response to metabolic demands. Once maximal myocardial oxygen extraction (~75%) has been reached, additional metabolic demands must be met with increases in myocardial blood flow.[13] Increases in heart rate and contractility can augment cardiac output, and vasodilatory metabolites from the myocardium decrease microcirculatory arteriolar resistance to enhance coronary blood flow (CBF).[13] Thus, the microcirculation plays a pivotal role to ensure coronary perfusion matches myocardial oxygen demand.

Pathobiology of Coronary Microvascular Disease

Coronary microvascular disease has been broadly classified as microvascular dysfunction (1) in the absence of obstructive coronary artery disease (CAD) or myocardial diseases, (2) in the presence of myocardial disease, (3) in the presence of obstructive CAD, or (4) from an iatrogenic cause.[14] A variety of mechanisms can contribute to structural or functional abnormalities of the microcirculation.[15,16] In patients without obstructive atherosclerosis or myocardial diseases, the pathogenesis of microvascular disease may include arteriolar remodeling and fibrosis, intimal proliferation, smooth muscle hypertrophy, or vessel rarefaction. Small vessel atherosclerosis, platelet activation and plugging,[17] or microembolization of thrombotic material in the setting of epicardial atherosclerotic disease may also contribute.[18] In the setting of myocardial disease, such as left ventricular hypertrophy, increased intramyocardial, left ventricular diastolic, and coronary venous pressures may also lead to increased resistance to microcirculatory flow.[19]

In addition to structural disorders of the microcirculation, functional abnormalities associated with impairment to the normal responses to neurohormonal and metabolic signaling can lead to impaired microcirculatory flow. This may include attenuated responses to or decreased synthesis of vasodilators such as nitric oxide.[20,21] Coronary microvascular spasm, with episodic increases in microvascular resistance and provocation of myocardial ischemia can also occur.[22]

Although the exact pathophysiology of CMD is uncertain, risk factors include older age, hypertension, dyslipidemia, diabetes mellitus, cigarette smoking, and chronic inflammatory disorders, including systemic lupus erythematosus and rheumatoid arthritis.[23–28] Additional investigation is needed to identify modifiable risk factors to prevent development of microcirculatory disease.

Assessing the Microcirculation in the Catheterization Laboratory

Unlike the epicardial coronary arteries, coronary microcirculation cannot be directly visualized. Thus, assessments are largely based on parameters of microcirculatory flow. Coronary flow reserve (CFR), the original integrated measure of coronary epicardial flow and microvascular function, is defined as the ratio of hyperemic CBF to CBF at rest. Normal coronary arteries can augment blood flow greater than 4-fold at maximal hyperemia, whereas a CFR less than 2 to less than 2.5 in the absence of epicardial coronary disease is abnormal and reflects microvascular dysfunction (**Table 1**).[5,6]

Table 1
Invasively derived measures to assess coronary microvascular dysfunction

Technique	Measurement Method	Normal Value	Comments
CFR	Doppler or Thermodilution	>2.0–2.5	• Requires hyperemia • Not specific for microvascular disease • Affected by resting hemodynamics and coronary epicardial stenosis • Predicts long-term MACE
IMR	Thermodilution (Bolus dose)	<25	• Requires hyperemia • Specific to the coronary microcirculation • Less variable than CFR despite change in hemodynamics • Requires correction (Yong) in the presence of significant epicardial stenosis • Predicts long-term death and heart failure readmissions in patients with STEMI • May predict graft dysfunction early after orthotopic heart transplant
hMR	Doppler	≤2	• Specific to the coronary microcirculation • Technical challenges of optimal Doppler signal acquisition
RRR	Doppler or thermodilution	<1.7–3.5	• Superior to CFR for prognosis
mMR	Doppler	Not defined	• Measured during wave-free period window of diastole and does not require hyperemia • Limited data on prognostic value
R_{micro}	Thermodilution (continuous infusion)	< 500 WU	• Strong agreement with PET-derived coronary flow • Saline infusion induces hyperemia • Accuracy in obstructive coronary artery disease is not well defined • Equipment not available in the United States
MRR	Thermodilution (continuous infusion)	Not defined	• Novel index • Specific to microvasculature; corrected for epicardial conductance • Independent of autoregulation and myocardial mass • Requires validation

Invasive evaluation of CFR can be performed in the catheterization laboratory using thermodilution or Doppler-based assessment of CBF. The intracoronary Doppler guidewire, first developed in the late 1980s, contains a piezoelectric ultrasound transducer mounted at the tip to measure CBF velocity.[29] The current generation of wire (FloWire or ComboWire XT, Phillips, Amsterdam, Netherlands) can measure the average peak velocity (APV) of CBF at a specific location using a commercially available console with dedicated software (ComboMap, Philips Volcano). Coronary APV is typically measured at rest, and then again after induction of hyperemia with the administration of a nonendothelial-dependent vasodilator such as adenosine. Doppler-derived CFR is typically simplified as the ratio of the hyperemic APV to the APV measured at rest. To estimate CBF, the vessel diameter (D) at the site of APV measurement can be determined using quantitative coronary angiography, and flow can then be calculated by the formula: $CBF = 0.5 \times APV \times (D2\ \pi)/4$.[29] In response to an infusion of acetylcholine, an endothelial-dependent vasodilator, CBF typically increases substantially. Augmentation of CBF by less than 50% in the presence of acetylcholine is abnormal and in the absence of significant epicardial coronary constriction indicates that endothelial dependent microvascular dysfunction may be present.[30,31]

In contrast to Doppler-based measures that measure coronary velocity at a single location, coronary thermodilution techniques assesses flow based on temperature changes across the vessel. This technique requires 3 mL bolus injections of room temperature saline through the guide catheter, with a distal thermistor on a coronary pressure-wire recording temperatures in the coronary artery (PressureWire X, Abbott Vascular, Abbott Park, IL USA). The shaft of this wire acts as a proximal thermistor. The speed of change of the distal temperature (relative to the proximal temperature) is used to calculate the mean transit time (T_{mn}), which is inversely proportional to coronary flow according to the principles of indicator dilution theory.

Doppler and thermodilution approaches to measurement of coronary flow each have limitations. Doppler-derived measures of coronary flow velocity assume that flow at the transducer is parallel, laminar, and parabolic, and may not remain constant at different wire positions.[32] Indeed, animal and human studies have demonstrated significant variability in Doppler wire measurements,[33] and Doppler measurements tend to be technically more challenging, require more time for data acquisition, and have a steeper learning curve.[34,35] Although coronary thermodilution is somewhat easier to obtain, it can be significantly impacted by changes in guide catheter position during administration of saline boluses. In an early porcine model, thermodilution-derived CFR correlated better with absolute flow measured by an external coronary flow probe than did the Doppler wire-derived CFR.[36] However, in a study of 98 vessels in 40 consecutive patients, Doppler-derived CFR correlated more closely with PET-derived CFR than thermodilution-derived CFR.[37] Ultimately, both techniques are considered to be valid in the assessment of the coronary microcirculation (see Table 1).

Unfortunately, CFR is not specific to microcirculation and is affected by epicardial coronary stenosis and resting hemodynamics. In the absence of obstructive epicardial disease, a reduced CFR can reflect increased microcirculatory resistance to flow, an abnormal response to the standard vasodilatory stimulus, or increased resting coronary flow before vasodilator administration. Among patients with INOCA, high resting flow is more common in women, younger patients, and patients with fewer cardiovascular risk factors, and may represent a distinct pathologic condition.[38]

Microvascular resistance indices offer an alternative method to interrogate the microcirculation.[39] The index of microcirculatory resistance (IMR), first reported in 2003, is a thermodilution-based measure that reflects the minimal achievable resistance of the microcirculation with endothelial-independent vasodilators (see **Table 1**).[32] IMR is based on Ohm's law, which states that the potential difference across an ideal conductor is proportional to the current through the conductor (Voltage = current × resistance). Applying this to coronary physiology, the microcirculation acts as a conductor, the voltage is analogous to the difference in pressure across the microvasculature (mean distal coronary pressure [P_d] – coronary venous pressure [P_v]), and current is myocardial flow ($1/T_{mn}$). Because P_v is usually negligible, IMR may be calculated by the formula: $IMR = P_d \times T_{mn}$. A normal value of IMR has been reported to be lesser than 25,[40–42] with higher values reported in the right coronary artery (RCA), perhaps due to longer vessel length and larger diameters accounting for a somewhat prolonged T_{mn}.[42]

Yet, there are some situations in which IMR must be interpreted with caution. In the presence of a significant coronary stenosis, collateral flow to the vessel of interest may increase the coronary wedge pressure (Pw). Thus, coronary thermodilution may underestimate flow and IMR may overestimate resistance.[43] To account for collateral flow, the following formula has been proposed: $IMR = Pa \times T_{mn} \times ([P_d - P_w]/[P_a - P_w])$.[43] Because P_w are not routinely measured, a correction factor for IMR has been derived and validated from experimental data with P_w measured during proximal vessel balloon occlusions.[44,45] Corrected IMR can be calculated using Yong's modification (corrected $IMR = Pa \times T_{mn} \times [(1.35 \times Pd/Pa) - 0.32]$) during hyperemia.

There are several benefits to IMR, which remains stable in the presence of increasing epicardial stenosis,[43] and is relatively independent of resting hemodynamics.[46] Variability in IMR is lower than that of CFR, despite changes in heart rate, blood pressure, and contractility.[46] Finally, IMR is a highly reproducible measure over time, with low interobserver variability despite manual injection of saline boluses.[47,48]

Microcirculatory resistance can also be determined using a guidewire with a Doppler ultrasound transducer and simultaneous distal coronary pressure monitoring. The Doppler-derived hyperemic microvascular resistance (hMR) is analogous to IMR and is defined as the ratio of mean distal pressure to the Doppler-derived APV (see **Table 1**).[49] An hMR of 2 or greater is generally considered to be abnormal. In patients with INOCA, hMR less than 1.9 predicted recurrent chest pain in one study, although in another, a threshold of 2.5 or greater provided the highest sensitivity and specificity to detect CMR-determined microvascular disease or abnormal invasive CFR.[34,50] A related measure, the minimal microvascular resistance (mMR), was proposed as the ratio of hyperemic distal coronary pressure and hyperemic APV measured during wave-free period window of diastole, when microvascular resistance is at its lowest.[51] Although conceptually attractive, mMR requires further study.

The resistive reserve ratio (RRR), another recently developed microcirculatory parameter, is calculated as the ratio of baseline microvascular resistance to hMR, with higher values indicating greater vasodilatory capacity of the microcirculation (see **Table 1**).[52,53] Thresholds for abnormal RRR are not well established but have been proposed between less than 1.7 and 3.5 in various populations and with both Doppler and Thermodilution-derived resistance measures.[54–56] In a study of 1692 patients with INOCA, Doppler-derived RRR of less than 2.62 was associated with mortality and was superior to CFR to predict long-term survival.[57] Low RRR was also associated with long-term outcomes in cohorts with acute MI and CAD undergoing revascularization.[55,56]

Continuous thermodilution is another emerging technique to assess the microcirculation.[58] Temperature changes associated with intracoronary saline infusion, administered at a known rate through a dedicated monorail infusion catheter, can be measured in the distal coronary with a thermistor on a pressure-sensing coronary wire to calculate absolute coronary flow (Q). Q can be derived as $Q = 1.08 \times T_i/T \times Q_i$, where T_i is the temperature of saline as it exits the catheter, T is the temperature of the blood in the distal coronary during the steady-state infusion, and Q_i is the saline infusion rate (in milliliter per minute).[59,60] Based on Ohm's law, absolute microvascular resistance $(R = P_d/Q)$, measured in Woods units (WU), can be obtained. Slow coronary infusions of saline (typically 8–10 mL/min) are used to assess baseline resistance at rest, whereas hyperemia is induced at higher saline infusion rates (15–25 mL/min).[61] Continuous thermodilution Q has strong agreement with PET-derived coronary flow,[62] absolute resistance greater than 500 WU is the optimal threshold to identify patients with an IMR of 25 or greater,[63] and both absolute flow and resistance are associated with angina.[64]

Based on absolute flow from continuous thermodilution measures, the microvascular resistance reserve (MRR) has been proposed as an index specific for the microvasculature, independent of autoregulation and myocardial mass, and corrected for epicardial conductance. MRR can be defined as the ratio of the pure microvascular resistance at rest because it would exist in the absence of epicardial disease affecting microcirculatory autoregulation, to the mMR measured during hyperemia. Although the derivation of the formula for MRR is beyond the scope of this review, in practice, MRR can be calculated as the CFR divided by fractional flow reserve (FFR), corrected for coronary driving pressures as follows: MRR = (CFR/FFR) $\times$ ($P_{a\ at\ rest}/P_{a\ at\ hyperemia}$).[65] This conceptually elegant and promising new measure of microcirculatory function requires additional validation.

Practical Approach to Invasive Microcirculatory Assessment

Before testing, patients should be advised to abstain from caffeine intake to ensure appropriate responses to hyperemic agents. When combined with acetylcholine or ergonovine reactivity testing, patients should also withhold long-acting nitrates, calcium channel blockers, and beta-blockers for 48 hours before testing. Coronary angiography should be performed to assess for epicardial coronary stenosis and myocardial bridges. Coronary microvascular testing should be performed using a guiding catheter (preferably 6 or greater French) that is stably engaged in the coronary ostium, after administration of intracoronary nitroglycerin and systemic anticoagulation.

To measure thermodilution-based CFR and IMR, a coronary pressure–temperature sensor guidewire (Pressure Wire, Abbott Vascular) should be introduced into the guide, and residual contrast media flushed with saline. Pressure waveforms should be equalized with the pressure sensor at the tip of the guide catheter. Next, the temperature and pressure sensor should be advanced to the distal two-thirds of the left anterior descending (LAD) artery, approximately 8 to 10 cm into the circumflex and placed in a large obtuse marginal branch or dominant distal vessel, or in the distal RCA before the bifurcation of the posterior descending artery. A 3-way stopcock and a 3-mL syringe should be connected to the manifold. Next, 3 mL boluses of room-temperature saline should be briskly injected through the guide catheter to determine T_{mn} at rest. Measurements are performed in triplicate. If there is less than 30% variability between the measurements, the T_{mn} value that deviates most significantly from the mean value should be replaced. Once assessment of baseline flow has been completed, hyperemia is induced with intravenous adenosine (140 mcg/kg/min), or with a bolus of intracoronary papaverine (10–20 mg). Once maximal hyperemia has been achieved, typically ~2 minutes after initiation of intravenous adenosine, 3 mL boluses of room temperature saline should again be briskly injected through the guide. CFR can be calculated as the ratio of T_{mn} at rest to T_{mn} at hyperemia; IMR is the product of T_{mn} and P_d at hyperemia. Nonhyperemic pressure ratios and FFR should also be assessed to determine significance of any angiographically intermediate epicardial lesions. RRR can be calculated as the ratio of baseline to hMR ($T_{mn\ at\ rest} \times P_{d\ at\ rest}$)/IMR.

Doppler-based measurements of CFR and hMR follow a similar sequence. After intracoronary nitroglycerin, a 0.014″ coronary guidewire with a pressure sensor and Doppler crystal (ComboWire XT, Philips Volcano) should be positioned parallel to the vessel, away from the vessel wall, and manipulated to obtain a stable maximal Doppler flow signal. APV is measured at rest and again with maximal hyperemia, as previously described. The CFR is calculated as the ratio of hyperemic APV to resting APV. The hMR is calculated as the hyperemic P_d divided by the hyperemic APV. To assess endothelial dependent microvascular function, CBF at rest and during acetylcholine infusions can be estimated from Doppler-derived APV and luminal dimensions from quantitative coronary angiography.

Clinical Implications of Microcirculatory Disease

Microvascular disease in ischemia with nonobstructive coronary arteries

Nearly 50% of patients who present with chest pain have angiographically normal or nonobstructive epicardial coronary arteries (<50% stenosis) by angiography.[2,3,66] A comprehensive approach to the diagnosis of INOCA, including testing for microvascular disease, can improve the care of these patients (**Fig. 2**). In the Coronary Microvascular Angina (CorMicA) trial, 151 patients underwent blinded assessment of coronary microvascular function and provocative testing for coronary artery spasm; participants were randomly assigned to disclosure of the results or usual care.[6] Overall, microvascular angina was identified in 52% of patients, coronary spasm was identified in 20%, and mixed microvascular and spasm diagnosis was present in 17%, with no discernible cause identified in the remaining 11%.[67] Although noncardiac chest pain was presumed in 60% to 65% of participants before randomization, the results

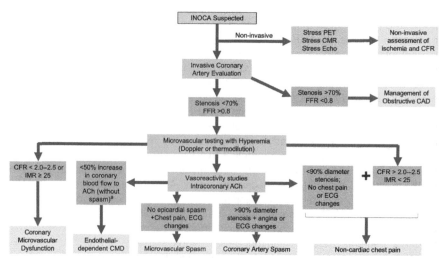

Fig. 2. Diagnostic pathway for the invasive assessment of patients with INOCA. [a]Assessed with Doppler APV and coronary diameter via quantitative coronary angiography to determine coronary blood flow at rest and with ACh. Ach, acetylcholine; CAD, coronary artery disease; CFR, coronary flow reserve; CFVR, coronary flow velocity reserve; CMD, coronary microvascular disease; CMR, cardiovascular magnetic resonance; ECG, electrocardiogram; FFR, fractional flow reserve; IMR, index for microvascular resistance; INOCA, ischemia with nonobstructive coronary arteries; PET, positron emission tomography.

of testing improved diagnostic certainty, reduced the number of patients inappropriately diagnosed with noncardiac chest pain, and impacted therapy in the overwhelming majority of patients in the intervention group. Although similar at baseline, patients assigned to disclosure of coronary functional testing had significantly better Angina Summary Scores and quality of life at 6 months and 1 year compared with the control group.[6,68] This trial provides compelling data in support of invasive microvascular testing to guide therapy and improve symptoms in INOCA (see **Fig. 2**). Additional studies to evaluate the clinical benefit of microvascular testing without coronary spasm testing are currently underway (iCorMICA NCT04674449).

Although outcomes are more favorable than patients with obstructive disease, INOCA is associated with excess major adverse cardiovascular events compared with reference populations without IHD.[69] Data from Women's Ischemia Syndrome Evaluation registry indicate that CFR of less than 2.3 is associated with increased risks of major adverse cardiovascular events (MACE) in patients with INOCA.[31,70] In a multicenter international study of INOCA patients with microvascular angina, the annual incidence of the composite of MACE was 7.7%.[71] In a study-level meta-analysis, CMD was associated with 5-fold greater odds for major adverse cardiovascular events compared with patients without CMD.[72] Thus, novel therapies to reduce the risk of MACE in patients with microvascular disease are urgently needed.

Impact of Coronary Microvascular Dysfunction in Myocardial Infarction and Percutaneous Coronary Intervention

In patients with acute myocardial infarction (MI), distal embolization of thrombotic material can lead to the "no-reflow phenomenon," characterized by myocardial tissue hypoperfusion in the presence of a patent epicardial coronary artery. No-reflow, mediated by microvascular disease, is a strong predictor for adverse outcomes post-MI.[73] Quantitative assessment of the coronary microcirculation provides additional insights into MI severity and outcomes. In patients with ST segment elevation MI (STEMI), IMR postpercutaneous coronary intervention (PCI) correlates with myocardial injury, echocardiographic wall motion abnormalities,[74] myocardial viability by PET,[75] and myocardial salvage by cardiac magnetic resonance (CMR).[48] Although IMR correlates with microvascular obstruction by CMR imaging overall,[76] discordances between the 2 measures are reported in up to a third of cases.[77] Yet, in a cohort of 253 patients undergoing primary PCI for STEMI with a median follow-up of 2.8 years, elevated IMR of 40 or greater immediately after revascularization was associated with a 2-fold excess hazard of long-term death or rehospitalization for heart failure, and a 4-fold excess hazard of mortality.[78] The Doppler-derived resistance index, hMR, has also been associated with outcomes after STEMI.[35] Similarly, in patients who presented with NSTEMI and underwent PCI, post-PCI elevated IMR greater than 27 was an independent predictor of MACE over a median follow-up of 21 months.[79]

Even in stable patients undergoing PCI, a high baseline IMR is an independent risk factor for periprocedural MI. Among patients undergoing PCI of simple LAD lesions, pre-PCI IMR of 27 or greater, was independently associated with a 23-fold increase in the risk of periprocedural MI.[80] Furthermore, in a cohort of 572 patients undergoing successful PCI for stable IHD, post-PCI IMR was independently associated with major adverse cardiovascular events at follow-up.[81]

SUMMARY

The coronary microcirculation represents the next frontier in the diagnosis and treatment of coronary artery disease. Recognition of the importance of coronary physiology has expanded our understanding of IHD and European and American societal guidelines now recommend comprehensive assessment of microvascular function in patients with INOCA.[7,8] Recent advances in invasive techniques and technologies to quantify microcirculatory CBF and resistance are vital to the comprehensive evaluation of coronary artery disease. Additional studies are needed to determine optimal therapies for patients with coronary microcirculatory disease in various cardiac disease states.

CLINICS CARE POINTS

- Coronary microvascular dysfunction is an important, and often under-appreciated, cause of angina and ischemia that can be diagnosed invasively based on an abnormally low coronary flow reserve (CFR) and/or an elevated index of microcirculatory resistance (IMR).

ACKNOWLEDGMENTS

Dr N.R. Smilowitz is supported, in part, by the National Heart, Lung, And Blood Institute of the National Institutes of Health, United States under Award Number K23HL150315.

DISCLOSURE

Dr N.R. Smilowitz serves on an advisory board for Abbott Vascular. The remainder of the authors report no financial relationships or conflicts of interest regarding the content herein.

REFERENCES

1. Tsao CW, Aday AW, Almarzooq ZI, et al. Heart Disease and Stroke Statistics-2022 Update: A Report From the American Heart Association. Circulation 2022. https://doi.org/10.1161/CIR.0000000000001052. CIR0000000000001052.
2. Patel MR, Peterson ED, Dai D, et al. Low diagnostic yield of elective coronary angiography. N Engl J Med 2010;362(10):886–95.
3. Shaw LJ, Shaw RE, Merz CN, et al. Impact of ethnicity and gender differences on angiographic coronary artery disease prevalence and in-hospital mortality in the American College of Cardiology-National Cardiovascular Data Registry. Circulation 2008;117(14):1787–801.
4. Bairey Merz CN, Pepine CJ, Walsh MN, et al. Ischemia and No Obstructive Coronary Artery Disease (INOCA): Developing Evidence-Based Therapies and Research Agenda for the Next Decade. Circulation 2017;135(11):1075–92.
5. Ong P, Camici PG, Beltrame JF, et al. International standardization of diagnostic criteria for microvascular angina. Int J Cardiol 2018;250:16–20.
6. Ford TJ, Stanley B, Good R, et al. Stratified Medical Therapy Using Invasive Coronary Function Testing in Angina: The CorMicA Trial. J Am Coll Cardiol 2018; 72(23 Pt A):2841–55.
7. Gulati M, Levy PD, Mukherjee D, et al. 2021 AHA/ACC/ASE/CHEST/SAEM/SCCT/SCMR Guideline for the Evaluation and Diagnosis of Chest Pain: A Report of the American College of Cardiology/American Heart Association Joint Committee on Clinical Practice Guidelines. Circulation 2021;144(22):e368–454.
8. Kunadian V, Chieffo A, Camici PG, et al. An EAPCI Expert Consensus Document on Ischaemia with Non-Obstructive Coronary Arteries in Collaboration with

European Society of Cardiology Working Group on Coronary Pathophysiology & Microcirculation Endorsed by Coronary Vasomotor Disorders International Study Group. Eur Heart J 2020;41(37):3504–20.

9. Padro T, Manfrini O, Bugiardini R, et al. ESC Working Group on Coronary Pathophysiology and Microcirculation position paper on 'coronary microvascular dysfunction in cardiovascular disease. Cardiovasc Res 2020;116(4):741–55.

10. Wilson RF, Marcus ML, White CW. Prediction of the physiologic significance of coronary arterial lesions by quantitative lesion geometry in patients with limited coronary artery disease. Circulation 1987;75(4):723–32.

11. Camici PG, d'Amati G, Rimoldi O. Coronary microvascular dysfunction: mechanisms and functional assessment. Nat Rev Cardiol 2015;12(1):48–62.

12. Diez-Delhoyo F, Gutierrez-Ibanes E, Loughlin G, et al. Coronary physiology assessment in the catheterization laboratory. World J Cardiol 2015;7(9):525–38.

13. Duncker DJ, Bache RJ. Regulation of coronary blood flow during exercise. Physiol Rev 2008;88(3):1009–86.

14. Camici PG, Crea F. Coronary microvascular dysfunction. N Engl J Med 2007; 356(8):830–40.

15. Crea F, Camici PG, Bairey Merz CN. Coronary microvascular dysfunction: an update. Eur Heart J May 2014;35(17):1101–11.

16. Lanza GA, Crea F. Primary coronary microvascular dysfunction: clinical presentation, pathophysiology, and management. Circulation 2010;121(21):2317–25.

17. Lanza GA, Andreotti F, Sestito A, et al. Platelet aggregability in cardiac syndrome X. Eur Heart J 2001;22(20):1924–30.

18. Kleinbongard P, Heusch G. A fresh look at coronary microembolization. Nat Rev Cardiol 2021. https://doi.org/10.1038/s41569-021-00632-2.

19. Cecchi F, Olivotto I, Gistri R, et al. Coronary microvascular dysfunction and prognosis in hypertrophic cardiomyopathy. N Engl J Med 2003;349(11):1027–35.

20. Mills I, Fallon JT, Wrenn D, et al. Adaptive responses of coronary circulation and myocardium to chronic reduction in perfusion pressure and flow. Am J Physiol 1994;266(2 Pt 2):H447–57.

21. Egashira K, Inou T, Hirooka Y, et al. Impaired coronary blood flow response to acetylcholine in patients with coronary risk factors and proximal atherosclerotic lesions. J Clin Invest 1993;91(1):29–37.

22. Ong P, Athanasiadis A, Borgulya G, et al. Clinical usefulness, angiographic characteristics, and safety evaluation of intracoronary acetylcholine provocation testing among 921 consecutive white patients with unobstructed coronary arteries. Circulation 2014;129(17):1723–30.

23. Recio-Mayoral A, Mason JC, Kaski JC, et al. Chronic inflammation and coronary microvascular dysfunction in patients without risk factors for coronary artery disease. Eur Heart J 2009;30(15):1837–43.

24. Hirata K, Kadirvelu A, Kinjo M, et al. Altered coronary vasomotor function in young patients with systemic lupus erythematosus. Arthritis Rheumatism 2007;56(6): 1904–9.

25. Di Carli MF, Charytan D, McMahon GT, et al. Coronary circulatory function in patients with the metabolic syndrome. J Nucl Med 2011;52(9):1369–77.

26. Dayanikli F, Grambow D, Muzik O, et al. Early detection of abnormal coronary flow reserve in asymptomatic men at high risk for coronary artery disease using positron emission tomography. Circulation 1994;90(2):808–17.

27. Laine H, Raitakari OT, Niinikoski H, et al. Early impairment of coronary flow reserve in young men with borderline hypertension. J Am Coll Cardiol 1998;32(1):147–53.

28. Lee BK, Lim HS, Fearon WF, et al. Invasive evaluation of patients with angina in the absence of obstructive coronary artery disease. Circulation 2015;131(12): 1054–60.

29. Doucette JW, Corl PD, Payne HM, et al. Validation of a Doppler guide wire for intravascular measurement of coronary artery flow velocity. Circulation 1992; 85(5):1899–911.

30. Sara JD, Widmer RJ, Matsuzawa Y, et al. Prevalence of Coronary Microvascular Dysfunction Among Patients With Chest Pain and Nonobstructive Coronary Artery Disease. JACC Cardiovasc Interv 2015;8(11):1445–53.

31. AlBadri A, Bairey Merz CN, Johnson BD, et al. Impact of Abnormal Coronary Reactivity on Long-Term Clinical Outcomes in Women. J Am Coll Cardiol 2019; 73(6):684–93.

32. Fearon WF, Balsam LB, Farouque HM, et al. Novel index for invasively assessing the coronary microcirculation. Circulation 2003;107(25):3129–32.

33. Barbato E, Aarnoudse W, Aengevaeren WR, et al. Validation of coronary flow reserve measurements by thermodilution in clinical practice. Eur Heart J 2004; 25(3):219–23.

34. Williams RP, de Waard GA, De Silva K, et al. Doppler Versus Thermodilution-Derived Coronary Microvascular Resistance to Predict Coronary Microvascular Dysfunction in Patients With Acute Myocardial Infarction or Stable Angina Pectoris. Am J Cardiol 2018;121(1):1–8.

35. de Waard GA, Fahrni G, de Wit D, et al. Hyperaemic microvascular resistance predicts clinical outcome and microvascular injury after myocardial infarction. Heart 2018;104(2):127–34.

36. Fearon WF, Farouque HM, Balsam LB, et al. Comparison of coronary thermodilution and Doppler velocity for assessing coronary flow reserve. Circulation 2003; 108(18):2198–200.

37. Everaars H, de Waard GA, Driessen RS, et al. Doppler Flow Velocity and Thermodilution to Assess Coronary Flow Reserve: A Head-to-Head Comparison With [(15)O]H2O PET. JACC Cardiovasc Interv 2018;11(20):2044–54.

38. Nardone M, McCarthy M, Ardern CI, et al. Concurrently Low Coronary Flow Reserve and Low Index of Microvascular Resistance Are Associated With Elevated Resting Coronary Flow in Patients With Chest Pain and Nonobstructive Coronary Arteries. Circ Cardiovasc Interv 2022. https://doi.org/10.1161/CIRCINTERVENTIONS.121. 011323.

39. Wilson RF, Wyche K, Christensen BV, et al. Effects of adenosine on human coronary arterial circulation. Circulation 1990;82(5):1595–606.

40. Luo C, Long M, Hu X, et al. Thermodilution-derived coronary microvascular resistance and flow reserve in patients with cardiac syndrome X. Circ Cardiovasc Interv 2014;7(1):43–8.

41. Solberg OG, Ragnarsson A, Kvarsnes A, et al. Reference interval for the index of coronary microvascular resistance. Eurointervention 2014;9(9):1069–75.

42. Lee JM, Layland J, Jung JH, et al. Integrated physiologic assessment of ischemic heart disease in real-world practice using index of microcirculatory resistance and fractional flow reserve: insights from the International Index of Microcirculatory Resistance Registry. Circ Cardiovasc Interv 2015;8(11):e002857.

43. Aarnoudse W, Fearon WF, Manoharan G, et al. Epicardial stenosis severity does not affect minimal microcirculatory resistance. Circulation 2004;110(15):2137–42.

44. Yong AS, Layland J, Fearon WF, et al. Calculation of the index of microcirculatory resistance without coronary wedge pressure measurement in the presence of epicardial stenosis. JACC Cardiovasc Interv 2013;6(1):53–8.

45. Layland J, MacIsaac AI, Burns AT, et al. When collateral supply is accounted for epicardial stenosis does not increase microvascular resistance. Circ Cardiovasc Interv 2012;5(1):97–102.
46. Ng MK, Yeung AC, Fearon WF. Invasive assessment of the coronary microcirculation: superior reproducibility and less hemodynamic dependence of index of microcirculatory resistance compared with coronary flow reserve. Circulation 2006;113(17):2054–61.
47. Pagonas N, Gross CM, Li M, et al. Influence of epicardial stenosis severity and central venous pressure on the index of microcirculatory resistance in a follow-up study. Eurointervention 2014;9(9):1063–8.
48. Payne AR, Berry C, Doolin O, et al. Microvascular Resistance Predicts Myocardial Salvage and Infarct Characteristics in ST-Elevation Myocardial Infarction. J Am Heart Assoc 2012;1(4):e002246.
49. Chamuleau SA, Siebes M, Meuwissen M, et al. Association between coronary lesion severity and distal microvascular resistance in patients with coronary artery disease. American Journal of Physiology Heart and Circulatory Physiology 2003;285(5):H2194–200.
50. Sheikh AR, Zeitz CJ, Rajendran S, et al. Clinical and coronary haemodynamic determinants of recurrent chest pain in patients without obstructive coronary artery disease - A pilot study. Int J Cardiol 2018;267:16–21.
51. de Waard GA, Nijjer SS, van Lavieren MA, et al. Invasive minimal Microvascular Resistance Is a New Index to Assess Microcirculatory Function Independent of Obstructive Coronary Artery Disease. J Am Heart Assoc 2016;5(12). https://doi.org/10.1161/JAHA.116.004482.
52. Scarsini R, De Maria GL, Borlotti A, et al. Incremental Value of Coronary Microcirculation Resistive Reserve Ratio in Predicting the Extent of Myocardial Infarction in Patients with STEMI. Insights from the Oxford Acute Myocardial Infarction (Ox-AMI) Study. Cardiovasc revascularization Med : including Mol interventions 2019;20(12):1148–55.
53. Layland J, Carrick D, McEntegart M, et al. Vasodilatory capacity of the coronary microcirculation is preserved in selected patients with non-ST-segment-elevation myocardial infarction. Circ Cardiovasc Interv 2013;6(3):231–6.
54. Corcoran D, Young R, Adlam D, et al. Coronary microvascular dysfunction in patients with stable coronary artery disease: The CE-MARC 2 coronary physiology sub-study. Int J Cardiol 2018;266:7–14.
55. Maznyczka AM, Oldroyd KG, Greenwood JP, et al. Comparative Significance of Invasive Measures of Microvascular Injury in Acute Myocardial Infarction. Circ Cardiovasc Interv 2020;13(5):e008505.
56. Lee SH, Lee JM, Park J, et al. Prognostic Implications of Resistive Reserve Ratio in Patients With Coronary Artery Disease. J Am Heart Assoc 2020;9(8):e015846.
57. Toya T, Ahmad A, Corban MT, et al. Risk Stratification of Patients With NonObstructive Coronary Artery Disease Using Resistive Reserve Ratio. J Am Heart Assoc 2021;10(11):e020464.
58. Aarnoudse W, Van't Veer M, Pijls NH, et al. Direct volumetric blood flow measurement in coronary arteries by thermodilution. J Am Coll Cardiol 2007;50(24):2294–304.
59. Jansen TPJ, Konst RE, Elias-Smale SE, et al. Assessing Microvascular Dysfunction in Angina With Unobstructed Coronary Arteries: JACC Review Topic of the Week. J Am Coll Cardiol 2021;78(14):1471–9.

60. Xaplanteris P, Fournier S, Keulards DCJ, et al. Catheter-Based Measurements of Absolute Coronary Blood Flow and Microvascular Resistance: Feasibility, Safety, and Reproducibility in Humans. Circ Cardiovasc Interv 2018;11(3):e006194.

61. De Bruyne B, Adjedj J, Xaplanteris P, et al. Saline-Induced Coronary Hyperemia: Mechanisms and Effects on Left Ventricular Function. Circ Cardiovasc Interv 2017;10(4). https://doi.org/10.1161/CIRCINTERVENTIONS.116.004719.

62. Everaars H, de Waard GA, Schumacher SP, et al. Continuous thermodilution to assess absolute flow and microvascular resistance: validation in humans using [15O]H2O positron emission tomography. Eur Heart J 2019;40(28):2350–9.

63. Rivero F, Gutierrez-Barrios A, Gomez-Lara J, et al. Coronary microvascular dysfunction assessed by continuous intracoronary thermodilution: A comparative study with index of microvascular resistance. Int J Cardiol 2021;333:1–7.

64. Konst RE, Elias-Smale SE, Pellegrini D, et al. Absolute Coronary Blood Flow Measured by Continuous Thermodilution in Patients With Ischemia and Nonobstructive Disease. J Am Coll Cardiol 2021;77(6):728–41.

65. De Bruyne B, Pijls NHJ, Gallinoro E, et al. Microvascular Resistance Reserve for Assessment of Coronary Microvascular Function: JACC Technology Corner. J Am Coll Cardiol 2021;78(15):1541–9.

66. Patel MR, Dai D, Hernandez AF, et al. Prevalence and predictors of nonobstructive coronary artery disease identified with coronary angiography in contemporary clinical practice. Am Heart J 2014;167(6):846–852 e2.

67. Ford TJ, Yii E, Sidik N, et al. Ischemia and No Obstructive Coronary Artery Disease: Prevalence and Correlates of Coronary Vasomotion Disorders. Circ Cardiovasc Interv 2019;12(12):e008126.

68. Ford TJ, Stanley B, Sidik N, et al. 1-Year Outcomes of Angina Management Guided by Invasive Coronary Function Testing (CorMicA). JACC Cardiovasc Interv 2020;13(1):33–45.

69. Jespersen L, Hvelplund A, Abildstrom SZ, et al. Stable angina pectoris with no obstructive coronary artery disease is associated with increased risks of major adverse cardiovascular events. Eur Heart J 2012;33(6):734–44.

70. Pepine CJ, Anderson RD, Sharaf BL, et al. Coronary microvascular reactivity to adenosine predicts adverse outcome in women evaluated for suspected ischemia results from the National Heart, Lung and Blood Institute WISE (Women's Ischemia Syndrome Evaluation) study. J Am Coll Cardiol 2010;55(25):2825–32.

71. Shimokawa H, Suda A, Takahashi J, et al. Clinical characteristics and prognosis of patients with microvascular angina: an international and prospective cohort study by the Coronary Vasomotor Disorders International Study (COVADIS) Group. Eur Heart J 2021;42(44):4592–600.

72. Gdowski MA, Murthy VL, Doering M, et al. Association of Isolated Coronary Microvascular Dysfunction With Mortality and Major Adverse Cardiac Events: A Systematic Review and Meta-Analysis of Aggregate Data. J Am Heart Assoc 2020;9(9):e014954.

73. Ndrepepa G, Tiroch K, Fusaro M, et al. 5-year prognostic value of no-reflow phenomenon after percutaneous coronary intervention in patients with acute myocardial infarction. J Am Coll Cardiol 2010;55(21):2383–9.

74. Fearon WF, Shah M, Ng M, et al. Predictive value of the index of microcirculatory resistance in patients with ST-segment elevation myocardial infarction. J Am Coll Cardiol 2008;51(5):560–5.

75. Lim HS, Yoon MH, Tahk SJ, et al. Usefulness of the index of microcirculatory resistance for invasively assessing myocardial viability immediately after primary angioplasty for anterior myocardial infarction. Eur Heart J 2009;30(23):2854–60.

76. Carrick D, Haig C, Ahmed N, et al. Comparative Prognostic Utility of Indexes of Microvascular Function Alone or in Combination in Patients With an Acute ST-Segment-Elevation Myocardial Infarction. Circulation 2016;134(23):1833–47.
77. De Maria GL, Alkhalil M, Wolfrum M, et al. Index of Microcirculatory Resistance as a Tool to Characterize Microvascular Obstruction and to Predict Infarct Size Regression in Patients With STEMI Undergoing Primary PCI. JACC Cardiovasc Imaging 2019;12(5):837–48.
78. Fearon WF, Low AF, Yong AS, et al. Prognostic value of the Index of Microcirculatory Resistance measured after primary percutaneous coronary intervention. Circulation 2013;127(24):2436–41.
79. Murai T, Yonetsu T, Kanaji Y, et al. Prognostic value of the index of microcirculatory resistance after percutaneous coronary intervention in patients with non-ST-segment elevation acute coronary syndrome. Catheter Cardiovasc Interv 2018; 92(6):1063–74.
80. Ng MK, Yong AS, Ho M, et al. The index of microcirculatory resistance predicts myocardial infarction related to percutaneous coronary intervention. Circ Cardiovasc Interv 2012;5(4):515–22.
81. Nishi T, Murai T, Ciccarelli G, et al. Prognostic Value of Coronary Microvascular Function Measured Immediately After Percutaneous Coronary Intervention in Stable Coronary Artery Disease: An International Multicenter Study. Circ Cardiovasc Interv 2019;12(9):e007889.

The Role of Psychology in Pediatric Rheumatic Diseases

William S. Frye, PhD, BCB, ABPP[a],*, Diana Milojevic, MD[b]

KEYWORDS

• Pediatric psychology • Rheumatic disease • Juvenile arthritis • Interdisciplinary care

KEY POINTS

• Youth with pediatric rheumatic diseases (PRDs) experience a complex disease course, which can be difficult to manage and lead to psychosocial impairments and functional challenges.
• Pediatric psychologists are equipped to address many of the concerns seen within the management of PRDs.
• Integration of pediatric psychologists into PRD treatment or interdisciplinary clinics can be beneficial in overcoming barriers youth with PRDs experience and improving quality of life.

Pediatric rheumatic diseases (PRDs) are chronic conditions caused by disorders of the immune system and characterized by systemic inflammation (several organs in the body are affected) and/or local inflammation (only specific organs, frequently joints, are affected). Different rheumatic diseases are more prevalent in children at certain ages, although pediatric rheumatologists care for children from the first year of life through early adulthood. It has been estimated that more than 300,000 children in the United States have a chronic rheumatic disease.[1]

Inflammation seen in rheumatic conditions is caused by the immune system attacking its own body, which can be triggered by defects in either the specific immune system (ie, autoimmune diseases) or the nonspecific "primitive" or "naïve" immune system (ie, autoinflammatory diseases). Autoimmune diseases include systemic lupus

Disclosures.
This article previously appeared in *Pediatric Clinics* volume 69 issue 5 October 2022.
Funding: No funding, grants, or other support were received for this study.
Conflicts of interest/Competing interests: Dr W.S. Frye serves as an expert panelist for the Juvenile Arthritis Foundation.
a Department of Psychology, Johns Hopkins All Children's Hospital, 880 6th Street South, Suite 460, St Petersburg, FL 33701, USA; b Department of Medicine, Johns Hopkins All Children's Hospital, 601 5th Street South, Suite 502, Street, St Petersburg, FL 33701, USA
* Corresponding author.
E-mail address: wfrye1@jhmi.edu

erythematosus (SLE), most forms of juvenile idiopathic arthritis (JIA), juvenile dermatomyositis, different types of scleroderma, and some types of vasculitis (blood vessel inflammation). Examples of autoinflammatory diseases include periodic fever syndromes, some types of vasculitis (eg, Behcet's disease), some types of systemic arthritis, macrophage activation syndrome, and several rare, more recently described genetic disorders characterized by chronic inflammation. Although these are classified as two distinct groups of diseases, most of the autoimmune and autoinflammatory diseases share pathologic features and symptoms.

Our understanding of these disorders and immune mechanisms has evolved tremendously over the last 20 years and brought a number of new autoimmune and autoinflammatory diseases to our attention. Some of these diseases have been poorly understood and inadequately treated in the past, whereas some were never seen by rheumatologists because of the disease causing early death in childhood. However, with advancements in knowledge of basic science immunology and genetics, as well as diagnostic tools (eg, laboratory tests, imaging), these conditions are now readily identified. These advancements have resulted in an explosion of new treatments including "biologicals," which, unlike past medications, decrease inflammation by attacking specific targets in the immune system rather than causing broad immunosuppression with potentially more severe side effects on the body. The scenes from the twentieth-century pediatric rheumatology clinics of children in wheelchairs with severe musculoskeletal deformities affecting basic activities of daily living are largely gone. Indeed, the diagnosis of a rheumatic disease in a child today is no longer a sentence to a life with a severe physical disability or an early death. What they still experience; however, is a life with a chronic disease, most commonly without a promise of a cure, often with an unpredictable disease course despite the patient's and providers' best efforts.

DIFFICULTIES FOR YOUTH WITH PEDIATRIC RHEUMATIC DISEASES

The chronic nature and unpredictability of rheumatic disease course are features of PRDs that can be difficult for both the patient and their family to accept and can cause significant life disruption. As the disease often affects more than one organ, numerous organ-specific specialists are involved in care, causing numerous hospital visits and disruption of school life for children and work for parents. Patients' and families' reactions to the diagnosis may differ over time, as the child grows and family dynamics change. There may be denial at the time of the diagnosis, which can potentially lead to unnecessary harm from delaying treatment or interventions. Later, there may be a feeling of "defeat" when treatments were followed correctly, but the disease relapsed nonetheless, which can be detrimental to the patient/physician relationship and future compliance. Throughout a youth's disease journey, there are several concerns that are commonly seen and can obstruct management of PRDs.

Pharmacotherapy and Adherence

One of the mainstays of treating rheumatic conditions is the use of long-term pharmacotherapy such as disease-modifying antirheumatic drugs, immunosuppressive agents, or biological drugs to ameliorate symptoms.[2] Although these pharmacotherapies can halt disease process, medications must be regularly taken to be effective. Nonadherence to medications can lead to deleterious health outcomes and uncontrolled disease process and can be especially challenging for this population. Specifically, studies reviewing adherence rates to pharmacotherapy for JIA and SLE have described overall treatment adherence as inadequate.[3] Although nonadherence to

PRD medications can occur due to a host of known and unknown reasons, researchers often describe forgetting medication, medication refusal, complexity of regimen, unwanted side-effects, perceived disease severity, lack of perceived benefit or loss of medication effect over time, cost, and access to care as potential explanations.[4–6]

Cognitive Impairment

Cognitive impairment is a common comorbidity in PRDs, which has a potential impact upon executive functions, memory, and concentration.[7–9] The pathogenic mechanisms leading to cognitive decline in individuals with rheumatic disease are unknown; however, there are several proposed factors including chronic systemic inflammatory process of disease, long-term use of glucocorticoid steroids, or chemotherapy agents such as methotrexate that may also have effects on the developing brain.[10] Executive functions are a particularly important factor when considering one's ability to remain adherent to medications and medical regimen, as well as an adolescents' ability to academically perform or engage in functional behavior.[11,12]

Pain Management

Pain is a symptom accompanying many PRDs that can debilitate normal life functioning and lead to distressed mood. Approximately 86% of youth with PRDs such as JIA are reported to experience pain.[13,14] Acute pain in PRDs is often related to local inflammation as part of the disease process. Although many youth with PRDs experience acute pain as part of the sequalae of active disease, they may also experience continued pain after the acute process is gone. Such is the case with chronic pain syndromes including amplified musculoskeletal pain syndrome (AMPS), in which youth who are in disease remission continue to experience pain without the presence of inflammatory process. Regardless of pain's etiology, many youth find pain to be functionally impairing and emotionally distressing, especially when pharmacotherapy treatments for their acute disease process are unable to provide relief. In fact, many of the medications that assist with inflammation and active disease process, such as biological drugs and immunosuppressive agents, are ineffective for chronic pain syndromes.[15,16] This can be a distressing situation for both families and providers as these medications are requested by families given their previous benefit, but are not appropriate for chronic pain management. Uncontrolled chronic pain despite inactive disease process can also lead to confusion, disrupted mood, and decreased functioning.[17]

Functional Disability

Youth with PRDs commonly experience increased functional disability and reduced quality of life (QoL) compared with healthy peers.[18,19] Functioning is especially impacted in youth with PRDs experiencing pain, who are found to be less likely to attend school, engage in sports, be physically active, or socially engage with their peers.[20–22] Such functional changes can have a compounding impact on youth. Although social support and engagement in physical activity is recommended to buffer the deleterious effects of chronic illness, youth who are unable to regularly attend school or engage in sports, groups, or other peer activities will have less social contact and may see peer support diminish.[23] Reduced functional behavior and socialization can lead to social isolation and peer rejection,[24] which may further impact mood and reinforce avoidance of social activities. In addition, reduced functioning and decreased use of joints and muscles can result in deconditioning, which can increase pain scores when youth with PRDs become more active, furthering the cycle of functional disability and impaired mood.[25]

Mood

Within patients who have rheumatic conditions, increased rates of anxiety and depression have been found when compared with healthy controls throughout the lifespan.[26] This impact upon mental health is apparent in youth. According to the Arthritis Foundation, almost two-thirds of youth with JIA reported having issues with anxiety, and almost half reported struggling with depression.[27] This is consistent with findings across PRDs, in which adolescents show higher rates of mental health disorders such as depression and anxiety than healthy peers.[28,29] Unfortunately, as symptoms of depression or anxiety worsen, youth with PRDs experience decreased health-related QoL and functional disability.[30,31] This can create a negative loop in which patients engage in less activity, experience increased pain, and subsequently develop feelings of sadness and helplessness.[32,33]

Mood impairments in PRDs are not solely triggered by functional disability and pain. Researchers have posited many reasons for why mood may be disrupted including the psychological burden of chronic illness, physical effects from disease damage, treatment-related side effects, and unpredictability of symptoms and disease course.[28,33,34] Illness uncertainty in particular is common among chronic illnesses and has a negative impact on coping, anxiety, and emotional adjustment.[35,36] As part of typical disease course, youth with PRDs often experience unpredictability of symptom flares and periods of quiescence, which can lead to feelings of lacking control of one's disease or uncertainty regarding management and outcome.

Changes in mood and functioning can also have a profound impact on families of youth with PRDs. In qualitative studies examining parents of youth with JIA, parents endorse confusion, emotional turmoil, guilt, worries, anger, helplessness, and frustration related to the disease and the process of caring for a child with JIA.[34,37] These emotions were often related to not understanding JIA, difficulty managing the disease, and feeling sorrow for their child's discomfort. Parents in these studies described how diseases such as JIA can impact the entire family unit and leave everyone feeling physically and emotionally drained. Even siblings of patients with JIA were noted to have difficulty understanding the illness, having difficult seeing their sibling in pain, and feeling frustrated or angry due to having less attention from their parents or less time together as an entire family.

INCLUSION OF PSYCHOLOGY IN INTERDISCIPLINARY CARE

Given the strong relationships between rheumatic conditions, disordered mood, and reduced QoL, it has been recommended that physicians treating patients with rheumatologic conditions integrate assessment and treatment of mood concerns into regular clinical practice.[38] One way this is conducted in pediatric rheumatology clinics is through the inclusion of a psychologist as part of an interdisciplinary team. In fact, there are many ways psychology has been integrated into treating the multifaceted concerns of youth with chronic illness.

Psychology's Role in Adherence

Psychologists are providers that can assist in leading interventions to improve treatment adherence in youth with PRDs. A combination of behavioral (eg, problem-solving, parent training) and educational (eg, providing instruction or teaching related to illness or treatment) interventions to improve adherence is recommended, as these have provided better health outcomes for patients with chronic illness.[39] Interventions that include social support, social skills training, family therapy, or other psychosocial targets may also be beneficial in improving adherence.[40] Psychologists can use these multicomponent interventions to target adherence to medication, physical activity recommendations, or other aspects of interdisciplinary care. In addition to these interventions, motivational interviewing is a patient-centered approach which focuses upon the patient's intrinsic motivation to change and a collaborative interaction style to help the patient understand their goals, reasons for change, and barriers.[41] A recent review of the literature suggests motivational interviewing appears to be a promising intervention to address nonadherence and improve QoL, and is well received by adolescents and young adults.[42] Psychologists may consider using motivational interviewing techniques to form a collaborative relationship with patients that allows for intrinsic change to improve adherence. A review of helpful and unhelpful motivational interviewing questions to assess adherence can be found within the practice implications of Schaefer and Kavookjian.[42]

Psychology's Role in Cognitive Decline

Pediatric neuropsychologists are frequently embedded within hospital systems to provide brief or comprehensive evaluations and diagnose cognitive and behavioral concerns related to a child's neurological profile. One way they can serve youth with PRDs is by offering neuropsychology testing to determine how neurological functioning may be impacted. Much like testing for late effects in cancer, baseline and repeat neuropsychological testing at age of onset, repeated during grade school, and college, can help determine cognitive impact or decline.[43] By identifying and addressing cognitive concerns, these psychologists can assist families in obtaining school accommodations and provide recommendations to help youth functional behavior. Identifying and addressing cognitive concerns can also help resolve barriers to adherence, subsequently leading to better disease management and improved QoL.

Psychology's Role in Pain Management

An often-unrecognized area in which psychologists can aid patients with PRDs is pain management. Pain is defined as both an emotional and physical process, regardless of etiology. Our current understanding of pain neuroscience describes our pain experience as a culmination of several parts of the brain, including our limbic system and emotional state.[44] The influence of emotional state, fear of pain, and the belief that pain can be controlled or changed are all aspects of youth's pain experience in which psychologists can help intervene. In both acute and chronic pain processes, psychologists can assist youth in learning relaxation and coping skills that calm the body's response to pain and reduce pain perception. Skills may include teaching diaphragmatic breathing, progressive muscle relaxation, imagery, meditation, or mindfulness strategies. Although these skills can reduce pain perception, they are also intended to serve as strategies that increase patients' self-efficacy for returning to functional activities. In the case of chronic pain conditions such as AMPS, psychologists can play multiple roles. As part of treatment, psychologists can teach skills to help patients find comfort while in pain and adjust to changes that have occurred in their life. A component of building self-efficacy related to managing chronic pain is education on chronic pain versus acute pain. With the assistance of a rheumatologist or other provider assessing disease progression, psychologists can help provide education upon how pain can persist despite having no active rheumatic disease process. Specifically, explaining sensitization of the nervous system and how, even though a child may still experience pain, chronic pain is not indicative of danger or harmful to their body. This explanation may allow patients to believe they have the ability to control aspects of their pain, subsequently reducing fear of pain and pain experience. As part of this education, providers should note that disruptions in mood do not cause pain, however, can influence and maintain chronic pain. In many pain conditions without obvious visible symptoms, such as AMPS or juvenile fibromyalgia, well-meaning providers invalidate patients by stating that pain is due to anxiety or "in the child's head." Proper psychoeducation on the relationship between pain and mood may reconcile some of these incorrect and invalidating remarks.

Psychology's Role in Functional Behavior

Consistent with the treatment of pain, pediatric psychologists can assist in improving functional behaviors by teaching youth coping skills and increasing their self-efficacy to improve functioning. These skills are intended to improve youths' management of both pain and mood, allowing for increased functioning. As previously mentioned, improving adherence can lead to decreased disease activity, decreasing pain, and allowing youth to engage in more functional behaviors.

Throughout a child's disease journey, families may have difficulties as they balance protecting their child from the outcomes of poor disease management while allowing their child to build medical self-efficacy and autonomy as a young adult. Although support and supervision of a child's medical regimen is frequently required, too much enmeshment and protectiveness can lead to negative outcomes.[45] Psychologists have the ability to assess family structure and dynamics, provide interventions that involve the entire family unit, and help teach caregivers how to respond to their children in ways that allow for promotion of functioning and management of their disease, rather than fostering the child's dependence on their parents. These strategies can include rewarding adherence and functional behaviors or encouraging steps toward independent disease management.

As these youth grow to become young adults with rheumatic disease, they continue to face many of the same challenges as during their adolescence, though often with less support. Psychologists can serve as part of the team assisting in transitioning pediatric patients to adult care by having frank discussions with families about the transition process, assessing for barriers and progress toward transition, and connecting families with social work for assistance with vocational and educational planning.

In addition to adjusting to general changes in life, psychologists are also equipped to assist youth in changes that occur socially. Psychologists can serve as a support system and guide youth who are navigating social changes or attempting to reintegrate into school or other peer activities. Part of this work can occur through teaching coping skills or using cognitive-behavioral therapy (CBT) to address worried thoughts or fears youth may have when returning to functional activities. For youth who have been away from their peers for long periods or feel they generally lack interpersonal skills, psychologists can work with them to develop scripts to explain their condition or absence, role play worrisome interactions, or teach social skills that may improve confidence.

Psychology's Role in Mood and Coping

At its core, the field of psychology is known for the treatment of mood concerns. When working with youth with rheumatic conditions, psychologists often apply therapies such as CBT to challenge unhelpful thinking patterns and assist patients in improving mood and functioning.[46] Within PRDs, CBT often focuses upon restructuring unhelpful thoughts about physical illness, encourages social and other functional activities, and prevents learned helplessness that can occur from disease unpredictability and has shown positive effects on QoL and mood.[47] Given the chronicity of rheumatic conditions, psychologists can help youth with adjustment to symptoms at different developmental phases and teach coping strategies to improve mood or functioning. Although these skills may not be expected to remove all symptoms that limit function, they can teach youth ways to better control their pain and improve self-efficacy in their own disease management. In the case of illness uncertainty, families often cite the lack of information about PRDs and treatment options as major concerns.[48] These concerns may be ameliorated by providing information about the pathophysiology and treatment of PRDs in the early stages of the disease process, as well as having a trained professional, such as a psychologist, help treat the emotional aspects of illness uncertainty.

SUMMARY

PRDs are a heterogeneous group of diseases which have similar characteristics of chronic, episodic, and unpredictable disease course that can greatly impact the patient and patient's family life in multiple areas of mood and functioning. Providers should consider psychosocial complexities as part of managing active disease process when working with youth with PRDs. Pediatric psychologists are well-equipped to assess cognitive impairment and emotional distress, and provide empirically based interventions addressing adherence to treatment, pain management, improving functional disability, and regulating mood. These interventions can then be adjusted and adapted to the unique needs of patients with PRDs depending on their ever-changing psychosocial functioning and disease course. Referring patients with PRDs to psychology can be part of regular holistic practice. Providers may also choose to integrate a pediatric psychologist into an interdisciplinary rheumatology clinic, allowing them to assess psychosocial concerns, jointly develop a conceptualization and plan with a rheumatologist, and provide a targeted intervention. Providing this style of comprehensive disease management can address the complex needs of patients with PRDs, help obtain favorable disease outcomes, and deliver quality care.

CLINICS CARE POINTS

- Integration of pediatric psychologist into interdisciplinary care for youth with pediatric rheumatic diseases (PRDs) can assist in addressing psychosocial concerns and holistic disease management.

- Early involvement of pediatric psychologists in the care of youth with PRDs can allow for monitoring and intervention throughout disease course and address problems that may occur at different stages of development.

- Psychological interventions should be adapted to a patient's unique psychosocial needs, functional impairments, disease trajectory, and age.

REFERENCES

1. Arthritis Foundation. News Blog. Juvenile Arthritis (JA). Available at: https://www.arthritis.org/diseases/juvenile-arthritis. Accessed January 28, 2021.
2. Cavallo S, Brosseau L, Toupin-April K, et al. Ottawa panel evidence-based clinical practice guidelines for structured physical activity in the management of juvenile idiopathic arthritis. Arch Phys Med Rehabil 2017;98(5):1018–41.

3. De Achaval S, Suarez-Almazor ME. Treatment adherence to disease-modifying antirheumatic drugs in patients with rheumatoid arthritis and systemic lupus erythematosus. Int J Clin Rheumtol 2010;5(3):313.
4. Favier LA, Taylor J, Rich KL, et al. Barriers to adherence in juvenile idiopathic arthritis: a multicenter collaborative experience and preliminary results. J Rheumatol 2018;45(5):690–6.
5. Pelajo CF, Sgarlat CM, Lopez-Benitez JM, et al. Adherence to methotrexate in juvenile idiopathic arthritis. Rheumatol Int 2012;32(2):497–500.
6. Rapoff MA. Adherence to pediatric medical regimens. 2nd edition. London: Springer; 2010.
7. Meade T, Manolios N, Cumming SR, et al. Cognitive impairment in rheumatoid arthritis: a systematic review. Arthritis Care Res 2018;70(1):39–52.
8. Oláh C, Schwartz N, Denton C, et al. Cognitive dysfunction in autoimmune rheumatic diseases. Arthritis Res Ther 2020;22(1):78.
9. Sood A, Raji MA. Cognitive impairment in elderly patients with rheumatic disease and the effect of disease-modifying anti-rheumatic drugs. Clin Rheumatol 2020; 40(4):1221–31.
10. Katchamart W, Narongroeknawin P, Phutthinart N, et al. Disease activity is associated with cognitive impairment in patients with rheumatoid arthritis. Clin Rheumatol 2019;38(7):1851–6.
11. Bagner DM, Williams LB, Geffken GR, et al. Type 1diabetes in youth: the relationship between adherence and executive functioning. Child Health Care 2007; 36(2):169–79.
12. Cortés Pascual A, Moyano Muñoz N, Quilez Robres A. The relationship between executive functions and academic performance in primary education: Review and meta-analysis. Front Psychol 2019;10:1582.
13. Arnstad ED, Rypdal V, Peltoniemi S, et al. Early self-reported pain in juvenile idiopathic arthritis as related to long-term outcomes: results from the Nordic Juvenile Idiopathic Arthritis Cohort Study. Arthritis Care Res 2019;71(7):961–9.
14. Bromberg MH, Connelly M, Anthony KK, et al. Self-reported pain and disease symptoms persist in juvenile idiopathic arthritis despite treatment advances: an electronic diary study. Arthritis Rheumatol 2014;66(2):462–9.
15. Howard RF, Wiener S, Walker SM. Neuropathic pain in children. Arch Dis Child 2014;99(1):84–9.
16. Palermo TM, Eccleston C, Lewandowski AS, et al. Randomized controlled trials of psychological therapies for management of chronic pain in children and adolescents: an updated meta-analytic review. Pain 2010;148(3):387–97.
17. Liossi C, Howard RF. Pediatric chronic pain: biopsychosocial assessment and formulation. Pediatrics 2016;138(5):e20160331.
18. Jones JT, Cunningham N, Kashikar-Zuck S, et al. Pain, fatigue, and psychological impact on health-related quality of life in childhood-onset lupus. Arthritis Care Res 2016;68(1):73–80.
19. Müller-Godeffroy E, Lehmann H, Küster RM, et al. Quality of life and psychosocial adaptation in children and adolescents with juvenile idiopathic arthritis and reactive arthritis. Z Rheumatol 2005;64(3):177–87.
20. Milatz F, Klotsche J, Niewerth M, et al. Participation in school sports among children and adolescents with juvenile idiopathic arthritis in the German National Paediatric Rheumatologic Database, 2000–2015: results from a prospective observational cohort study. Pediatr Rheumatol Online J 2019;17(1):1.

21. Limenis E, Grosbein HA, Feldman BM. The relationship between physical activity levels and pain in children with juvenile idiopathic arthritis. J Rheumatol 2014; 41(2):345–51.
22. Rebane K, Ristolainen L, Relas H, et al. Disability and health-related quality of life are associated with restricted social participation in young adults with juvenile idiopathic arthritis. Scand J Rheumatol 2019;48(2):105–13.
23. Bailey R. Physical education and sport in schools: a review of benefits and outcomes. J Sch Health 2006;76(8):397–401.
24. Kashikar-Zuck S, Lynch AM, Graham TB, et al. Social functioning and peer relationships of adolescents with juvenile fibromyalgia syndrome. Arthritis Rheum 2007;57(3):474–80.
25. Gualano B, Bonfa E, Pereira RMR, et al. Physical activity for paediatric rheumatic diseases: standing up against old paradigms. Nat Rev Rheumatol 2017;13(6): 368–79.
26. McWilliams LA, Clara IP, Murphy PD, et al. Associations between arthritis and a broad range of psychiatric disorders: findings from a nationally representative sample. J Pain 2008;9(1):37–44.
27. Arthritis Foundation. News Blog. Improving Mental Health for Kids with Juvenile Arthritis. Available at: http://blog.arthritis.org/news/improving-mental-health-kids-juvenile-arthritis/. Accessed December 6, 2021.
28. Fair DC, Rodriguez M, Knight AM, et al. Depression and anxiety in patients with juvenile idiopathic arthritis: current insights and impact on quality of life, a systematic review. Open Access Rheumatol 2019;11:237–52.
29. Knight A, Weiss P, Morales K, et al. Depression and anxiety and their association with healthcare utilization in pediatric lupus and mixed connective tissue disease patients: a cross-sectional study. Pediatr Rheumatol Online J 2014;12:42.
30. Donnelly C, Cunningham N, Jones JT, et al. Fatigue and depression predict reduced health-related quality of life in childhood-onset lupus. Lupus 2018; 27(1):124–33.
31. Hoff AL, Palermo TM, Schluchter M, et al. Longitudinal relationships of depressive symptoms to pain intensity and functional disability among children with disease-related pain. J Pediatr Psychol 2006;31(10):1046–56. https://doi.org/10.1093/jpepsy/jsj076.
32. Tarakci E, Yeldan I, Mutlu EK, et al. The relationship between physical activity level, anxiety, depression, and functional ability in children and adolescents with juvenile idiopathic arthritis. Clin Rheumatol 2011;30(11):1415–20.
33. El-Najjar AR, Negm MG, El-Sayed WM. The relationship between depression, disease activity and physical function in juvenile idiopathic arthritis patients in Zagazig University Hospitals–Egypt. Egypt. Rheumatol 2014;36(3):145–50.
34. Gómez-Ramírez O, Gibbon M, Berard R, et al. A recurring rollercoaster ride: a qualitative study of the emotional experiences of parents of children with juvenile idiopathic arthritis. Pediatr Rheumatol Online J 2016;14(1):13.
35. Johnson LM, Zautra AJ, Davis MC. The role of illness uncertainty on coping with fibromyalgia symptoms. Health Psychol 2006;25(6):696.
36. Van Pelt JC, Mullins LL, Carpentier MY, et al. Brief report: illness uncertainty and dispositional self-focus in adolescents and young adults with childhood-onset asthma. J Pediatr Psychol 2006;31(8):840–5.
37. Yuwen W, Lewis FM, Walker AJ, et al. Struggling in the dark to help my child: parents' experience in caring for a young child with juvenile idiopathic arthritis. J Pediatr Nurs 2017;37:e23–9.

38. Anyfanti P, Gavriilaki E, Pyrpasopoulou A, et al. Depression, anxiety, and quality of life in a large cohort of patients with rheumatic diseases: common, yet under-treated. Clin Rheumatol 2016;35(3):733–9.
39. Graves MM, Roberts MC, Rapoff M, et al. The efficacy of adherence interventions for chronically ill children: a meta-analytic review. J Pediatr Psychol 2010;35(4): 368–82.
40. Kahana S, Drotar D, Frazier T. Meta-analysis of psychological interventions to promote adherence to treatment in pediatric chronic health conditions. J Pediatr Psychol 2008;33(6):590–611.
41. Miller WR, Rollnick S. Motivational interviewing. New York: Guilford Press; 1991.
42. Schaefer MR, Kavookjian J. The impact of motivational interviewing on adherence and symptom severity in adolescents and young adults with chronic illness: a systematic review. Patient Educ Couns 2017;100(12):2190–9.
43. Annett RD, Patel SK, Phipps S. Monitoring and assessment of neuropsychological outcomes as a standard of care in pediatric oncology. Pediatr Blood Cancer 2015;62(Suppl 5):S460–513.
44. Bushnell MC, Ceko M, Low LA. Cognitive and emotional control of pain and its disruption in chronic pain. Nat Rev Neurosci 2013;14(7):502–11.
45. Hann-Moorison D. Maternal enmeshment: the chosen child. SAGE Open 2012; 2(4). https://doi.org/10.1177/2158244012470115.
46. Butler AC, Chapman JE, Forman EM, et al. The empirical status of cognitive-behavioral therapy: a review of meta-analyses. Clin Psychol Rev 2006;26(1): 17–31.
47. Rubinstein TB, Davis AM, Rodriguez M, et al. Addressing mental health in pediatric rheumatology. Curr Treat Options Rheum 2018;4(1):55–72.
48. Pearce C, Newman S, Mulligan K. Illness uncertainty in parents of children with juvenile idiopathic arthritis. ACR Open Rheumatol 2021;3(4):250–9.

Newer Immunosuppressants for Rheumatologic Disease
Preoperative Considerations

Ye Rin Koh, MD, Kenneth C. Cummings III, MD, MS*

KEYWORDS

- Rheumatic diseases • Perioperative period • Biologic therapy
- Medication therapy management

KEY POINTS

- Many new targeted therapies are available for patients with rheumatic diseases.
- Knowledge of the mechanisms, risks, and pharmacokinetics of these agents is necessary for optimal perioperative management.
- Choosing how to manage these agents for each patient involves balancing infectious (and other) risks with the very real risk of disease flares.

INTRODUCTION

Preoperative stratification of risk factors and optimizing comorbidities can pose many challenges for anesthesiologists. Perioperative management of inflammatory rheumatic disease (IRD) requires further investigation due to lack of evidence and difficulties in conducting prospective trials in this context. IRDs affect soft tissues, muscles, joints, and bones and include rheumatoid arthritis (RA), psoriatic arthritis (PsA) ankylosing spondylitis (AS), juvenile idiopathic arthritis (JIA), and systemic lupus erythematosus (SLE).

With disease progression, joint replacement surgeries, including total hip arthroplasties (THA) and total knee arthroplasties (TKA), are often an inevitable course of treatment in patients with IRD and have been shown to be successful in treating and improving quality of life. Accordingly, over 30% of patients with rheumatic disease will require surgery within 30 years of diagnosis.[1] One key consideration in these patients is minimizing the risk of prosthetic joint infections (PJI) and delayed wound healing which are devastating complications that require long-term antibiotic therapy and eventually prosthetic joint removal. Inflammatory arthritis confers increased risk of infection following both THA and TKA.[2,3] PJIs have a mortality rate as high as 18% and therefore, prevention is of utmost importance.

This article previously appeared in *Anesthesiology Clinics* volume 42 issue 1 March 2024.
Anesthesiology Institute, Cleveland Clinic, 9500 Euclid Avenue, E-31, Cleveland, OH 44195, USA
* Corresponding author. 9500 Euclid Avenue, E-31, Cleveland, OH 44195.
E-mail address: cummink2@ccf.org

This increased risk of complications is due to (1) the inflammatory nature of the disease, (2) associated cardiovascular comorbidities, and (3) the use of immunosuppressant medications. However, interruption in antirheumatic therapy has also been associated with increased risk of disease flare. Therefore, one of the biggest questions that arise for anesthesiologists, rheumatologists, and orthopedic surgeons is the perioperative management of antirheumatic medications.[4] Perioperative management of antirheumatic therapy is a careful balance between minimizing risk of PJI and delayed wound healing while also preventing disease flare. Although significant advancements in antirheumatic therapy have been made over the past few decades, many questions remain about the proper perioperative management of these patients.

Corticosteroids are widely used for a variety of diseases to suppress inflammation and regulate the body's immune system. However, steroids have significant long-term side effects. Due to concerns for its safety profile, nonsteroidal therapy began to garner attention. To minimize these effects, disease-modifying antirheumatic drugs (DMARDs) such as methotrexate, azathioprine, and sulfasalazine are used. They have been shown to be more effective but also have their own toxicities. More recently, better mechanistic understanding of disease processes led to the development of targeted immunotherapy such as small molecule modulators, monoclonal antibodies, and recombinant/fusion proteins. These agents are highly effective but carry their own risks as well.

This review will provide an overview of the variety of immunosuppressive therapies for IRD and perioperative recommendations based on recent evidence with emphasis some of the more novel medications. **Table 1** provides a list of drug classes and specific examples.

Traditional Agents

1. Corticosteroids

Corticosteroids have been a major component of immunosuppressive therapy for a variety of autoimmune and inflammatory diseases. However, their use is limited by significant side effects with chronic use including surgical site infections, impaired wound

Table 1
Types of biologics

Class	Type of Molecule	Examples
CD20 antagonist	Chimeric antibody (30%–35% murine)	Rituximab
TNF-alpha inhibitor	Chimeric antibody (30%–35% murine)	Infliximab
	Chimeric antibody (<10% murine)	Certolizumab
	Human monoclonal antibody	Adalimumab
		Golimumab
	Fusion protein	Etanercept
IL-1 antagonist	Human monoclonal antibody	Canakinumab
	Fusion protein	Rilonacept
IL-2 antagonist	Chimeric antibody (<10% murine)	Daclizumab
IL-4 antagonist	Human monoclonal antibody	Dupilumab
IL-6 receptor antagonist	Chimeric antibody (<10% murine)	Tocilizumab
Immune checkpoint inhibitor	Human monoclonal antibody	Ipilimumab
		Nivolumab
	Chimeric antibody (<10% murine)	Pembrolizumab
BLyS inhibitor	Human monoclonal antibody	Belimumab
Costimulation inhibitor	Fusion protein	Abatacept

healing, hemodynamic instability secondary to steroid induced adrenal insufficiency, Cushing syndrome, and gastrointestinal (GI) bleeding from ulcers. Steroids have a dose dependent increase in postoperative infections and readmission with prednisone doses greater than 10 mg/d[5] Compared to biologics, glucocorticoids had a higher risk of adverse events (including hospitalized infections, PJI, and 30 day readmission).

Stress dose steroids are often administered perioperatively but their efficacy is unclear due to lack of evidence demonstrating hemodynamic instability and the unknown dose threshold that induces suppression of the hypothalamic–pituitary–adrenal axis. The American College of Rheumatology/American Association of Hip and Knee Surgeons (ACR/AAHKS) guidelines recommended that patients take their daily dose of steroids rather than receiving a stress dose on the day of surgery.[6] Preferably, steroids should be tapered to less than 20 mg before surgery. If unable to taper to less than 15 mg due to disease flare, physicians should take extra precautions to avoid increasing risk of infections.

2. Methotrexate

Methotrexate (MTX) was first introduced in the 1940s for chemotherapy before it became commonly used to treat RA and psoriasis in the 1950s. It is continually used for a variety of autoimmune and inflammatory diseases including RA, psoriasis, JIA, SLE, inflammatory bowel disease (IBD), vasculitis, and many other connective tissue disorders.[7] MTX inhibits purine and pyrimidine synthesis resulting in reduced T-cell proliferation. It has the best efficacy-to-toxicity ratio among the DMARDs and is generally well tolerated. The most common side effect is GI upset and rarely can cause bone marrow suppression, pulmonary injury, and hepatotoxicity. Among the DMARDs, the perioperative recommendations for MTX are best established. It has been shown not to increase risk of infections[8] and continuation decreases the risk of disease flares.[9] Therefore, the ACR/AHHKS guidelines recommend MTX to be continued perioperatively.[6]

3. Leflunomide

Leflunomide (LEF) is a nonbiologic DMARD that prevents lymphocyte proliferation by inhibiting dihydroorotate dehydrogenase (DHODH) necessary for pyrimidine synthesis.[10] It is also used to treat PsA, JIA, dermatomyositis, and SLE. There have been conflicting results about the infectious risk from perioperative use of this drug.[11,12] At this time, the ACR/AAHKS guidelines state that perioperative continuation of LEF is safe in patients without risk factors (such as history of recurrent infections or prior PJIs).[6]

Common side effects of LEF include nausea, diarrhea, and liver injury. LEF has also rarely been associated with pancytopenia, interstitial lung disease and pneumonitis. For this reason, it is contraindicated in patients with hepatic and pulmonary diseases. Liver enzymes, complete blood counts (CBC), and blood pressure should be monitored in patients on LEF therapy. Due to teratogenic effects, LEF is also contraindicated during pregnancy.

4. Mercaptopurine

6-Mercaptopurine (6-MP) is an antimetabolite that prevents proliferation of T lymphocytes by inhibiting intracellular purine synthesis. Nausea, abdominal pain, aphthous ulcers, and bone marrow suppression are common side effects of 6-MP. It has also been shown to cause hepatotoxicity and rarely liver cancers (including hepatocellular carcinoma and hepatosplenic T-cell lymphoma). For this reason, CBC and liver enzymes should be monitored in patients on therapy.

Many studies have shown that perioperative continuation of 6-MP for patients with inflammatory bowel disease undergoing elective surgery does not increase morbidity or infectious complications.[13,14] According to ACR/AAHKS guidelines, 6-MP should be continued perioperatively for patients with severe IRD but, due to its toxicities, should be held 1 week before surgery for nonsevere IRD.[6]

5. Sulfasalazine

Sulfasalazine is a DMARD that is used to treat RA, JIA, and ulcerative colitis. Other off label uses include AS, Crohn's disease, and PsA. Sulfasalazine can cause nausea, vomiting, dyspepsia, and skin rashes. Rarely it can also cause pancytopenia, liver, and renal injury. Therefore, CBC, serum creatinine, and liver enzymes should be monitored in patients on sulfasalazine therapy. Unlike other DMARDs, it is not teratogenic. Perioperative continuation of sulfasalazine is not associated with increased risk of infections[15] and the ACR/AHHKS guidelines recommend perioperative continuation of sulfasalazine in patients with no risk factors.[6]

6. Hydroxychloroquine

Well-known as an antimalarial drug, hydroxychloroquine has been shown to have immunomodulatory properties and is now used to treat a variety of rheumatic diseases including RA and SLE. However, its mechanism as an immunosuppressant is not well understood. Hydroxychloroquine has low immunosuppressive potency compared with other DMARDs and due its favorable toxicity profile, it has been thought to be safe to continue perioperatively.[8,16] Therefore, the ACR/AHHKS guidelines recommend perioperative continuation of sulfasalazine in patients with no risk factors.[6]

New Oral Disease-Modifying Antirheumatic Drugs

1. Phosphodiesterase type 4 inhibition

Apremilast is a novel oral DMARD that is FDA approved for treating PsA, plaque psoriasis, and oral ulcers in Behcet's disease. It is a selective PDE4 inhibitor that works in the innate immune system by increasing cAMP and decreasing inflammatory mediators including IL-2, TNF-alpha, and interferon (IFN)-gamma. The most common side effects include GI (primarily nausea, diarrhea, and rarely weight loss). For this reason, the patients' weight should be monitored carefully during therapy.[17] Rarely, apremilast has been shown to be associated with psychiatric conditions such as depression and suicidal ideations. Apremilast is relatively well tolerated with high safety profile and low risk of infections.[18] ACR/AHHKS guidelines recommend perioperative continuation of apremilast with the exception of patients with a history of recurrent/severe infections or prior PJI.[6] In high-risk patients, it can be held 3 days before surgery based on its half-life of 6 to 9 hours.[4]

2. Janus kinase inhibitors

Tofacitinib is the first oral Janus kinase (JAK) inhibitor developed to treat RA. Tofacitinib preferentially inhibits JAK3/JAK1 and downstream production of inflammatory cytokines including IL-2 that are essential for lymphocyte function.[19] It is currently approved for treatment of RA, PsA, ulcerative colitis (UC), and polyarticular JIA. Tofacitinib has a black box warning against serious infections, malignancies, and lymphoma. Due to the risk of opportunistic infections (with cytomegalovirus [CMV], Epstein-Barr virus [EBV], BK virus, tuberculosis [TB]) patients should be tested for active/latent TB before initiating treatment and monitored for TB routinely while receiving therapy. JAK inhibitors are also known to increase the risk of thromboembolic disease and therefore should be used with caution in patients with increased cardiovascular risk. Some of the more common side effects include infections (urinary and respiratory tract), pancytopenia, hepatotoxicity, and hyperlipidemia. Blood counts, lipid panels, and liver enzymes should be monitored while on therapy. Concurrent use with strong immunosuppressants and biologic agents are not recommended. Patients should not receive live vaccinations before and during therapy as well. Tofacitinib was originally recommended to be held a week before surgery but, due to rapid offset of clinical effect, current guidelines recommend holding JAK inhibitors 3 days before surgery.[6]

Biologics/recombinant Proteins

1. Emapalumab

Macrophage activation syndrome-hemophagocytic lymphohistiocytosis (MAS-HLH) is a life-threatening dysregulation of the immune system seen in patients with rheumatic disease due to uncontrolled activation and exaggerated responses of cytotoxic T cells producing massive amounts of interferon gamma. It is most frequently associated with systemic JIA and adult onset Still disease. Emapalumab is a monoclonal antibody that inhibits interferon gamma and the first targeted therapy that was approved for the treatment of HLH in rheumatic disease. Clinically presents with fever, hepatosplenomegaly, cytopenia, liver dysfunction, coagulation abnormalities, and eventually progresses to multiorgan failure. In the past, MAS has been treated with high-dose glucocorticoids and cyclosporin. Emapalumab is extremely effective for treating MAS, especially in patients who fail standard therapy.[20,21] The 2 most common side effects are infections and hypertension. Infusion-related reactions and fever are other frequent side effects that have been reported as well.[22]

2. Immune checkpoint inhibitors

Immune checkpoints are T-cell surface proteins involved in downregulating T-cell activity and regulating the immune system. Examples include cytotoxic T lymphocyte antigen 4 (CTLA-4), programmed death protein 1 (PD1), and PD1 ligand (PDL1). Immune checkpoints may be overexpressed on the surface of tumor cells to downregulate and evade the immune system.[23] Targeted therapy against these immune checkpoints has shown great promise in treating cancer. Ipilimumab is a CTLA4 inhibitor that is administered every 3 weeks for a total of 4 doses. Therapy with PD-1/PDL1 inhibitors can vary between 1 week and every 2 to 3 weeks.

Nivolumab is a monoclonal antibody against PD1 that is FDA approved for a variety of cancers including melanoma, esophageal cancer, urethral cancer, and non-small cell lung cancer. Pembrolizumab is another monoclonal antibody against PD1 that is indicated for various cancers including melanoma, non-small cell lung cancer, and advanced breast and uterine cancers.

However, immune checkpoint inhibitors are also associated with significant side effects. The incidence of immune-related side effects is greater with anti-CTLA4 therapy compared with anti-PD1 therapy. The GI tract, skin, and endocrine system are affected most but less commonly these agents can also affect the pulmonary, cardiac, and neurologic system.[24] The GI system is the most affected and can present with diarrhea, enterocolitis, and hepatitis.[25] Immune-related endocrine dysfunction can present with pituitary dysfunction, adrenal insufficiency, and hypothyroidism. Therefore, anesthesiologists should check electrolyte levels and assess thyroid and adrenal function.[26] Immune-related cardiac toxicity is rare with an incidence of less than 1%. Myocarditis is the most common cardiac complication but heart failure, cardiomyopathy, and conduction abnormalities may also be seen.[27,28] Anesthesiologists should make sure to assess for cardiac symptoms and review appropriate testing (such as electrocardiography, echocardiography, and possibly biomarkers) before surgery. Pneumonitis is the most common pulmonary complication and therefore respiratory symptoms should be assessed preoperatively to evaluate the need for steroid therapy.[29,30]

3. TNF alpha inhibitors

TNF alpha inhibitors (infliximab, adalimumab, certolizumab, and golimumab) are monoclonal antibodies that decrease inflammation by binding and inhibiting TNF alpha, a proinflammatory molecule involved in activating host cell responses leading to neutrophil recruitment and initiating inflammatory responses. TNF alpha inhibitors are used to treat a variety of inflammatory and autoimmune diseases including psoriasis, RA, PsA, and IBD.[31] Etanercept is a recombinant fusion protein combining the TNF receptor with the Fc portion of the IgG1 antibody. Like the previously mentioned antibodies, it also inhibits the activity of TNF alpha but does so by acting as a "decoy" receptor, binding TNF alpha and preventing its biological activity.

Infliximab was the first anti-TNF antibody that was used to treat chronic inflammatory and autoimmune diseases. The side effects of infliximab are well known, the most common being infection. Other adverse reactions include hypersensitivity reactions, infections (hepatitis B virus [HBV], opportunistic infection, and TB reactivation), malignancies, lupus like syndrome, pancytopenia, demyelinating disorders, congestive heart failure, and hepatotoxicity.[32] There are contradictory results regarding the association between perioperative continuation of tumor necrosis factor (TNF) alpha inhibitors with postoperative complications. Results range from increased infectious risk to decreased risk and improved wound healing.

Guidelines vary for the perioperative management for TNF alpha inhibitors and treatment should be individualized. The optimal individualized strategy is based on a combination of anti-TNF half-life and bioavailability. In general, the effects of anti-TNF alpha inhibitors disappear approximately after 4 to 5 half-lives and the timing of preoperative interruption of therapy depends on each medication's half-life and dosing regimen.[33,34] Witrand and colleagues[35] demonstrated that discontinuing treatment 5 half-lives before surgery does not increase the risk of complications. Postoperative complications increased by 13% with infliximab if given within 2 to 5 half-lives before orthopedic surgeries. Therefore, majority guidelines recommend stopping infliximab 4 to 5 weeks before elective surgery. The half-life of infliximab is 9.5 days, adalimumab 10 to 20 days, etanercept 3.5 to 5.5 days, golimumab 14 days, and certolizumab 14 days.[36] Based on these data, one group recommends that infliximab should be discontinued 21 to 39 days before surgery.[34] Because of its long half-life, this is equivalent to less than 1 dose of infliximab that should be held. Etanercept should be held 7 to 14 days, adalimumab 56 days, and golimumab 4 weeks before surgery.

Similarly, the ACR/AHHKS guidelines recommend scheduling surgery after the end of the dosing cycle to ensure that there is minimal drug left in the system.[6] For infliximab, hold medication 5 weeks before surgery if the patient is taking it every 4 weeks. For adalimumab, hold 3 weeks prior and for etanercept, hold 2 weeks before surgery.

To prevent a disease flare postoperatively, therapy should be resumed as soon as it is deemed safe from the surgical standpoint. The process of wound healing is often completed 2 weeks postoperatively and some use this as a general guideline as to when to restart therapy. However, for specific medications a combination of the half-life and mechanism of action can be used to provide guidance. In general, infliximab is recommended to be restarted 3 to 4 weeks, etanercept 12 days, and ada-limumab 56 days postoperatively.[34]

4. IL-1 inhibitors

Interleukin-1 (IL-1) and its receptor are strong inflammatory activators that can induce fever and acute phase reactions by stimulating production of IL-6 at higher doses. For this reason, IL-1 receptor antagonists are used to treat diseases mediated by excessive IL-1 such as hereditary autoinflammatory disease, cryopyrin associated periodic syndromes (CAS), and monogenic period fever syndrome that often present with recurrent febrile episodes. Rilonacept is a fusion protein incorporating the IL-1 receptor bound to the Fc region of human IgG1. This binds to IL-1, preventing its biologic effects. It is the first and only FDA approved medication for recurrent pericarditis and CAS. In addition to immunosuppression and risk of infections, other common side effects include injection reactions, upper respiratory tract infections, and joint and muscle aches.[37]

IL-1 is also a major cartilage destructive cytokine. Anakinara, which is a recombinant IL-1 receptor antagonist, has been used to decrease cartilage destruction in RA. Other off label use of anakinra includes idiopathic juvenile arthritis and other autoimmune arthritic diseases (adult onset still disease and macrophage activation syndrome). Common side effects of anakinra include local skin reactions, GI upset, headache, arthralgias, and increased risk of infections. More severe side effects include TB reactivation, neutropenia, and hypersensitivity reactions.[38] Therefore, blood counts should be monitored regularly while on therapy. Anakinara is taken daily and has a half-life of 4 to 6 hours. According to ACR/AHHKS guidelines, anakinra should be held 2 days before surgery.

5. IL-6 inhibitors

IL-6 is a proinflammatory cytokine released in response to infection and injuries. It is also a key mediator of chronic inflammation. IL-6 is highly expressed during the active phases of RA and has been shown to induce osteoclast differentiation, explaining its destructive effects on cartilage.[39,40] Tocilizumab is a human monoclonal antibody against the IL-6 receptor.[41] It has been shown to successfully treat a variety of inflammatory diseases including COVID-19 and cancer patients with cytokine release syndrome.[42,43] As other biologics, the ACR/AHHKS guidelines recommend scheduling surgery the week after the end of the dosing cycle: Hold tocilizumab 2 weeks before surgery in patients who take it subcutaneously every week and hold it 5 weeks before surgery in patients who receive tocilizumab therapy intravenously every 4 weeks. Side effects of tocilizumab include bowel perforation,[44] neutropenia/thrombocytopenia,[45] hepatotoxicity,[46] hypersensitivity reactions,[47] and reactivation of latent TB and opportunistic infections.[48]

6. CD-20 inhibitors

Rituximab (RTX) is a monoclonal antibody against CD20 on B lymphocytes. B lymphocytes play a large role in the pathogenesis of a variety of autoimmune diseases such as RA by secreting proinflammatory cytokines, activating T lymphocytes, and acting as antigen-presenting cells (APCs).[34] CD20 is expressed by 95% of B lymphocytes in non-Hodgkin's lymphoma and was first monoclonal antibody that was approved for treating that disease. It is now used for patients with RA who are intolerant or had inadequate response to anti-TNF therapy.[49] RTX is FDA approved for treating hematologic cancers (including non-Hodgkin's lymphoma, diffuse large B-cell lymphoma, B-cell acute lymphocytic leukemia, and chronic lymphocytic leukemia) and a variety of autoimmune diseases (including RA, SLE, idiopathic thrombocytopenic purpura, vasculitis and chronic autoinflammatory polyneuropathy).[50] There is growing evidence that it could be effective in treating vasculitis and connective tissue diseases.[51]

Hypogammaglobulinemia is a well-known side effect of RTX therapy, and clinical trials have demonstrated that the rate of serious infections increases with RTX therapy.[52,53] However, there is little evidence about the risk of postoperative infections when continuing RTX therapy as the effects of RTX therapy can last up to 1 year after discontinuing treatment.[51] However, the risk of postoperative complications including surgical site infection (SSI) following orthopedic surgery in patients receiving rituximab has been shown to be similar to those receiving anti-TNF therapy.[15]

For IRD patients undergoing elective orthopedic surgeries, surgery should be scheduled after the end of the dosing interval; for instance, surgery should be scheduled on the fifth month for patients taking RTX every 4 months. Therapy should be resumed 14 days following surgery at which point wound healing has been completed. For severe SLE, surgery should be scheduled in the last month of the dosing cycle; for instance, if the patient is taking RTX every 4 months, then surgery should be scheduled in the fourth month to avoid skipping doses.

7. Alpha4beta7 integrin antibodies

Vedolizumab is an antibody against alpha4beta7 integrin that is currently FDA approved for the treatment for UC and Crohn's disease. Its efficacy in treating IBD is due to better safety profile and gut selectivity. Although biologic therapy has played a role in controlling the disease process, surgical intervention continues to be a part of the treatment plan for a majority of patients with IBD. Perioperative management of vedolizumab is not well established, and there are conflicting studies regarding the association of perioperative continuation of vedolizumab and postoperative infections.[54,55] It has been difficult to study vedolizumab's association with postoperative infections in patients with Crohn's disease because the majority of patients are already on multiple therapies, making it difficult to isolate the effects of vedolizumab from other agents. Common side effects include nasopharyngitis, headaches, arthralgias, nausea, and fatigue. Vedolizumab has been associated with more severe side effects such as infusion-related reactions, hypersensitivity reactions, infections, rarely progressive multifocal leukoencephalopathy (PML), and hepatotoxicity. As other with biologics, the ACR/AAHKS guidelines recommend elective surgeries to be scheduled at the end of the dosing cycle and restarted 14 days after surgery.[6]

8. B-cell activating factor

Belimumab is the first targeted therapy and only biologic agent that is FDA approved for the treatment of SLE and lupus nephritis. It is a human monoclonal antibody against B lymphocyte stimulator (BLyS) and mostly used as adjunct therapy for patients with SLE who are already receiving standard therapy. BlyS is essential for B-cell maturation and survival. Overexpression of BlyS can cause production of autoreactive B lymphocytes that can lead to variety of autoimmune diseases including SLE. Therefore, targeted therapy against BlyS such as belimumab can be used to control the disease process in autoimmune disorders.[56]

Side effects of belimumab include infections, infusion reactions, hypersensitivity reactions, headache, nausea, and fatigue. Psychiatric complications including suicidal tendency, PML, and malignancies have also been reported. Belimumab is generally well tolerated and as other biologics, recommended to undergo surgery at the end of the dosing cycle. ACR/AHHKS guidelines recommend continuing belimumab perioperatively for severe SLE in patients taking it subcutaneously weekly and taking it on the fourth week for those taking it intravenously every month. For nonsevere SLE, surgery should be scheduled the week after the end of the dosing cycle.[6] For instance, surgery should be scheduled on the fifth week following the last dose for those taking it every month.

9. Costimulation blockade

Abatacept (CTLA4-Ig) is a dimeric fusion protein that targets the interaction between T lymphocytes (CD28) and receptors (CD80/CD86) on APCs to modulate the costimulatory signal required for T-cell activation involved in joint swelling and damage. It is currently approved for patients with moderate-severe RA refractory to DMARDs and TNF-alpha inhibitors.[57] It is also used for treating JIA, PsA, and prophylaxis for graft-versus-host disease. One study by Nishida and colleagues[58] found no increase in SSI or delayed wound healing when abatacept was discontinued an average of 16 days before surgery (ranging between 8 and 21 days before the surgery depending on the patients' condition). There was also no difference in adverse outcomes when intravenous abatacept therapy was held 2 weeks before surgery versus 1 month (1 dosing interval) before surgery.[59] Therapy is recommended to be resumed a week after the process of wound healing is complete (approximately 3 weeks postoperatively).

The half-life of abatacept is 14 days and recommended to be held 2 to 3 weeks before surgery to prevent risk of flare. Abatacept can be administered intravenously every month or subcutaneously every week. The ACR/AHHKS guidelines recommend scheduling surgery on the fifth week following last dose (for monthly IV dosing) or the 2nd week following the last dose (for weekly subcutaneous dosing).

SUMMARY

Therapeutic options for patients with IRDs have greatly expanded in recent years. In addition to traditional medications like corticosteroids and the early DMARDs, today's armamentarium includes small-molecule immune modulators, recombinant fusion proteins, and monoclonal antibodies. Although very effective, these agents carry significant risks that affect perioperative care. Although there are published guidelines for the perioperative management of most of these agents, an individualized approach to each patient, balancing known risks and benefits, remains the most prudent course.

CLINICS CARE POINTS

- The optimal perioperative management of therapies for IRDs is a challenge for clinicians. Joint replacement surgeries are an inevitable course of treatment with disease progression and have been shown to be successful in treating and improving quality of life. However, patients with IRD are already at increased risk for serious postoperative complications (especially prosthetic joint infections and delayed wound healing) which have a high mortality rate in that population. Perioperative management of antirheumatic therapy requires careful balance between the risk of infections and the risk of prompting disease flares.

- Because of their extensive effects on various organ systems, corticosteroid use has decreased. Because of risk of adrenal suppression from exogenous steroid administration, perioperative stress dose steroids have been administered but there continues to be conflicting data regarding the dose and efficacy of giving supraphysiologic doses of steroids.

- The introduction of DMARDs including methotrexate, sulfasalazine, mercaptopurine, hydroxychloroquine leflunomide, and aprelimast revolutionized the treatment of rheumatic disease. These agents successfully delay disease progression while avoiding the side effects resulting from steroids. Generally, these steroid-sparing DMARDs are safe and recommended to continue throughout the perioperative period to avoid disease flares. JAK inhibitors are recommended to be held 3 days before surgery.

- As knowledge of these diseases' pathophysiology improved, direct targeted immunotherapy against specific parts of the inflammatory pathways such as small molecule modulators, monoclonal antibodies, and recombinant/fusion proteins were developed. Biologics are recommended to be held preoperatively and elective surgeries are recommended to be scheduled the week after the end of the last dosing cycle.

DISCLOSURE

The authors have no financial relationships to disclose.

REFERENCES

1. Da Silva E, Doran MF, Crowson CS, et al. Declining use of orthopedic surgery in patients with rheumatoid arthritis? Results of a long-term, population-based assessment. Arthritis Care Res 2003;49(2):216–20.
2. Richardson SS, Kahlenberg CA, Goodman SM, et al. Inflammatory Arthritis Is a Risk Factor for Multiple Complications After Total Hip Arthroplasty: A Population-Based Comparative Study of 68,348 Patients. J arthroplasty 2019; 34(6):1150–4.e1152.
3. Ravi B, Croxford R, Hollands S, et al. Increased Risk of Complications Following Total Joint Arthroplasty in Patients With Rheumatoid Arthritis. Arthritis Rheumatol 2014;66(2):254–63.
4. Gualtierotti R, Parisi M, Ingegnoli F. Perioperative Management of Patients with Inflammatory Rheumatic Diseases Undergoing Major Orthopaedic Surgery: A Practical Overview. Adv Ther 2018;35(4):439–56.
5. George MD, Baker JF, Winthrop K, et al. Risk of Biologics and Glucocorticoids in Patients With Rheumatoid Arthritis Undergoing Arthroplasty: A Cohort Study. Ann Intern Med 2019;170(12):825–36.
6. Goodman SM, Springer BD, Chen AF, et al. American College of Rheumatology/ American Association of Hip and Knee Surgeons Guideline for the Perioperative Management of Antirheumatic Medication in Patients With Rheumatic Diseases Undergoing Elective Total Hip or Total Knee Arthroplasty. Arthritis Care Res (Hoboken) 2022;74(9):1399–408.
7. Weinblatt ME. Methotrexate in rheumatoid arthritis: a quarter century of development. Trans Am Clin Climatological Assoc 2013;124:16–25.
8. Härle P, Straub RH, Fleck M. Perioperative management of immunosuppression in rheumatic diseases–what to do? Rheumatol Int 2010;30(8):999–1004.
9. Loza E, Martinez-Lopez JA, Carmona L. A systematic review on the optimum management of the use of methotrexate in rheumatoid arthritis patients in the perioperative period to minimize perioperative morbidity and maintain disease control. Clin Exp Rheumatol 2009;27(5):856–62.
10. Fox RI, Herrmann ML, Frangou CG, et al. Mechanism of action for leflunomide in rheumatoid arthritis. Clin Immunol (Orlando, Fla) 1999;93(3):198–208.
11. Fuerst M, Möhl H, Baumgärtel K, et al. Leflunomide increases the risk of early healing complications in patients with rheumatoid arthritis undergoing elective orthopedic surgery. Rheumatol Int 2006;26(12):1138–42.

12. Bongartz T, Halligan CS, Osmon DR, et al. Incidence and risk factors of prosthetic joint infection after total hip or knee replacement in patients with rheumatoid arthritis. Arthritis Rheum 2008;59(12):1713–20.
13. Kumar A, Auron M, Aneja A, et al. Inflammatory bowel disease: perioperative pharmacological considerations. Mayo Clinic Proc 2011;86(8):748–57.
14. Colombel JF, Loftus EV Jr, Tremaine WJ, et al. Early postoperative complications are not increased in patients with Crohn's disease treated perioperatively with in- fliximab or immunosuppressive therapy. Am J Gastroenterol 2004;99(5):878–83.
15. den Broeder AA, Creemers MC, Fransen J, et al. Risk factors for surgical site in- fections and other complications in elective surgery in patients with rheumatoid arthritis with special attention for anti-tumor necrosis factor: a large retrospective study. The J Rheumatol 2007;34(4):689–95.
16. Borgas Y, Gülfe A, Kindt M, et al. Anti-rheumatic treatment and prosthetic joint infection: an observational study in 494 elective hip and knee arthroplasties. BMC Musculoskelet Disord 2020;21(1):410.
17. Kavanaugh A, Gladman DD, Edwards CJ, et al. Long-term experience with apre- milast in patients with psoriatic arthritis: 5-year results from a PALACE 1-3 pooled analysis. Arthritis Res Ther 2019;21(1):118.
18. Strober BE. New Therapies for Psoriasis. Semin Cutan Med Surg 2016;35(4s): S71–3.
19. Wollenhaupt J, Silverfield J, Lee EB, et al. Safety and efficacy of tofacitinib, an oral janus kinase inhibitor, for the treatment of rheumatoid arthritis in open- label, longterm extension studies. The J Rheumatol 2014;41(5):837–52.
20. Vallurupalli M, Berliner N. Emapalumab for the treatment of relapsed/refractory hemophagocytic lymphohistiocytosis. Blood 2019;134(21):1783–6.
21. Benedetti FD, Grom AA, Brogan PA, et al. Efficacy and safety of emapalumab in macrophage activation syndrome. Ann Rheum Dis 2023;82(6):857–65.
22. Al-Salama ZT. Emapalumab: First Global Approval. Drugs 2019;79(1):99–103.
23. Liu J, Chen Z, Li Y, et al. PD-1/PD-L1 Checkpoint Inhibitors in Tumor Immuno- therapy. Front Pharmacol 2021;12:731798.
24. Kottschade LA. Incidence and Management of Immune-Related Adverse Events in Patients Undergoing Treatment with Immune Checkpoint Inhibitors. Curr Oncol Rep 2018;20(3):24.
25. Stucci S, Palmirotta R, Passarelli A, et al. Immune-related adverse events during anticancer immunotherapy: Pathogenesis and management. Oncol Lett 2017; 14(5):5671–80.
26. Byun DJ, Wolchok JD, Rosenberg LM, et al. Cancer immunotherapy - immune checkpoint blockade and associated endocrinopathies. Nat Rev Endocrinol 2017;13(4):195–207.
27. Moslehi JJ, Salem JE, Sosman JA, et al. Increased reporting of fatal immune checkpoint inhibitor-associated myocarditis. Lancet (London, England) 2018; 391(10124):933.
28. Ganatra S, Neilan TG. Immune Checkpoint Inhibitor-Associated Myocarditis. The oncologist 2018;23(8):879–86.
29. Khunger M, Rakshit S, Pasupuleti V, et al. Incidence of Pneumonitis With Use of Programmed Death 1 and Programmed Death-Ligand 1 Inhibitors in Non-Small Cell Lung Cancer: A Systematic Review and Meta-Analysis of Trials. Chest 2017;152(2):271–81.
30. Lewis AL, Chaft J, Girotra M, et al. Immune checkpoint inhibitors: a narrative re- view of considerations for the anaesthesiologist. Br J Anaesth 2020;124(3): 251–60.

31. Koons K, Plotas V, Tichansky DS, et al. The safety of elective surgery with concurrent use of immunosuppresants. Glob Surg 2017;3(2):1–4.
32. Melsheimer R, Geldhof A, Apaolaza I, et al. Remicade(®) (infliximab): 20 years of contributions to science and medicine. Biologics : Targets Ther 2019;13:139–78.
33. Corrao S, Pistone G, Arnone S, et al. Safety of etanercept therapy in rheumatoid patients undergoing surgery: preliminary report. Clin Rheumatol 2007;26(9): 1513–5.
34. Rezaieyazdi Z, Sahebari M, Khodashahi M. Preoperative Evaluation and Management of Patients Receiving Biologic Therapies. The Arch bone Jt Surg 2019;7(3):220–8.
35. Ruyssen-Witrand A, Gossec L, Salliot C, et al. Complication rates of 127 surgical procedures performed in rheumatic patients receiving tumor necrosis factor alpha blockers. Clin Exp Rheumatol 2007;25(3):430–6.
36. Franco AS, Iuamoto LR, Pereira RMR. Perioperative management of drugs commonly used in patients with rheumatic diseases: a review. Clinics (Sao Paulo, Brazil) 2017;72(6):386–90.
37. Hoffman HM, Throne ML, Amar NJ, et al. Efficacy and safety of rilonacept (interleukin-1 Trap) in patients with cryopyrin-associated periodic syndromes: results from two sequential placebo-controlled studies. Arthritis Rheum 2008;58(8): 2443–52.
38. Mahamid M, Mader R, Safadi R. Hepatotoxicity of tocilizumab and anakinra in rheumatoid arthritis: management decisions. Clin Pharmacol : Adv Appl 2011; 3:39–43.
39. Romano M, Sironi M, Toniatti C, et al. Role of IL-6 and its soluble receptor in induction of chemokines and leukocyte recruitment. Immunity 1997;6(3):315–25.
40. Kotake S, Sato K, Kim KJ, et al. Interleukin-6 and soluble interleukin-6 receptors in the synovial fluids from rheumatoid arthritis patients are responsible for osteoclast-like cell formation. J bone mineral Res : official J Am Soc Bone Mineral Res 1996;11(1):88–95.
41. Maini RN, Taylor PC, Szechinski J, et al. Double-blind randomized controlled clinical trial of the interleukin-6 receptor antagonist, tocilizumab, in European patients with rheumatoid arthritis who had an incomplete response to methotrexate. Arthritis Rheum 2006;54(9):2817–29.
42. Interleukin-6 Receptor Antagonists in Critically Ill Patients with Covid-19. New Engl J Med 2021;384(16):1491–502.
43. Maude SL, Barrett D, Teachey DT, et al. Managing cytokine release syndrome associated with novel T cell-engaging therapies. Cancer J (Sudbury, Mass) 2014;20(2):119–22.
44. Strangfeld A, Richter A, Siegmund B, et al. Risk for lower intestinal perforations in patients with rheumatoid arthritis treated with tocilizumab in comparison to treatment with other biologic or conventional synthetic DMARDs. Ann Rheum Dis 2017;76(3):504–10.
45. Moots RJ, Sebba A, Rigby W, et al. Effect of tocilizumab on neutrophils in adult patients with rheumatoid arthritis: pooled analysis of data from phase 3 and 4 clinical trials. Rheumatology 2016;56(4):541–9.
46. Alfreijat M, Habibi M, Bhatia P, et al. Severe hepatitis associated with tocilizumab in a patient with rheumatoid arthritis. Rheumatology 2013;52(7):1340–1.
47. Park EH, Lee EY, Shin K, et al. Tocilizumab-induced anaphylaxis in patients with adult-onset Still's disease and systemic juvenile idiopathic arthritis: a case-based review. Rheumatol Int 2020;40(5):791–8.

48. Pawar A, Desai RJ, Solomon DH, et al. Risk of serious infections in tocilizumab versus other biologic drugs in patients with rheumatoid arthritis: a multidatabase cohort study. Ann Rheum Dis 2019;78(4):456–64.
49. Sibilia J, Gottenberg J-E, Mariette X. Rituximab: A new therapeutic alternative in rheumatoid arthritis. Joint Bone Spine 2008;75(5):526–32.
50. Lee SJ, Chinen J, Kavanaugh A. Immunomodulator therapy: monoclonal antibodies, fusion proteins, cytokines, and immunoglobulins. The J Allergy Clin Immunol 2010;125(2 Suppl 2):S314–23.
51. Buch MH, Smolen JS, Betteridge N, et al. Updated consensus statement on the use of rituximab in patients with rheumatoid arthritis. Ann Rheum Dis 2011;70(6):909–20.
52. Emery P, Fleischmann R, Filipowicz-Sosnowska A, et al. The efficacy and safety of rituximab in patients with active rheumatoid arthritis despite methotrexate treatment: results of a phase IIB randomized, double-blind, placebo-controlled, dose-ranging trial. Arthritis Rheum 2006;54(5):1390–400.
53. Cohen SB, Emery P, Greenwald MW, et al. Rituximab for rheumatoid arthritis refractory to anti-tumor necrosis factor therapy: Results of a multicenter, randomized, double-blind, placebo-controlled, phase III trial evaluating primary efficacy and safety at twenty-four weeks. Arthritis Rheum 2006;54(9):2793–806.
54. Poylin VY, Serrato JC, Pastrana Del Valle J, et al. Vedolizumab does not increase perioperative surgical complications in patients with inflammatory bowel disease, cohort study. Intest Res 2022;20(1):72–7.
55. Lightner AL, Edward VL Jr, McKenna NP, et al. Vedolizumab in the Perioperative Management of Inflammatory Bowel Disease. Curr Drug Targets 2019;20(13):1317–22.
56. Srivastava A. Belimumab in systemic lupus erythematosus. Indian J Dermatol 2016;61(5):550–3.
57. Blair HA, Deeks ED. Abatacept: A Review in Rheumatoid Arthritis. Drugs 2017;77(11):1221–33.
58. Nishida K, Nasu Y, Hashizume K, et al. Abatacept management during the perioperative period in patients with rheumatoid arthritis: report on eight orthopaedic procedures. Mod Rheumatol 2014;24(3):544–5.
59. George MD, Baker JF, Winthrop K, et al. Timing of Abatacept Before Elective Arthroplasty and Risk of Postoperative Outcomes. Arthritis Care Res 2019;71(9):1224–33.

Moving?

Make sure your subscription moves with you!

To notify us of your new address, find your **Clinics Account Number** (located on your mailing label above your name), and contact customer service at:

Email: journalscustomerservice-usa@elsevier.com

800-654-2452 (subscribers in the U.S. & Canada)
314-447-8871 (subscribers outside of the U.S. & Canada)

Fax number: 314-447-8029

Elsevier Health Sciences Division
Subscription Customer Service
3251 Riverport Lane
Maryland Heights, MO 63043

*To ensure uninterrupted delivery of your subscription, please notify us at least 4 weeks in advance of move.